T0291086

50 Pharmacotherapy Studies Every Palliative Practitioner Should Know

50 STUDIES EVERY DOCTOR SHOULD KNOW

50 Studies Every Doctor Should Know: The Key Studies that Form the Foundation of Evidence Based Medicine, Revised Edition
Michael E. Hochman

50 Studies Every Internist Should Know
Kristopher Swiger, Joshua R. Thomas, Michael E. Hochman, and Steven Hochman

50 Studies Every Neurologist Should Know
David Y. Hwang and David M. Greer

50 Studies Every Pediatrician Should Know
Ashaunta T. Anderson, Nina L. Shapiro, Stephen C. Aronoff, Jeremiah Davis, and Michael Levy

50 Imaging Studies Every Doctor Should Know
Christoph I. Lee

50 Studies Every Surgeon Should Know
SreyRam Kuy, Rachel J. Kwon, and Miguel A. Burch

50 Studies Every Intensivist Should Know
Edward A. Bittner

50 Studies Every Palliative Care Doctor Should Know
David Hui, Akhila Reddy, and Eduardo Bruera

50 Studies Every Psychiatrist Should Know
Ish P. Bhalla, Rajesh R. Tampi, and Vinod H. Srihari

50 Studies Every Anesthesiologist Should Know
Anita Gupta, Michael E. Hochman, and Elena N. Gutman

50 Studies Every Ophthalmologist Should Know
Alan D. Penman, Kimberly W. Crowder, and William M. Watkins, Jr.

50 Studies Every Urologist Should Know
Philipp Dahm

50 Studies Every Obstetrician and Gynecologist Should Know
Constance Liu, Noah Rindos, and Scott Shainker

50 Studies Every Doctor Should Know: The Key Studies that Form the Foundation of Evidence-Based Medicine 2nd Edition
Michael E. Hochman and Steven D. Hochman

50 Studies Every Occupational Therapist Should Know
Elizabeth A. Pyatak and Elissa S. Lee

50 Studies Every Vascular Surgeon Should Know
Julien Al Shakarchi

50 Studies Every Global Health Provider Should Know
Andrea Walker, Anup Agarwal, and Yogesh Jain

50 Studies Every Orthopaedic Surgeon Should Know
Kapil Sugand and Hani B. Abdul-Jabar

50 Studies Every Neonatologist Should Know
John Zupancic, Susanne Hay, Roger F. Soll, Barbara Schmidt, and Haresh Kirpalani

50 Pharmacotherapy Studies Every Palliative Practitioner Should Know
Mary Lynn McPherson, Mellar P. Davis, Alexandra L. McPherson, Ryan Costantino, and Eduardo Bruera

50 Pharmacotherapy Studies Every Palliative Practitioner Should Know

EDITED BY

Mary Lynn McPherson, Mellar P. Davis, Alexandra L. McPherson, Ryan Costantino, & Eduardo Bruera

SERIES EDITOR

Michael E. Hochman

OXFORD
UNIVERSITY PRESS

OXFORD
UNIVERSITY PRESS

Oxford University Press is a department of the University of Oxford. It furthers the University's objective of excellence in research, scholarship, and education by publishing worldwide. Oxford is a registered trade mark of Oxford University Press in the UK and certain other countries.

Published in the United States of America by Oxford University Press
198 Madison Avenue, New York, NY 10016, United States of America.

Library of Congress Cataloging-in-Publication Data
Names: McPherson, Mary Lynn M., editor. | Davis, Mellar P., editor. |
McPherson, Alexandra L., editor. | Costantino, Ryan, editor. |
Bruera, Eduardo, editor.
Title: 50 pharmacotherapy studies every palliative practitioner should know /
[edited by] Mary Lynn McPherson, Mellar P. Davis, Alexandra L. McPherson,
Ryan Costantino & Eduardo Bruera.
Other titles: Fifty pharmacotherapy studies every palliative practitioner should know |
50 studies every doctor should know (Series)
Description: New York, NY : Oxford University Press, [2025] |
Series: Fifty studies every doctor should know series |
Includes bibliographical references and index.
Identifiers: LCCN 2023056781 (print) | LCCN 2023056782 (ebook) |
ISBN 9780197770337 (paperback) | ISBN 9780197770351 (epub) |
ISBN 9780197770368
Subjects: MESH: Drug Therapy—methods | Palliative Care |
Pain Management—methods | Palliative Medicine—methods | Clinical Trials as Topic
Classification: LCC R726.7 (print) | LCC R726.7 (ebook) |
NLM WB 310 | DDC 616.02/9—dc23/eng/20240229
LC record available at https://lccn.loc.gov/2023056781
LC ebook record available at https://lccn.loc.gov/2023056782

DOI: 10.1093/med/9780197770337.001.0001

This material is not intended to be, and should not be considered, a substitute for medical or other professional advice. Treatment for the conditions described in this material is highly dependent on the individual circumstances. And, while this material is designed to offer accurate information with respect to the subject matter covered and to be current as of the time it was written, research and knowledge about medical and health issues is constantly evolving and dose schedules for medications are being revised continually, with new side effects recognized and accounted for regularly. Readers must therefore always check the product information and clinical procedures with the most up-to-date published product information and data sheets provided by the manufacturers and the most recent codes of conduct and safety regulation. The publisher and the authors make no representations or warranties to readers, express or implied, as to the accuracy or completeness of this material. Without limiting the foregoing, the publisher and the authors make no representations or warranties as to the accuracy or efficacy of the drug dosages mentioned in the material. The authors and the publisher do not accept, and expressly disclaim, any responsibility for any liability, loss, or risk that may be claimed or incurred as a consequence of the use and/or application of any of the contents of this material.

Printed by Marquis Book Printing, Canada

FSC
www.fsc.org
MIX
Paper | Supporting responsible forestry
FSC® C103567

CONTENTS

CONTRIBUTORS

Jennifer Allen, MD
Chief, Division of Palliative Medicine and Hospice Lehigh Valley Health Network

Deborah Araya, PA-C MA, MS
Palliative Care Physician Assistant University of Maryland Charles Regional Medical Center

Ryan Baldeo, MPAS, MSPC, PA-C, FAAHPM
Physician Assistant, Division of Palliative Medicine, Department of Medicine, Mayo Clinic Arizona Assistant Professor in Palliative Medicine, Mayo Clinic College of Medicine

Alan Patrick Baltz, MD
Assistant Professor, Department of Internal Medicine, Division of Hematology and Oncology, University of Arkansas for Medical Sciences Winthrop P. Rockefeller Cancer Institute

Ashley Barlow, PharmD, BCOP
Assistant Scientific Director, AbbVie

Nina M. Bemben, PharmD, BCPS

Bavna Bhagavat, MD
Internal Medicine Resident Physician, Loyola University Medical Center

Dwight Blair, MD
Fellow, Division of Palliative Care Medical University of South Carolina

Joshua Borris, PharmD, MS, BCGP
MedStar Harbor Hospital, Palliative Care Pharmacist

Joni Brinker, MSN/MHA, RN, WCC
Clinical Nurse Educator, Hospice Optum Pharmacy Services

Eduardo Bruera, MD
Professor and Chair Department of Palliative, Rehabilitation and Integrative Medicine, The University of Texas MD Anderson Cancer Center

Gary T. Buckholz, MD, MNDS, FAAHPM
Clinical Professor of Medicine and Family Medicine; Doris Howell Palliative Care Service

Joan Cain, MSN, FNP-BC, ACHPN
Nurse Practitioner in the department of Palliative care and General Internal Medicine Medical University of South Carolina (MUSC)

Kirstin L. Campbell, MD
Assistant Professor of Pediatrics, Pediatric Palliative Care, Medical University of South Carolina

Elizabeth Capano, AGPCNP-BC, ACHPN
Nurse Practitioner, Division of Geriatrics and Palliative Medicine Weill Cornell Medicine

Alex Choi, MD
Assistant Professor, Yale Palliative Care Program, Department of Medicine, Yale School of Medicine

Daniel Cogan, MSN
Nurse Practitioner Calvary Hospital

Ryan C. Costantino, PharmD, MS, BCPS
Branch Chief, Data Science & Innovation Enterprise Intelligence & Data Solutions Program Management Office

Constance Dahlin, MSN, ANP-BC, ACHPN, FPCN, FAAN
Adjunct Faculty
Graduate Studies in Palliative Care
University of Maryland Baltimore
Palliative Nurse Practitioner
Salem Hospital
Consultant Center to Advance Palliative Care

Mellar P. Davis, MD, FCCP, FAAHPM
Director of Palliative Medicine Research, Geisinger Medical Center Geisinger Medical Center

Jennifer L. Derrick, MD
Instructor of Hospice and Palliative Medicine Mayo Clinic Health System

Susan DeSanto-Madeya, PhD, MSN-CNS, RN, FPCN, FAAN
Professor and Miriam Weyker Endowed Chair for Palliative Care University of Rhode Island, College of Nursing

Sandra DiScala, PharmD, BCPS, FAAHPM
Clinical Pharmacist Practitioner West Palm Beach VAHCS

Laura Elisabeth Gressler, MS, PhD
Assistant Professor, Department of Pharmacy Practice University of Arkansas for Medical Sciences

Jeffrey Fudin, BS, Pharm.D., FCCP, FASHP, FFSMB (Deceased)
Founder and CEO, Remitigate Therapeutics,
Director PGY2 Pain Residency
Stratton VA Medical Center

Alexander Gamble, MD
Clinical Assistant Professor of Medicine Stanford University

Brian Gans, MD
Palliative Care Physician, Dignity Health Cancer Institute

Elizabeth A. Higgins, MD
Professor of Internal Medicine and Palliative Care Attending, Department of Internal Medicine MUSC

Sydney Taylor Israel, PharmD, BCPS
Palliative Care Clinical Pharmacy Specialist University of Maryland Medical Center

Allison E. Jordan, MD, CCMS, NBC-HWC, FAAHPM
Psychiatrist, BJC HealthCare

Katherine M. Juba, PharmD
Associate Professor of Pharmacy Practice St. John Fisher University

Arif Kamal, MD, MBA, MHS
Associate Professor of Medicine Duke Cancer Institute

Alyssa Langi, MSN, CRNP, ACHPN
Palliative Spine Radiation Nurse, Practitioner University of Pennsylvania

Natalie M. Latuga, PharmD, BCPS
Hospice & Palliative Care Buffalo

Debra L. Luczkiewicz, MD
Hospice & Palliative Care Buffalo

Jimi S. Malik, MD
Assistant Professor, Division of Palliative Medicine, Department of Family and preeventive medicine, Emory University School of Medicine

Kristina Marchand, MD
Hospice & Palliative Care Fellow University of California

Emily J. Martin, MD, MS, FAAHPM
Director, UCLA Palliative Care and Assistant Clinical Professor, Department of Medicine, University of California

Meredith Maxwell, MD
Assistant Professor of Family and Preventative Medicine Division of Palliative Medicine, Emory University

Kevin McGehrin, MD
Neurologist and Palliative Care Physician The Neuron Clinic

Alexandra L. McPherson, PharmD, MPH
Palliative Care Clinical Pharmacy Specialist, Department of Medicine MedStar Washington Hospital Center

Mary Lynn McPherson, PharmD, PhD, FAAHPM
Professor and Executive Director, Advanced Post-Graduate Education in Palliative Care Executive Program Director, Graduate Studies in Palliative Care Department of Pharmacy Practice, Sciences, and Health Outcomes University of Maryland School of Pharmacy

Ambereen K. Mehta, MD, MPH, FAAHPM
Associate Professor of Palliative Care, Departments of Medicine and Neurology Johns Hopkins School of Medicine

Sarah Stayer, MD, MPH
Fellowship Program Director of Hospice and Palliative Medicine University of Texas at Austin Dell Medical School

Lydia Mis, BSPharm, PharmD, BCOP
Clinical Oncology Pharmacy Specialist Duke University Hospital

Laura Morrison, MD
Associate Professor, Yale Palliative Care Program, Department of Medicine, Yale School of Medicine

Balakrishnan Natarajan, MD
Chief Medical Officer, AccentCare; visiting faculty, University of Maryland-Baltimore; Clinical Adjunct Faculty, Northwestern University Feinberg School of Medicine, Chicago College of Osteopathic Medicine of Midwestern University

Cindy Nguyen, PharmD, MPH, MS, BCPS
Clinical Pharmacy Specialist, Division of Palliative Care Medstar Georgetown University Hospital

Jessica Nymeyer, MBA, MSN, AGACNP-BC, ACHPN
Palliative Care Nurse Practitioner Calvary Hospital

Judith A. Paice, PhD, RN, FAAN, FASCO
Director, Cancer Pain Program, Division of Hematology/ Oncology Northwestern University; Feinberg School of Medicine

Shila Pandey, DNP, AGPCNP-BC, ACHPN
Nurse Practitioner, Supportive Care Service; Memorial Sloan Kettering

Ravi Pathak, MD
Assistant Professor
Department of Anesthesiology
Division of Palliative Medicine, Department of Family & Preventive Medicine
Emory University School of Medicine

J. Keais Pope, MD
Assistant Medical Director, Hospice of the Foothills, Prisma Health

Bridget McCrate Protus, PharmD, MLIS, BCGP, CDP
Director of Drug Information, Optum Hospice Pharmacy Services

Tammie E. Quest, MD
Director, Emory Palliative Care Center
Professor, Emory University School of Medicine
Departments of Family and Preventive Medicine and Emergency Medicine

Anne Rohlfing, MD
Assistant Professor of Medicine, Adult Palliative Care Service Columbia University Irving Medical Center

Elizabeth Schack, GNP-BC
Senior Palliative Care Nurse Practitioner New York Presbyterian Hospital

Navendra Sing, MD, MPH
Assistant Professor of Clinical Medicine, Division of Geriatrics and Palliative Care, Weill Cornell Medical College

Abby Stevens, PharmD, MS, BCGP
Palliative Care Clinical Pharmacy Specialist MedStar Union Memorial Hospital

Scott A. Strassels, PharmD, PhD
Research Professor, Division of Pharmacy Atrium Health

Jefferson S. Svengsouk, MD, MBA
Professor of Emergency Medicine and Palliative Care, University of Rochester Medical Center

Paul Tatum, MD, MSPH, CMD, AGSF. FAAHPM
Professor of Palliative Medicine and Palliative Care Physician
Washington University in St. Louis and St. Louis VA Health Center

Sophia S. Urban, MD, MPH
Assistant Professor, Hospice and Palliative Care, Departments of Internal Medicine and Pediatrics Medical University of South Carolina

Vincent Jay Vanston, MD
Associate Professor of Medicine University of Pennsylvania Health System

Christine M. Vartan, PharmD, BCPS
Clinical Pharmacist Practitioner West Palm Beach VA Healthcare System

Lara Wahlberg, DNP, AGPCNP-BC, ACHPN
Clinical Professor
Coordinator of AGPCNP MS Specialization
Hunter-Bellevue School of Nursing
Hunter College of CUNY

Eric Widera, MD
Professor of Clinical Medicine, Division of Geriatrics, University of California San Franciso (UCSF), Director, Hospice and Palliative Care, San Francisco Veterans Affairs Health System

Crystal A. Wright, PharmD, BCPS, BCACP
Geriatrics and Palliative Care Clinical Pharmacy Specialist, Pharmacy Department Kaiser Foundation Health Plan of Georgia

David S. Wu, MD, FAAHPM
Associate Professor, Johns Hopkins School of Medicine
Director, Johns Hopkins Bayview Palliative Care Program
2023 Circle of Life Award, American Hospital Association

Angela Yeh, DO
Assistant Clinical Professor, Department of Medicine, University of California

Ali John Zarrabi, MD
Assistant Professor Family and Preventive Medicine, Division of Palliative Medicine, Emory University

Cheng Zeng, DO
Palliative care physician, The Southeast Permanente Medical Group

1

Low-Dose Neuroleptics for Treating Delirium

DEBORAH ARAYA

> Symptoms of delirium in medically hospitalized AIDS patients may be treated efficaciously with few side effects by using low-dose neuroleptic (haloperidol or chlorpromazine). Lorazepam alone appears to be ineffective and associated with treatment-limiting adverse effects.
>
> —BREITBART ET AL.[1]

Research Question: Are haloperidol, chlorpromazine, or lorazepam effective for treating delirium in hospitalized patients with HIV/AIDS, and if so, what is the optimal strength?

Funding: National Institute of Mental Health (NIMH)

Year Study Began: 1991

Year Study Published: 1996

Study Location: St. Luke's/Roosevelt Hospital Center

Who Was Studied: Hospitalized patients who met the criteria of the Centers for Disease Control and Prevention for AIDS and gave consent prior to development of delirium who subsequently developed a score of above 13 on the Delirium Rating Scale.[2]

Who Was Excluded: Patients with hypersensitivity to test drugs, underlying physiological disorder(s), seizure disorder, current treatment with chemotherapy in Kaposi sarcoma, withdrawal syndrome, anticholinergic delirium, or neuroleptic malignant syndrome and those already on test drugs were excluded from participation in the study.

How Many Patients: 30

Study Overview: This is a double-blind study in which 30 patients were randomized to 1 of 3 treatment arms. The patients gave consent to join the study prior to developing delirium. Neither the researchers nor the patients knew which of the 3 arms they were participating in. Medications were administered by pharmacists using a preestablished graduated protocol (Figure 1.1).

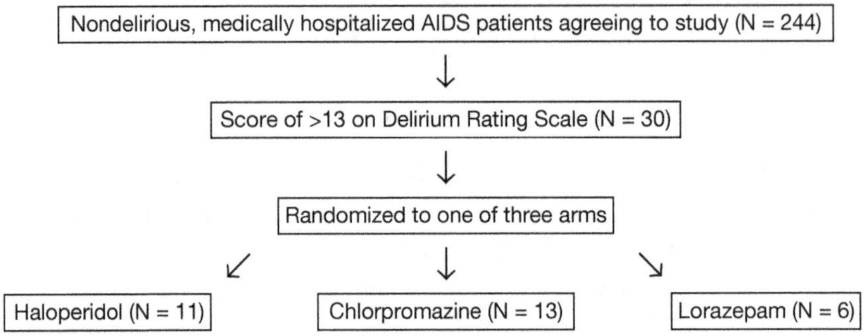

Figure 1.1. Summary of study design.

Study Intervention: Once delirium was identified the patient was monitored hourly. Each treatment arm had a graduated protocol for drug administration. If the patient's score on the Delirium Rating Scale was above 13, the assigned medication was titrated according to the protocol until the patient was stabilized. On day 2 a maintenance dose was started that equaled the amount of medication needed in 24 hours cut in half and administered in 2 doses. The maintenance continued for 6 days. The lorazepam arm was stopped midway through the study due to worsening of delirium with adverse side effects.

Follow-Up: 7 days

Endpoints:

Primary outcome: Mean Delirium Rating Scale score at onset, day 2, and end of treatment.

Secondary outcomes: Mean Mini-Mental State Examination score at onset, day 2, and end of treatment. Extrapyramidal Symptom Rating Scale scores measured at baseline prior to medication administration and during maintenance therapy.

RESULTS

- Low-dose haloperidol and chlorpromazine were effective in treating delirium, and by day 2 the mean Delirium Rating Scale score was below 13 (Table 1.1).
- Lorazepam was ineffective in treating delirium and did not lower the mean Delirium Rating Scale (Table 1.1).
- Haloperidol and chlorpromazine both showed improvement in cognitive status as measured by the Mini-Mental State examinations, while in the lorazepam group cognitive impairment increased (Table 1.1).
- Haloperidol and chlorpromazine showed low extrapyramidal side effects (Table 1.1).
- The lorazepam arm was discontinued midway through the study due to treatment-limiting adverse side effects, including a nonsignificant trend toward increased extrapyramidal side effects (Table 1.1).

Table 1.1 A SUMMARY OF THE STUDY'S KEY FINDINGS

	Haloperidol	**Chlorpromazine**	**Lorazepam**
Drug Dose			
Day 1	2.8	50.0	3.0
Maintenance	1.4	36.0	4.6
DRS			
Baseline	20.45	20.62	18.33
Day 2	12.45	12.08	17.33
P value	**< .001**	**< .001**	< .63
Endpoint	11.64	11.85	17.00
P value	< .43	< .81	< .81
M-MS			
Baseline	13.45	10.92	15.17
Day 2	17.27	18.31	12.67
P value	< .09	**< .001**	< .09
Endpoint	17.18	15.08	11.50
P value	< .96	< .04	< .60
ESRS			
Baseline	7.00	7.42	5.54
Maintenance	5.54	5.08	12.20

Abbreviations: DSR, Delirium Rating Scale; ESRS, Extrapyramidal Symptom Rating Scale; M-MS, Mini-Mental Status.
Note: Maintenance is day 2 to endpoint.

Criticisms and Limitations:

- The study included only patients with AIDS from a single hospital setting. It is unclear if the results are applicable to patients with other disease states and in other settings.
- The study was underpowered to draw statistically robust conclusions.
- There was not a placebo arm in the trial because the authors felt it was unethical to have a placebo treatment arm; as a result, it is not possible to know whether the study medications were superior to no pharmacologic treatment at all.

Other Relevant Studies and Information:

- This study by Breitbart et al. spurred further research confirming the effectiveness of neuroleptics in treating delirium.[3–5]
- Use of higher-dose neuroleptics is more likely to result in extrapyramidal side effects.[6]
- A recent well-conducted placebo-controlled randomized trial of haloperidol and risperidone versus placebo failed to confirm the benefits of haloperidol in treating cancer-related delirium.[7] This places into question the benefits of haloperidol. The reproducibility of outcomes is much stronger evidence than a single positive trial.[8,9]

Summary and Implications: A double-blind trial comparing haloperidol, chlorpromazine, and lorazepam in the treatment of delirium in hospitalized patients with AIDS showed that haloperidol and chlorpromazine, but not lorazepam, are effective in the treatment of delirium. Guidelines currently recommend neuroleptics as the first-line pharmacologic therapy for delirium.

CLINICAL CASE: TREATMENT OF DELIRIUM IN A PATIENT WITH AIDS

Case History

The palliative care medical provider was asked to evaluate and make recommendations for a 68-year-old male patient with a past medical history of diabetes, hypertension, and AIDS who developed sudden onset of confusion on postoperative day 1 after undergoing an appendectomy. He refused to eat or take medications, stating someone was trying to poison him. He also refused to ambulate with physical therapy or use his incentive spirometer. His Delirium Rating Scale score was 15.

Is it reasonable to start him on a low-dose neuroleptic such as haloperidol?

Suggested Answer

The Breitbart et al. study demonstrated that while simultaneously searching for the cause of the delirium and providing the best supportive care, the palliative care provider can begin treating the patient with a low-dose neuroleptic such as haloperidol or chlorpromazine. This patient meets the criteria outlined in the double-blind trial of haloperidol, chlorpromazine, and lorazepam in the treatment of delirium in hospitalized AIDS patients.

References

1. Breitbart W, Marotta R, Platt MM, et al. A double-blind trial of haloperidol, chlorpromazine, and lorazepam in the treatment of delirium in hospitalized AIDS patients. *Am J Psychiatry*. 1996;153(2):231–237.
2. Trzepacz PT. The Delirium Rating Scale. Its use in consultation-liaison research. *Psychosomatics*. 1999;40(3):193–204.
3. Hu H, Deng W, Yang H. A prospective random control study: comparison of olanzapine and haloperidol in senile delirium. *Chongqing Med J*. 2004;8:1234–1237.
4. Breitbart W, Tremblay A, Gibson C. An open trial of olanzapine for the treatment of delirium in hospitalized cancer patients. *Psychosomatics*. 2002;43:175–182.
5. Kim KY, Bader GM, Kotlyar V, et al. Treatment of delirium in older adults with quetiapine. *J Geriatr Psychiatry Neurol*. 2003;16:29–31.
6. Boettger S, Friedlander M, Breitbart W, et al. Aripiprazole and haloperidol in the treatment of delirium. *Aust N Z J Psychiatry*. 2011;45:477–482.
7. Agar MR, Lawlor PG, Quinn S, et al. Efficacy of oral risperidone, haloperidol, or placebo for symptoms of delirium among patients in palliative care: a randomized clinical trial. *JAMA Intern Med*. 2017;177(1):34–42.
8. Goodman SN. A comment on replication, p-values and evidence. *Stat Med*. 1992;11(7):875–879.
9. Goodman SN, Fanelli D, Ioannidis JP. What does research reproducibility mean? *Sci Transl Med*. 2016;8(341):341ps12.

2

Dexamethasone in Addition to Metoclopramide for Chronic Nausea in Patients With Advanced Cancer

RYAN BALDEO AND JENNIFER L. DERRICK

> In this double-blind, parallel study we found that dexamethasone was not significantly better than placebo in the management of chronic nausea, appetite or fatigue in patients with advanced cancer.
>
> —Bruera et al.[1]

Research Question: What is the antiemetic effect of dexamethasone in patients with advanced cancer and chronic nausea refractory to metoclopramide.

Funding: The Brown Foundation, Houston, Texas, funded the study. The author, Florian Strasser, was supported by a grant from Swiss Cancer Research (BIL grant KFS 950-09-1999).

Year Study Began: 2003

Year Study Published: 2004

Study Locations:

1. Instituto Nacional de Cancerologia, Bogota, Colombia
2. Hospital Escala/Eva Peron-Rosario, Rosario, Argentina
3. Instituto Nacional del Cancer, Santiago, Chile
4. Institute for Oncology and Radiology of Serbia, Belgrade, Serbia
5. Unidad de Cuidados Paliativos, Buenos Aires, Argentina

Who Was Studied: Patients assessed to have normal cognition aged 16 years or older with advanced cancer (local recurrence or metastatic disease) and chronic nausea (defined as at least 2 weeks) rated as mild to moderate (defined as at least 3 out of 10 on self-reported numeric scale) despite 48 hours of treatment with metoclopramide (40–60 mg per 24-hour period).

Who Was Excluded: Patients were excluded if they had 1 or more of the following:

- Received chemotherapy and/or radiation therapy in the previous 4 weeks
- Received dexamethasone in the previous 4 weeks
- Treated with antiemetics other than metoclopramide in the previous 3 days
- Developed an acute complication such as sepsis, delirium, or excessive use of metoclopramide (defined as greater than 4 additional doses of 10 mg/day)

How Many Patients: 51

Study Overview: This is a double-blind, parallel study of 51 patients randomized to receive dexamethasone or placebo treatment for chronic nausea in addition to scheduled metoclopramide. Figure 2.1 provides a breakdown on the study's sample size. The duration of the treatment portion of the trial lasted 7 days. Symptom intensity assessment was completed at baseline and daily throughout the duration of the study. Well-being and quality-of-life assessments were completed at baseline and following completion of the intervention, on day 8. Toxicity and side effects were assessed and opioid and metoclopramide intake was monitored.

Study Intervention: All patients enrolled in this study received metoclopramide 10 mg every 4 hours for the duration of the study and were allowed extra doses of metoclopramide (10 mg every 1 hour as needed for excessive nausea). Patients were randomized to receive dexamethasone 10 mg twice daily or placebo twice daily at 8 AM and 2 PM for the duration of the study.

Follow-Up: 8 days

Endpoints:

Primary outcome: Therapeutic effect on chronic nausea.

Secondary outcomes: Impact of intervention on patient's pain, fatigue, appetite, and well-being/quality of life.

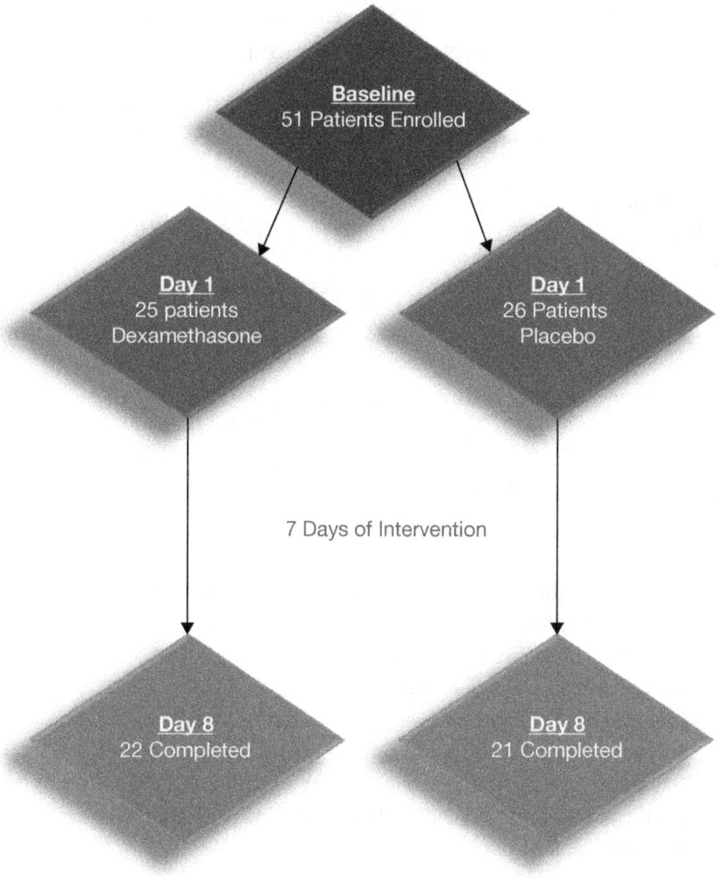

Figure 2.1. Randomization of patients in the study.

RESULTS

- In both the dexamethasone and placebo groups, the symptoms of nausea, appetite, and fatigue improved over the duration of the study, as noted in Table 2.1.
- Dexamethasone was not superior to placebo in improving symptoms of nausea, appetite, fatigue, pain, or well-being.
- Comparing dexamethasone to placebo, patients experienced a faster improvement in appetite by day 3. By day 8, improvement was comparable.
- Low pain intensity ratings throughout the duration of the study prohibited any conclusion on the impact of dexamethasone on pain.
- Patient well-being improved over the duration of the study in both the dexamethasone and placebo groups.

Table 2.1 MEAN INTENSITY OF NAUSEA, APPETITE, FATIGUE, AND PAIN AT BASELINE, DAY 3 AND DAY 8

Symptoms	Baseline Mean (SD)	Day 3 Mean (SD)	P^b	Day 8 Mean (SD)	P^c
Nausea					
Dexamethasone	8.0 (2.1)	3.5 (3.7)	<0.001	2.1 (3.0)	<0.001
Placebo	7.4 (2.3)	4.8 (3.7)	<0.001	2.0 (2.8)	<0.001
Appetite					
Dexamethasone	6.5 (3.3)	4.2 (3.4)	0.03	3.1 (3.7)	<0.001
Placebo	7.4 (3.1)	6.3 (3.4)	0.16	4.1 (3.1)	<0.001
Fatigue					
Dexamethasone	5.4 (3.5)	4.2 (3.8)	0.08	3.2 (3.6)	0.06
Placebo	5.7 (3.7)	4.0 (3.5)	0.09	3.0 (2.9)	0.01
Pain					
Dexamethasone	2.5 (2.9)	2.8 (3.1)	0.85	2.4 (3.4)	0.96
Placebo	3.1 (3.5)	2.1 (2.7)	0.08	2.8 (3.6)	0.49

a. Symptoms were evaluated using a 0 to 10 numerical scale, where 0 indicates the absence of the symptom and 10 indicates the worst possible symptom.
b. Paired *t* test, for change between baseline and Day 3
c. Paired *t* test, for change between baseline and Day 8.
Reprinted from *Journal of Pain and Symptom Management*, 28/4, E. Bruera, J. Ricardo Moyano, R. Sala, M. Antonieta Rico, S. Bosnjak, M. Bertolino, J. Willey, F. Strasser, J.L. Palmer, Dexamethasone in addition to metoclopramide for chronic nausea in patients with advanced cancer: a randomized controlled trial, 381–389, Copyright 2004, with permission from Elsevier.

- A total of 14 patients (27%) reported side effects: 6 in dexamethasone arm and 8 in placebo arm. Notable side effects included ankle edema, insomnia, and restlessness.

Criticisms and Limitations:

- Limitations of the study include a small sample size at the onset of the study further reduced by the inability of all enrolled patients to complete the study (51 patients enrolled, 43 completed). Thus, the study had limited power to detect meaningful differences.

Other Relevant Studies and Information:

- A second study by Mystakidou and colleagues that involved randomization between combinations of chlorpromazine, dexamethasone, metoclopramide, and tropisetron showed no benefit with the addition of dexamethasone to any of the combinations.[2]

- In a 2020 study, Navari et al. similarly looked at patients with advanced cancer experiencing chronic nausea. This study investigated the use of olanzapine daily compared to placebo. Olanzapine was effective in improving symptoms of nausea and vomiting. Similar to Bruera et al.'s study, patients were found to have improvement in appetite, fatigue, and overall well-being.[3]
- Bruera et al.'s study along with many other foundational studies for palliative treatment of nausea and vomiting in advanced cancer patients was used to develop current clinical practice guidelines in oncology.[4]
- The new Multinational Association of Supportive Care in Cancer guidelines recommend metoclopramide or haloperidol as first-line antiemetics and methotrimeprazine or olanzapine as second-line antiemetics. Third-line antiemetics are tropisetron and levosulpiride. There are no high-quality studies that support the use of combination antiemetics. Therefore, sequential trials of single antiemetic agents should be the standard approach to managing nausea and vomiting in advanced cancer.[5]

Summary and Implications: In this small, randomized, controlled study, dexamethasone was not superior to placebo in treatment of chronic nausea in patients with advanced cancer. Based on this and other research, major guidelines recommend metoclopramide or haloperidol as first-line antiemetics for this patient population.

CLINICAL CASE: SHOULD DEXAMETHASONE BE ADDED TO METOCLOPRAMIDE REGIMEN FOR CHRONIC NAUSEA?

Case History

A 70-year-old male with a past medical history significant for stage IV gastric adenocarcinoma (initially diagnosed 3 years prior as stage II, status post–partial gastrectomy) with metastases to the liver and peritoneum undergoing palliative-intent oncologic-directed therapies (last treatment 2 months prior) presents to the clinic with uncontrolled nausea and vomiting. He is averaging 2 emesis episodes per day for the last 3 weeks. He was initiated on metoclopramide 2 days ago with continued nausea and vomiting. Imaging studies obtained reveal no evidence of obstruction.

Should dexamethasone be added as an adjuvant for persistent nausea management?

Suggested Answer

Bruera et al.'s study reviewed dexamethasone compared to placebo in addition to ongoing metoclopramide for chronic nausea in patients with advanced cancer. This study found that dexamethasone was not superior to placebo for nausea control. Subjects in both groups had improvement in nausea, appetite, fatigue, and well-being.[1]

In the above case history, with persistent nausea on metoclopramide, this patient could be considered for an adjuvant agent. Based on Bruera et al.'s study, addition of dexamethasone is not recommended as symptoms similarly improved with or without the adjuvant dexamethasone while continuing metoclopramide.

References

1. Bruera E, Moyano JR, Sala R, et al. Dexamethasone in addition to metoclopramide for chronic nausea in patients with advanced cancer: a randomized controlled trial. *J Pain Symptom Manage.* 2004;28(4):381–388. doi:10.1016/j.jpainsymman.2004.01.009.
2. Mystakidou K, Befon S, Liossi C, Vlachos L. Comparison of the efficacy and safety of tropisetron, metoclopramide, and chlorpromazine in the treatment of emesis associated with far advanced cancer. *Cancer.* 1998;83(6):1214–1223.
3. Navari RM, Pywell CM, Le-Rademacher JG, et al. Olanzapine for the treatment of advanced cancer–related chronic nausea and/or vomiting. *JAMA Oncol.* 2020;6(6):895. doi:10.1001/jamaoncol.2020.1052.
4. Navari RM. Nausea and vomiting in advanced cancer. *Curr Treat Options Oncol.* 2020;21(2):1–10. doi:10.1007/s11864-020-0704-8.
5. Davis M, Hui D, Davies A, et al. MASCC antiemetics in advanced cancer updated guideline. *Support Care Cancer.* 2021;29(12):8097–8107.

3

Ibandronate Compared to Radiotherapy for Metastatic Bone Pain in Patients With Solid Tumors

ASHLEY BARLOW AND EDUARDO BRUERA

> A single infusion of ibandronate had outcomes similar to a single dose of radiotherapy for metastatic prostate bone pain. Ibandronate could be considered when radiotherapy is not available.
>
> —Hoskin et al.[1]

Research Question: Does a single infusion of ibandronate have similar efficacy in reduction of pain related to skeletal metastases for patients with metastatic prostate cancer compared to standard radiotherapy?

Funding: Sponsored by University College London; funding from Cancer Research UK. Roche Products Limited provided ibandronate free of charge.

Year Study Began: 2006

Year Study Published: 2015

Study Location: Multiple medical centers in the United Kingdom

Who Was Studied: Adults with a histological or cytological diagnosis of cancer and referral for palliative radiotherapy for localized bone pain with radiological bone metastasis confirmation using x-ray, isotope, computed tomography, or magnetic resonance scan; predicted life expectancy of > 3 months; and ability to comply with the pain chart and to participate in quality of life assessments. Initially patients with prostate, breast, and lung cancer were included, although due to limited enrollment in the breast and lung cohorts, they were subsequently removed from the analysis.

Who Was Excluded: Patients unable to receive radiotherapy or ibandronate because of renal failure, hypocalcemia, hypercalcemia, or known hypersensitivity to ibandronate or other bisphosphonates; allergy to aspirin; pregnancy or lactation; and any of the following previous treatments: radiotherapy with external beam to index site; high-dose chemotherapy; bisphosphonates within the previous 6 months; aminoglycoside antibiotics within 4 weeks of the study drug; change in systemic chemotherapy or hormone therapy within 4 weeks of trial entry; or any investigational drug within 30 days of study drug.

How Many Patients: 470

Study Overview: This is a multicenter, unblinded, phase 3, noninferiority trial in which 470 patients with prostate cancer and painful bony metastases from 58 centers were randomized to receive ibandronate or radiotherapy. Crossover between groups was allowed if response was not obtained within 4 weeks (Figure 3.1).

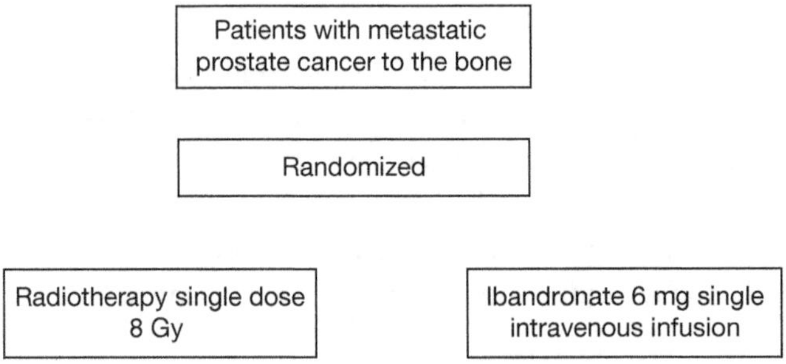

Figure 3.1. Summary of study design.

Study Intervention: Patients were randomly assigned in a 1:1 fashion to receive either ibandronate or localized radiotherapy. Ibandronate was administered as a single 6-mg intravenous infusion over 15 minutes. Radiotherapy was administered as a megavoltage external beam therapy delivered in a single dose of 8

Gy. The target volume covered the painful site with a margin of 3 cm or more and for a vertebral body a margin of 1 vertebra above and below. Subsequent treatments outside this window were allowed at the treating clinician's discretion, and crossover design was enabled in the setting where patients failed to respond in 4 weeks.

Follow-up: Median 11.7 months

Endpoints:

Primary outcome: Pain response at 4 weeks and 12 weeks compared to the baseline as measured by the World Health Organization (WHO) pain ladder and the Effective Analgesic Score (EAS). Patients reported their pain score based on the Brief Pain Inventory, a 10-point scale ranging from no pain (0) to severe pain (10), and detailed their analgesic use at baseline and then at 4, 8, 12, 26, and 52 weeks after treatment. Pain response was assessed by analgesic use and self-assessed pain score relative to baseline. The worst pain score was used in the primary analyses.

Secondary endpoints included long-term pain response at 26 and 52 weeks, quality of life at 4 and 12 weeks, crossover rates, bone complications, toxicity using Common Terminology Criteria for Adverse Events, and overall survival.

RESULTS

- There was no difference in the primary outcome of mean worst pain response at 4, 12, 26, or 52 weeks according to the WHO and EAS. Results were similar based on the per-protocol and intention-to-treat analysis (Tables 3.1 and 3.2).
- There was a more rapid initial response with radiotherapy when compared to ibandronate at 4 weeks, but this effect was not seen at 12 weeks.
- There was no overall difference in toxicity or quality of life between groups, although twice as many patients reported diarrhea in the radiotherapy arm as well as higher rates of nausea. This was balanced by a greater rate of other toxicities like fever and anorexia in the ibandronate arm.
- Overall survival was no different between study arms.

Table 3.1 TREATMENT EFFECTS AT 4 WEEKS

Pain Score Type	Individual IB (*n*)	RT (*n*)	Effect Size IB-RT (90% CI)	*P*
WHO RR	49.5 (182)	52.1 (175)	−3.7% (−12.4 to 5)	.49
EAS RR	52.7 (201)	60.2 (166)	−7.5% (−15.7 to 0.7)	.14
Mean EAS	1.16 (201)	−3.23 (191)	4.39 (−0.07 to 8.86)	.11
Median EAS	−0.02	−0.12	0.38 (0.02–1.44)	.04

Abbreviations: EAS, Effective Analgesic Score; IB, ibandronate; RR, response rate; RT, radiotherapy; WHO, World Health Organization.

Table 3.2 TREATMENT EFFECTS AT 12 WEEKS

Pain Score Type	Individual IB (*n*)	RT (*n*)	Effect Size IB-RT (90% CI)	*P*
WHO RR	56.1 (157)	49.4 (156)	6.7% (−2.6 to 16)	.24
EAS RR	56.7 (171)	60.2 (166)	−3.5% (−12.3 to 5.3)	.51
Mean EAS	−1.67 (171)	−0.19 (166)	−1.48 (−8.52 to 5.57)	.73
Median EAS	−0.06	−0.08	0.08 (−0.10 to 0.84)	.48

Abbreviations: EAS, Effective Analgesic Score; IB, ibandronate; RR, response rate; RT, radiotherapy; WHO, World Health Organization.

Criticisms and Limitations:

- Prior to this trial, radiotherapy had been the standard or care for management of painful bony metastases. The results from this trial show that ibandronate offers a convenient, equivalent alternative for those who are unable or unwilling to undergo radiotherapy.
- Crossover rates were high, 24% in the ibandronate arm versus 31% in the radiotherapy arm; therefore, it is difficult to determine the true effect of these strategies when used individually. In addition, the indication for crossover was not consistently correlated with symptom burden and could have been due to clinician preference, which results in difficulty in comparing efficacy versus treatment plan decisions made by clinicians.
- Due to the difference in nature between the 2 treatments, the study investigators could not be blinded, which may have introduced biases in the results.
- Given that the trial went on to exclude other patient populations that suffer from bony metastases due to low enrollment (lung and breast cancer), it is unknown if these results are generalizable to other disease states.

Other Relevant Studies and Information:

- Additional data on the use of ibandronate exists for patients with breast cancer, where rates of skeletal-related adverse events (SRAEs) were reduced by 20% when compared to placebo.[2]
- Positive data also exists for other nitrogen-containing bisphosphonates, zoledronic acid and pamidronate, which have demonstrated efficacy in the prevention of SRAEs in patients with breast and prostate cancer.
- Zoledronic acid has been studied for prevention of SRAEs and treatment of established painful bony metastases and has demonstrated efficacy in a wide array of disease states including hormone-refractory prostate cancer, breast cancer, multiple myeloma, or lung cancer and other solid tumors.[2] In a study of 24 patients with prostate cancer–related bone metastases, 75% had an improvement in pain score from the visual analog scale (VAS) to less than 4. The mean baseline score on the VAS was 7.8, which decreased to 3.6 after 1 month of treatment with zoledronic acid.[3]
- Zoledronic acid was compared head to head with pamidronate in a randomized double-blind trial of patients with metastatic breast cancer and multiple myeloma. The superiority of zoledronic acid was demonstrated in the reduction in the need for radiation therapy to the bone and rates of SRAEs compared to pamidronate, with no differences in the rates of adverse effects between treatment groups.[4]
- Following evidence from this and other studies, the National Comprehensive Cancer Center guidelines recommend bisphosphonates for the management of bone pain in the absence of an oncologic emergency.[5]

Summary and Implications: This large noninferiority randomized trial demonstrated that ibandronate was as effective as radiotherapy regarding pain scores, quality of life, and overall survival for the treatment of pain related to skeletal metastases in patients with prostate cancer. Based on this and other research, major guidelines now recommend bisphosphonates for the management of bone pain in patients with skeletal metastases.

CLINICAL CASE: WHO SHOULD BE CONSIDERED FOR BISPHOSPHONATE THERAPY?

Case History

A 72-year-old man with castrate-resistant prostate cancer presents with new-onset back pain and nonspecific shoulder pain. He states he has not had any recent falls or trauma to these areas. Further diagnostic workup reveals his cancer has progressed and he now has stage IV disease with widespread bony metastasis. He is experiencing depression due to inability to interact with his grandchildren or care for his wife due to the constant pain. The oncologist plans to initiate chemotherapy with cabazitaxel with prednisone in combination with the patient's androgen deprivation therapy for management of his metastatic disease. The patient has good renal function and dental health, and his lab values are within normal limits.

How should the patient's pain related to skeletal metastases be managed?

Suggested Answer

The trial comparing ibandronate to radiotherapy demonstrated that treatment options were noninferior with regard to pain control, quality of life, and overall survival. Given the patient in the above scenario is receiving concurrent chemotherapy to control his metastatic disease, the safety of radiotherapy with cabazitaxel has not been extensively studied and may increase his risk of myelosuppression depending on the site of radiation. Although radiotherapy may palliate symptoms more rapidly, this factor is not relevant in this case given that radiotherapy will have to be delayed until weeks after the patient has completed chemotherapy to minimize additive toxicities. In contrast, ibandronate 6 mg as an intravenous infusion would be able to be used concurrently with his chemotherapy without potentiating any treatment-related toxicities. Furthermore, the addition of a bisphosphonate has an added benefit in the ability to reduce future SRAEs such as fractures and maintain bone health while receiving corticosteroid treatment as a part of his prostate cancer treatment. Therefore, a bisphosphonate appears to be the ideal treatment option at the given time for this patient scenario, with the option to transition to radiotherapy if the patient does not respond to bisphosphonates or discontinues chemotherapy.

References

1. Hoskin P, Sundar S, Reczko K, et al. A multicenter randomized trial of ibandronate compared with single-dose radiotherapy for localized metastatic bone pain in prostate cancer. *JNCIJ*. 2015;107(10):djv197.
2. Costa L, Major PP. Effect of bisphosphonates on pain and quality of life in patients with bone metastases. *Nat Rev Clin Oncol*. 2009;6(3):163–174.
3. Fulfaro F, Leto G, Badalamenti G, et al. The use of zoledronic acid in patients with bone metastases from prostate carcinoma: effect on analgesic response and bone metabolism biomarkers. *J Chemother*. 2005;17(5):555–559.
4. Berenson JR, Rosen LS, Howell A, et al. Zoledronic acid reduces skeletal-related events in patients with osteolytic metastases. *Cancer*. 2001;91(7):1191–1200.
5. National Comprehensive Cancer Network. Adult Cancer Pain (Version 1.2020). https://www.nccn.org/professionals/physician_gls/pdf/pain.pdf. Accessed January 21, 2021.

4

Duloxetine for Cancer-Related Neuropathic Pain

ASHLEY BARLOW AND EDUARDO BRUERA

Additive Duloxetine for Cancer-Related Neuropathic Pain Nonresponsive or Intolerant to Opioid-Pregabalin Therapy: A Randomized Controlled Trial (JORTC-PAL08)

> The addition of duloxetine to opioid pregabalin combination therapy might have benefit in alleviating pain in patients [with chronic neuropathic pain] nonresponsive or intolerant to opioid-pregabalin combination therapy.
>
> —*Matsuoka et al.*[1]

Research Question: Can duloxetine reduce pain intensity of cancer-related neuropathic pain in patients who are nonresponsive or intolerant to opioid-pregabalin combination therapy?

Funding: Supported by the following grants: Sasakawa Memorial Health Foundation Research Grant (Grant No. 2013-A003), 2014–2016 Grant-in-Aid for Scientific Research (Grant-in-Aid for Young Scientists B; Grant No. 26860486), 2014 Health Labour Sciences Research Grant (Grant for Innovative Clinical Cancer Research: Multicenter Clinical Research Concerning the Development of Palliative Medicine for Severe Symptoms in Cancer Patients)

Research Team (H26-Innovative Cancer-General-056), and 2015–2017 Japan Agency for Medical Research and Development Award (Innovative Clinical Cancer Research)

Year Study Began: 2015

Year Study Published: 2019

Study Location: Japan

Who Was Studied: Patients suffering from definite or probable cancer pain (neuropathic or mixed), refractory to opioids and gabapentinoids, diagnosed according to the International Association for the Study of Pain algorithm. Patients required an average numerical rating scale (NRS) pain score in the preceding 24-hour period of ≥ 4 and a total Hospital Anxiety and Depression Scale (HADS) score of < 20 despite pregabalin ≥ 300 mg/day or intolerable side effects limiting pregabalin use.

Who Was Excluded: Patients with progressive paralysis, a known contraindication to use of duloxetine; depression; chemotherapy-induced peripheral neuropathy; or impaired cognitive function.

How Many Patients: 70

Study Overview: See Figure 4.1.

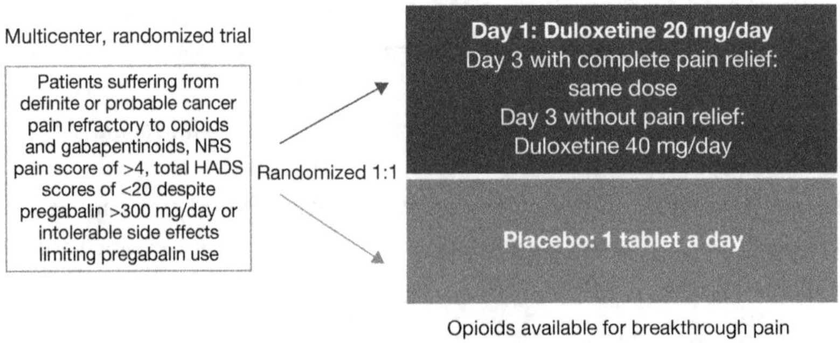

Figure 4.1. Study design overview.

Study Intervention: Eligible patients were randomly assigned on day 1 to either 1 capsule of duloxetine 20 mg/day or lactose (placebo). On day 3, patients who reported complete or substantial relief based on pain relief scale continued to receive the same dose; those without relief were increased to 2 capsules, equivalent to duloxetine 40 mg/day. Administration of previous coanalgesics remained unchanged throughout the study. Immediate-release opioids were available for breakthrough pain.

Follow-Up: Evaluations were performed at 4 time points: baseline (time of randomization), the day before the start of treatment, day 3 after starting treatment, and a final assessment performed on day 10 after starting treatment.

Endpoints:

Primary endpoints: Average pain intensity over 24 hours at day 10 as measured by Brief Pain Inventory (BPI)[7]-Item 5 and percentages of patients with 30% and 50% pain reduction from day 0.

Secondary endpoints: European Organization for Research and Treatment of Cancer QLQ-C15-PAL scores, frequency of daily rescue use, and adverse events (assessed by the Common Terminology Criteria for Adverse Events v.4.0, Japan Clinical Oncology Group version).

RESULTS

- Duloxetine was associated with modest but significant improvements in mean pain scores versus placebo (Table 4.1).

Table 4.1 ANALYSIS OF PAIN DURING THE TREATMENT PERIOD: BPI-ITEM 5 AND SENSITIVITY ANALYSIS

	Duloxetine (n = 34)	**Placebo (n = 33)**	**Difference in Means**	
Analysis	**Mean (90% CI), n**		**Mean (90% CI), n**	***t*-Test (One-Sided)**
CC	4.03 (3.33–4.74), 33	4.88 (4.37–5.38), 32	−0.84 (1.71–0.02)	0.053
BOCF	4.06 (3.37–4.74), 34	4.91 (4.41–5.41), 33	−0.85 (1.69–0.01)	0.048

Abbreviations: BOCF, baseline observation carried forward; BPI, Brief Pain Inventory; CC, case complete.

- At day 10, 44.1% of patients receiving duloxetine reported a pain improvement of > 30% versus 18.2% of patients receiving placebo, while 32.4% of patients receiving duloxetine reported pain improvement > 50% versus 3.0% (1/33) of patients receiving placebo (P = .002).

- No difference was observed in overall quality of life, physical function, or emotional function between the groups on day 10.
- Compared with placebo, patients receiving duloxetine demonstrated significantly better scores for pain ($P = .04$) though worse scores for appetite loss ($P = .001$) on day 10.
- More nausea and malaise were reported in patients receiving duloxetine compared to placebo.

Criticisms and Limitations:

- The dose of duloxetine (20–40 mg/day) was relatively low and could have been titrated to 60 mg/day. This may have limited the effectiveness of treatment since the dose was not optimized.
- The overall observation period was relatively short (i.e., 10 days) and may not have been sufficient to document the full effects of duloxetine versus placebo.
- This study has limited external validity given the small sample size and limited diversity in the population (confined to the Japanese population).

Other Relevant Studies and Information:

- Duloxetine is a serotonin norepinephrine reuptake inhibitor approved by the Food and Drug Administration (FDA) for painful diabetic neuropathy and has been reported in a randomized placebo-controlled phase 3 trial to be effective in reducing the pain associated with chemotherapy-induced peripheral neuropathy.[6]
- National Comprehensive Cancer Center guidelines that do not incorporate findings from this study indicate that adjuvant analgesics such as gabapentinoids should be trialed for cancer-associated peripheral neuropathy, with duloxetine reserved for those with chemotherapy-induced peripheral neuropathy.[7]

Summary and Implications: This small analysis suggests a modest but statistically significant benefit of duloxetine for cancer-associated peripheral neuropathy in patients refractory to opioids and gabapentinoids. While there is a need for further research on duloxetine for treating cancer-associated peripheral neuropathy, given the limited options for patients who are refractory to other medications, it is a treatment to consider.

CLINICAL CASE: NEUROPATHIC PAIN SECONDARY TO METASTATIC BREAST CANCER

Case History

NR is a 61-year-old female with metastatic breast cancer and leptomeningeal disease. Due to her sites of disease, she has been experiencing progressively worse numbness and tingling in her hands and feet. Her current pain regimen consists of morphine sulfate 80 mg every 12 hours and morphine immediate release 15 mg every 4 hours. She had a trial of gabapentin 300 mg 3 times daily but experienced severe drowsiness, fatigue, and peripheral edema that led her to decline further treatment with this agent. She presents to the clinic with depression associated with inability to achieve adequate control of her neuropathic pain to the point where she can no longer button her own clothes. What would be the next steps recommended for NR to achieve adequate pain control?

Suggested Answer

NR has significant neuropathic pain related to her leptomeningeal disease.[1,2] She has experienced limited pain relief in terms of neuropathic pain with her current opioid regimen, which is likely due to the lack of neurotransmitter modulation with morphine and therefore it does not target the pathogenesis of cancer-associated peripheral neuropathy.[1,7] Further uptitration of her morphine would provide limited and minimal benefit. Furthermore, the addition of gabapentin as recommended in the case was an appropriate next option; however, the toxicities this patient experienced are very common in practice and limit continued treatment with this agent. It could be plausible to start the patient at a lower dose of 300 mg at bedtime and retitrate more slowly; however, the patient is reluctant to retrialing therapy. The next ideal step for this patient would include the initiation of duloxetine 20 mg orally daily, with uptitration by 20 mg every 4–7 days based on tolerability until the patient reaches a dose of 60 mg/day. Duloxetine modulates by a different mechanism compared to opioids and is therefore able to synergize with these agents.[6,7] With regard to side effects, the patient should not experience drowsiness or peripheral edema as experienced with gabapentin but may experience nausea and anorexia. In this case, the patient can take the medication with food to limit nausea and uptitration can be slowed. A further benefit for the addition of duloxetine would be in the treatment of her depression since duloxetine is FDA approved for major depressive disorder.[7]

References

1. Amato AA, Collins MP. Neuropathies associated with malignancy. *Semin Neurol.* 1998;18(1):125–144.
2. Falah M, Schiff D, Burns TM. Neuromuscular complications of cancer diagnosis and treatment. *J Supp Oncol.* 2005;3(4):271–282.
3. Kelly JJ, Karcher DS. Lymphoma and peripheral neuropathy: a clinical review. *Muscle Nerve.* 2005;31(3):301–313.
4. Matsuoka H, Iwase S, Miyaji T, et al. Additive duloxetine for cancer-related neuropathic pain nonresponsive or intolerant to opioid-pregabalin therapy: a randomized controlled trial (Jortc-pal08). *J Pain Symptom Manage.* 2019;58(4):645–653.
5. Lavoie Smith EM, Pang H, Cirrincione C, et al. CALGB 170601: a phase III double blind trial of duloxetine to treat painful chemotherapy-induced peripheral neuropathy (CIPN). *J Clin Oncol.* 2012;30(suppl):Abstract CRA9013.
6. Cleeland CS, Ryan KM. Pain assessment: global use of the Brief Pain Inventory. *Ann Acad Med Singapore.* 1994;23(2):129–138.
7. Adult Cancer Pain. National Comprehensive Cancer Network Clinical Practice Guidelines in Oncology. Version 1, Feb 26 2021.

5

Methadone as a Coanalgesic

NINA M. BEMBEN

> In the absence of contraindications, an add-on trial of methadone should not be reserved as a last-line treatment, but might be worth considering earlier for patients presenting with cancer pain of high intensity, as safety and tolerability were good.
>
> —COURTEMANCHE ET AL.[1]

Research Question: How does adding low-dose methadone as a coanalgesic impact pain intensity in patients on palliative care with cancer?

Funding: Faculte de Pharmacie of the University of Montreal

Year Study Began: 2014

Year Study Published: 2016

Study Location: Centre Hospitalier de l'Universite de Montreal (CHUM), Montreal, Canada

Who Was Studied: Inpatients or outpatients followed by the palliative care team who were prescribed methadone as a coanalgesic for cancer pain.

Who Was Excluded: Patients who received methadone for opioid withdrawal, patients with hepatic impairment, those with a prognosis of < 7 days, and patients for whom < 7 days of data were available.

How Many Patients: 153

Study Overview: This cohort study included all patients followed by the palliative care team who received methadone as a coanalgesic for cancer pain between October 16, 2010, and May 19, 2014. Patients were included in either a prospective or retrospective arm, although only 7 patients were included in the prospective arm (Figure 5.1).

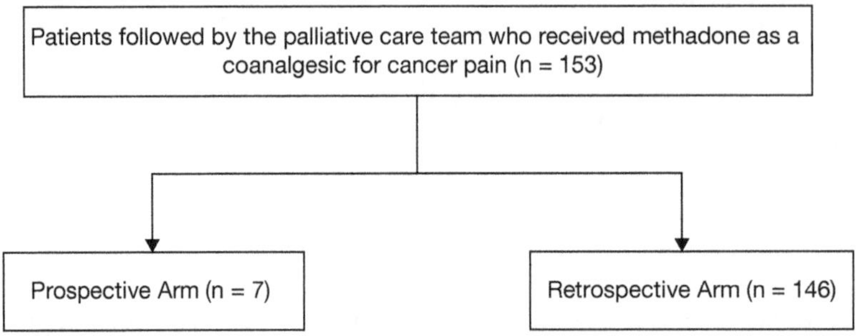

Figure 5.1. Summary of study design.

Study Intervention: All of the included patients received methadone as a coanalgesic for cancer pain. Pain intensity was assessed for study patients, as were changes in patients' use of other analgesics.

Follow-Up: A median of 32 days (interquartile range 17.8–60 days)

Endpoints:

Primary outcome: The proportion of patients who were significant and substantial responders to methadone as a coanalgesic, as measured by a reduction in pain intensity on the numeric rating scale (NRS) of ≥ 30% and ≥ 50%, respectively. The median time to significant or substantial response was also collected as a primary outcome.

Secondary outcomes: Daily dose of methadone and other opioids, dose of "as needed" opioids, adverse effects, quality of life, and global impression of change (reported by the patient and practitioner, prospectively).

RESULTS (TABLE 5.1)

- 49.3% of patients had at least a significant response (≥ 30% reduction in pain intensity) to methadone as a coanalgesic.
- 30% of patients had a substantial response (≥ 50% reduction in pain intensity) to methadone as a coanalgesic.

Table 5.1 SUMMARY OF KEY PRIMARY AND SECONDARY OUTCOMES

Outcome	Day 3	Day 7	Day 15	*Day 30*
Significant responder, (≥ 30% reduction in pain intensity) Number (%)	35 (36.8)	37 (42.1)	22 (36.7)	11 (36.7)
Substantial responder, (≥ 50% reduction in pain intensity) Number (%)	23 (24.2)	22 (25)	12 (20)	6 (20)
Daily dose of methadone (significant responders) Median (IQR)	3 mg (3–6 mg)	6 mg[a] (3–6 mg)	6 mg[a] (3–6 mg)	6 mg (3–21 mg)
Daily dose of methadone (substantial responders) Median (IQR)	3 mg (3–6 mg)	4 mg (3–6 mg)	6 mg (3–12 mg)	3 mg[a] (2–4 mg)

Abbreviation: IQR, interquartile range.
[a] Statistically significant difference between responders and nonresponders.

- The median time to significant response was 7 days.
- The daily doses of nonmethadone opioids and as-needed opioids were not significantly different between responders and nonresponders.
- Most responders to methadone did so within 7 days, and the response rate did not increase after 1 week.
- Increasing methadone dose did not increase analgesia.
- 90.4% of patients reported an adverse effect, with the most common being drowsiness (51.4%), confusion (27.4%), and constipation (24.7%).

Criticisms and Limitations:

- This study did not use a comparator, and the prospective arm enrolled only 7 patients. It is impossible to know if use of another coanalgesic or treatment strategy would have provided similar, or even better, analgesia.
- Interpretation of the study findings is limited by the large amount of missing data (NRS rating was not systemically recorded in provider progress notes and even after review of nursing notes was still absent, particularly beyond day 7).
- While 90.4% of patients reported an adverse effect, it is impossible to determine whether these adverse effects were due to methadone or the other opioid as patients continued their other opioid therapy.

Other Relevant Studies and Information:

- Limited data evaluating low-dose methadone as a coanalgesic exist; however, a 2019 review found a statistically significant improvement in analgesia in 4 of 7 included studies evaluating methadone as a coanalgesic in palliative medicine.[2] The remaining 3 studies did not address the statistical significance of improvement in analgesia.
- Expert consensus guidelines for the use of methadone in hospice and palliative care state that while there is limited, low-quality evidence, adjunctive methadone may be useful for patients who have poorly controlled pain, especially those with limited life expectancy due to the short time to first significant analgesic response.[3] The median time to response of 7 days demonstrated in this study provided support for the recommendation for use of methadone as a coanalgesic in patients with limited life expectancy.
- Using methadone as an adjuvant analgesic has not been evaluated to our knowledge in a randomized clinical trial, particularly in comparison to a complete conversion to methadone (evaluating both therapeutic response and toxicity). Additional research would be helpful to best identify situations where a partial versus complete conversion to methadone would be most advantageous.

Summary and Implications: This study supports the utility of methadone as a coanalgesic in palliative medicine, with nearly half (49%) of patients achieving at least a 30% reduction in pain intensity. With a median time to response of 7 days, adjuvant methadone is an important tool for patients with pain that is unresponsive to traditional first-line opioids, particularly among patients with a limited prognosis.

CLINICAL CASE: WHO IS A CANDIDATE FOR COANALGESIC METHADONE?

Case History

A 74-year-old woman with stage IV lung cancer is being followed by the palliative care team. She has been treated with long-acting morphine 50 mg twice daily and immediate-release morphine 15 mg every 3 hours as needed for breakthrough pain. She has been using 5 to 6 doses of breakthrough pain medication daily for the past 3 days. She reports receiving some relief from her breakthrough dose of morphine, which brings her pain to a 5/10, but it does not improve beyond that. At worst she rates the pain as 8/10. The palliative care team estimates her prognosis as in the range of days to weeks.

Is this patient a candidate for coanalgesic methadone?

Suggested Answer

The study by Courtemanche and colleagues evaluated methadone as a coanalgesic and found that 49% of patients achieved a reduction in pain intensity of at least 30% in a median of 7 days.

This patient is experiencing breakthrough pain despite an adequate dose of breakthrough morphine and is using 175–190 mg oral morphine daily. Coanalgesic methadone may significantly improve this patient's pain within her remaining life expectancy. The palliative care team should discuss the potential benefits and risks with this patient and her caregivers and ensure that an appropriate monitoring plan is in place.

References

1. Courtemanche F, Dao D, Gagne F, et al. Methadone as a coanalgesic for palliative care cancer patients. *J Palliat Med.* 2016;19(9):972–978.
2. Chalker C, O'Neill H, Cranfield F. Efficacy of low-dose and/or adjuvant methadone in palliative medicine. *BMJ Support Palliat Care.*2022;12(e6):e730–e735.
3. McPherson ML, Walker KA, Davis MP, et al. Safe and appropriate use of methadone in hospice and palliative care: expert consensus white paper. *J Pain Symptom Manage.* 2019;57(3):635–645.e4.

6

Methadone Versus Fentanyl for Nociceptive Cancer Pain

JOSHUA BORRIS AND SYDNEY TAYLOR ISRAEL

> Our study shows that treatment with methadone will not result in inferior pain relief in patients with nociceptive pain caused by head and neck cancer.
>
> —HAUMANN ET AL.[1]

Research Question: Is methadone inferior to fentanyl for treating radiation-induced nociceptive pain?

Funding: Maastricht University Medical Center

Year Study Began: 2011

Year Study Published: 2017

Study Location: Maastricht University Medical Center, Maastricht, the Netherlands

Who Was Studied: Patients with histologically proven head and neck cancer experiencing nociceptive pain due to radiation mucositis and with a numeric rating scale (NRS) pain score of $\geq$ 4 out of 10 who required oral opioids after trialing oral topical therapies.

Who Was Excluded: Patients who were not naïve to opioids, had recent surgery, were pregnant, had asthma or myasthenia gravis, or had contraindications to opioids.

How Many Patients: 82

Study Overview: This was an open-label, noninferiority, randomized controlled trial in which opioid-naïve patients with head and neck cancer were randomized to receive methadone or fentanyl (Figure 6.1). Randomization was stratified by accelerated radiotherapy, chemotherapy with radiotherapy, and bilateral versus unilateral treatment.

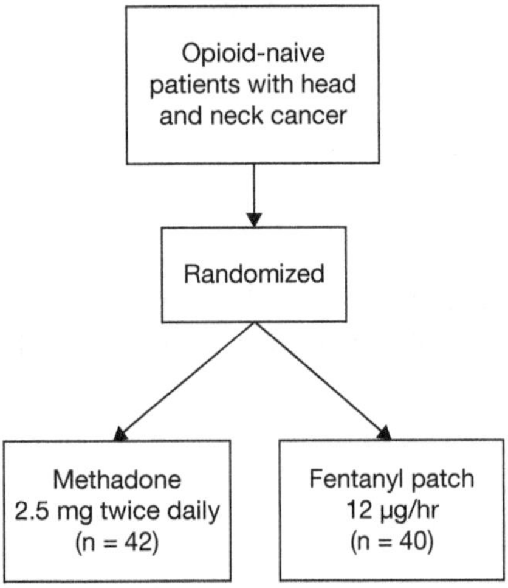

Figure 6.1. Summary of study subject randomization.

Study Intervention: One study arm was initiated on methadone 2.5 mg by mouth twice daily and the other study arm was initiated on fentanyl transdermal patch 12 µg/hour along with fentanyl 50 µg nasal spray or fentanyl 100 µg buccal tablet for breakthrough pain. Regimens for breakthrough pain could be used up to 6 times daily. If the subject reported using their breakthrough medication 4 times or more and the subject's average NRS pain score was > 4 at a follow-up visit, then the subject's baseline opioid dose was increased by 50%. If the subject's pain was perceived as acceptable, the baseline opioid dose was decreased by 30%. There was considerable loss to follow-up during the study, mainly due to no longer requiring opioids for pain control or due to intolerable side effects, leaving 24 patients in the fentanyl group and 16 patients in the methadone group by the end of the analysis period.

Follow-up: Evaluation at 1, 3, and 5 weeks

Endpoints:

Primary outcome: NRS pain score (with ≤ 50% decrease in NRS considered clinically significant).

Secondary outcomes: Pain interference (assessed on the Brief Pain Inventory [BPI]), opioid escalation index (mean increase of opioid dose), use of breakthrough opioid doses, global perceived effect (GPE), and side effects (Table 6.1).

Table 6.1 SUMMARY OF PRIMARY AND SECONDARY OUTCOMES FROM STUDY

Primary Outcome			
	Point Estimate (95% CI)[a]		**Difference (95% CI)**
NRS Pain Score			
Week 1	0.3 (−0.6 to 1.3)		Noninferior
Week 3	1.4 (0.1 to 2.7)		0.75 (−0.21 to 1.71)
Week 5	0.3 (−1.2 to 1.8)		Not significant
Secondary Outcomes			
	Methadone	**Fentanyl**	***P* Value**
Pain Interference			
Week 1	−7.55	−3.30	Not significant
Week 3	−9.58	−1.00	.023
Week 5	−12.63	−7.00	Not significant
Opioid Escalation Index			
Week 1	1.10	1.10	Not significant
Week 3	1.44	1.99	.0004
Week 5	1.50	2.32	.013

Abbreviation: NRS, numerical rating scale.

[a] Point estimates are approximations based on figure provided in the article.

RESULTS

There was no significance in use of breakthrough medication, GPE, or side effects.

Criticisms and Limitations:

- It was an open-label study.
- Single-center design limits external validity.
- Post hoc power analysis was only 45% for identifying a statistically significant difference of 1 point in the NRS.

- There was a significant loss to follow-up at the conclusion of the 5-week analysis, which may have biased the findings if drop-out was correlated with outcomes

Other Relevant Studies and Information:

- This trial was conducted simultaneously with a similar trial by the same authors that found methadone was superior to fentanyl in controlling neuropathic radiation-induced mucositis pain.[2]
- Haumann and colleagues analyzed the patients in these 2 trials to determine what characteristics were associated with a greater 1-week response to therapy and found that patients who recently had surgery were less likely to have treatment success. Patients who had greater baseline pain, were experiencing neuropathic pain, or were given methadone over fentanyl were more likely to experience treatment success. However, at 5 weeks, no characteristics were preferentially associated with treatment success.[3]
- The current study suggests methadone may also be effective for general radiotherapy-induced nociceptive pain.
- Two systematic reviews and 1 randomized controlled trial have compared the analgesic effect of methadone versus other opioids, but none suggested a difference in analgesia.[4–6]
- Efficacious nonopioid therapies for radiation-induced mucositis include topical doxepin, amitriptyline, diclofenac, and benzydamine.[7]

Summary and Implications: This small, open-label, randomized trial suggests that methadone is noninferior to fentanyl in controlling nociceptive radiation-induced mucositis pain. It also suggests that methadone and fentanyl have similar effects on pain interference and quality of life, with no significant differences in adverse events. Though this analysis was small and thus not definitive, it adds to the growing body of literature supporting the use of methadone as an analgesic for both nociceptive and neuropathic pain.

CLINICAL CASE: SHOULD METHADONE OR FENTANYL BE USED FOR THIS PATIENT?

Case History

A 54-year-old male with recently diagnosed stage IV head and neck cancer with metastases to the bone presents with worsening pain. The patient complains of a burning and stabbing pain in the back of his throat in addition to extremely sharp pains in his arms and spine. The attending asks your opinion about starting transdermal fentanyl in this patient. The patient is opioid naïve and is 5'11" and weighs 135 pounds. What dose of transdermal fentanyl would you recommend?

Suggested Answer

Clearly this is a trick question, because this patient is not an appropriate candidate for transdermal fentanyl. Per the labeling requirement, a patient must be opioid tolerant, defined as 60 mg/day or more of oral morphine equivalent for at least a week, and this patient is opioid naïve. Also, this patient is clearly cachectic and may not get the maximum benefit from transdermal fentanyl.[8] Alternately, methadone would be a reasonable opioid barring any precautions or contraindications. Assuming his QTc is normal, we could begin his methadone dose between 2 and 7.5 mg/day.[9] Because the patient has pain in his throat, it would be best to use the oral methadone solution, 10 mg/mL, to use the lowest volume possible. We could begin with methadone 2 mg orally every 12 hours (which would be a tiny volume) and insert it in the buccal cavity. We could also recommend morphine 20 mg/mL, 5 mg every 2 hours as needed for additional pain.

References

1. Haumann J, Kuijk SMJ van, Geurts JW, et al. Methadone versus fentanyl in patients with radiation-induced nociceptive pain with head and neck cancer: a randomized controlled noninferiority trial. *Pain Pract.* 2018;18(3):331–340.
2. Haumann J, Geurts JW, van Kuijk SMJ, Kremer B, Joosten EA, van den Beuken-van Everdingen MHJ. Methadone is superior to fentanyl in treating neuropathic pain in patients with head-and-neck cancer. *Eur J Cancer.* 2016;65:121–129.
3. Haumann J, van Kuijk SMJ, Joosten EA, van den Beuken-van Everdingen MHJ. The association between patient characteristics and opioid treatment response in neuropathic and nociceptive pain due to cancer. *J Palliat Med.* 2019;22(2):157–163.
4. Nicholson AB, Watson GR, Derry S, Wiffen PJ. Methadone for cancer pain. *Cochrane Database Syst Rev.* 2017;2:CD003971.
5. Haroutiunian S, McNicol ED, Lipman AG. Methadone for chronic non-cancer pain in adults. *Cochrane Database Syst Rev.* 2012;11:CD008025.
6. Mercadante S, Porzio G, Ferrera P, et al. Sustained-release oral morphine versus transdermal fentanyl and oral methadone in cancer pain management. *Eur J Pain.* 2008;12(8):1040–1046.
7. Christoforou J, Karasneh J, Manfredi M, et al. World Workshop on Oral Medicine VII: non-opioid pain management of head and neck chemo/radiation-induced mucositis: a systematic review. *Oral Dis.* 2019;25(S1):182–192.
8. Heiskanen T, Mätzke S, Haakana S, Gergov M, Vuori E, Kalso E. Transdermal fentanyl in cachectic cancer patients. *Pain.* 2009;144(1):218–222.
9. McPherson ML, Walker KA, Davis MP, et al. Safe and appropriate use of methadone in hospice and palliative care: expert consensus white paper. *J Pain Symptom Manage.* 2019;57(3):635–645.e4.

7

Improving Metastatic Bone Pain With Opioid Adjuvants

Low-Dose Antidepressants and Low-Dose Pregabalin

GARY T. BUCKHOLZ AND J. KEAIS POPE

> Low-dose pregabalin-antidepressant combinations with opioids were effective in the management of painful bone metastases without severe adverse effects.
>
> —NISHIHARA ET AL.[1]

Research Question: When combined together, can adjuvant, nonopioid medications, such as antiepileptics and antidepressants, effectively treat refractory metastatic bone pain?

Funding: None

Year Study Began: 2010

Year Study Published: 2013

Study Location: Multidisciplinary Pain Centre, Department of Orthopaedic Surgery, Kochi Medical School, Kochi University, Kohasu Aichi Medical School, Karimata, Nagakute-cho, Aichigun, Aichi Japan; Okocho, Nankoku, Kochi 783-8505, Japan

Who Was Studied: 37 adult Japanese patients with cancer in a pain clinic, all confirmed to have bone metastases refractory to opioids and nonsteroidal anti-inflammatory drugs (NSAIDs).

Who Was Excluded: It was noted that at day 7, pain control was not sufficient in 1 arm of the study, the pregabalin-only group, and thus those patients were then started on mirtazapine after day 7 and were withdrawn from the remainder of the study on days 10 and 14. No other exclusion criteria were directly addressed by the investigators.

How Many Patients: 37

Study Overview: This was a randomized controlled trial in which 37 oncology patients with bony metastasis were randomized to 1 of 3 groups (Figure 7.1):

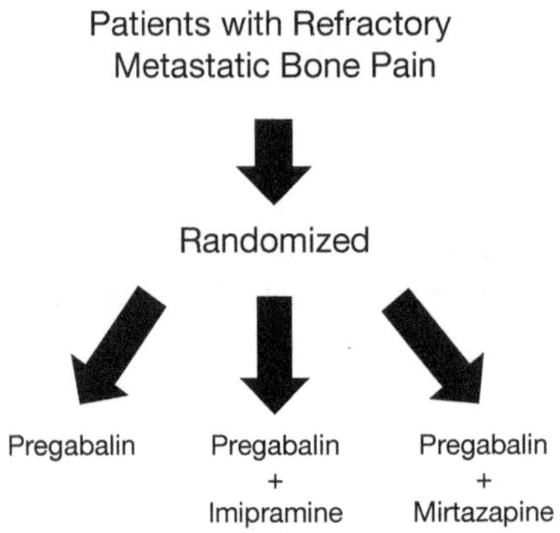

Figure 7.1. Study design.

1. Pregabalin monotherapy: P group
2. Pregabalin and imipramine: P-I group
3. Pregabalin and mirtazapine: P-M group

Study Intervention: Patients in all 3 groups received their usual standard opioid therapy, with rescue doses available as needed. Average oral morphine equivalents (OMEs) for all 3 groups was 55–60 mg/day. NSAIDs that were already prescribed were left unchanged. No new drugs were started during this time period. Glomerular filtration rate and QTc were measured prior to starting the study.

Patients randomized to each group were treated as follows:

1. P group: Pregabalin 50 mg orally every 8 hours
2. P-I group: Pregabalin 25 mg orally every 8 hours and imipramine 5 mg orally every 12 hours

3. P-M group: Pregabalin 25 mg orally every 8 hours and mirtazapine 7.5 mg orally every 12 hours

Follow-Up: 14 days

Endpoints:

Primary endpoint: Total pain score = average intensity of total pain over the previous 24 hours assessed on a 0–10 numerical scale

Secondary endpoint: Number of paroxysmal pain episodes in the previous 24 hours (shooting or lancinating pain)

RESULTS

- The total pain score and the number of paroxysmal pain episodes decreased on day 1 for all 3 groups after the start of medication, with a significantly greater pain reduction in the P-M group versus the P group.
- By day 7 it was determined that there was inadequate pain control in the P group, and patients in this study arm were started on mirtazapine and withdrawn from the remainder of the study.
- By day 14 it was demonstrated that the pain-relieving effects of the P-I and P-M groups were maintained for more than 1 week.
- Table 7.1 provides demographics and baseline characteristics of patients. Figures 7.2 and 7.3 show changes of pain scores and changes of daily paroxysmal pain episodes over time for each group.

Table 7.1 DEMOGRAPHICS AND BASELINE CHARACTERISTICS OF PATIENTS [A]

	P ($n = 12$)	**P-I** ($n = 12$)	**P-M** ($n = 13$)	***P* Value**
Age (year)	64 (47–71)	54 (40–77)	64 (37–72)	.4709
Sex (M/F)	8/4	8/4	8/5	.9538
Weight (kg)	54 (40–64)	53.5 (36–70)	50 (43–68)	.7877
Daily opioid dose[b] (mg/day)	60 (20–180)	55 (20–200)	60 (20–120)	.9342
Oxycodone SR	6	7	7	
Fentanyl Patch	6	5	6	

[a] Values are median (range) or number.

[b] Oral morphine equivalent.

Reprinted with permission from Nishihara M, Arai YC, Yamamoto Y, et al. Combinations of low-dose antidepressants and low-dose pregabalin as useful adjuvants to opioids for intractable, painful bone metastases. Pain Physician. 2013 Sep-Oct;16(5):E547–E552.

Criticisms and Limitations:

- Because there wasn't a true control group, it is not clear based on this study design that pain control was better with the medications than it would have been without any treatment.
- This was a small study limited to a single site in Japan with only 37 participants suffering from bony pain from cancer metastases, and thus the findings may not be more broadly generalizable to other situations.

Other Relevant Studies and Information:

- The authors are building on their previous work by showing that pain-reducing effects of low-dose antidepressants in combination with low-dose antiepileptics may occur faster and with a lower adverse effect profile compared to monotherapy, which may require higher doses and 2 or more weeks to achieve the desired response. Their previous work was with combining gabapentin and imipramine.[2]
- Both gabapentin and imipramine individually have evidence of being effective for neuropathic pain.[3]
- There is good evidence for tricyclic antidepressant medications assisting with neuropathic pain.[4] However, the authors utilized lower doses than

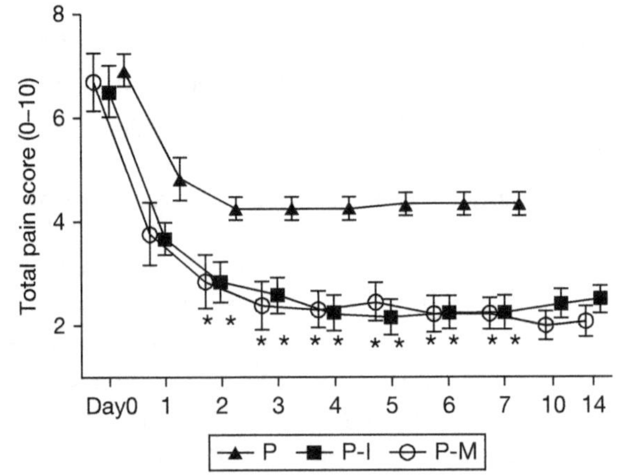

Figure 7.2. Changes of the total pain score. P, pregabalin; P-I, pregabalin–imipramine; P-M, pregabalin–mirtazapine. Error bar represents standard error of the mean (SEM), * $P < 0.05$ vs pregabalin.

Reprinted with permission from Nishihara M, Arai YC, Yamamoto Y, et al. Combinations of low-dose antidepressants and low-dose pregabalin as useful adjuvants to opioids for intractable, painful bone metastases. Pain Physician. 2013 Sep-Oct;16(5):E547–E552.

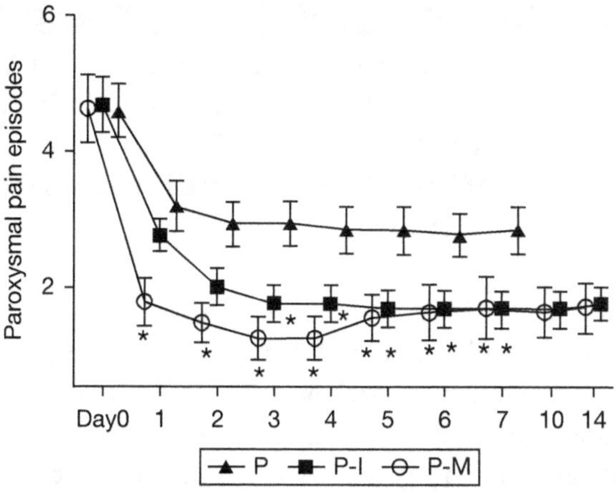

Figure 7.3. Changes of the daily paroxysmal pain episodes. P, pregabalin; P-I, pregabalin–imipramine; P-M, pregabalin–mirtazapine. Error bar represents standard error of the mean (SEM). * $P < 0.05$ vs pregabalin.
Reprinted with permission from Nishihara M, Arai YC, Yamamoto Y, et al. Combinations of low-dose antidepressants and low-dose pregabalin as useful adjuvants to opioids for intractable, painful bone metastases. Pain Physician. 2013 Sep-Oct;16(5):E547–E552.

supported in the literature, which may impact the mechanism of action with higher antihistaminergic and lower noradrenergic effects.

- The prior evidence for mirtazapine helping with pain is minimal at best. There is some evidence to suggest that mirtazapine might be helpful to treat pain in the setting of concomitant depression.
- Guidelines on the treatment of cancer pain have only minor sections describing treatment for cancer-related bone pain, and these primarily focus on radiotherapy, radiopharmaceuticals, bone-modifying agents, or procedural management. The only guideline specific to treatment of bone metastasis does not comment on use of antidepressants or anticonvulsants.[5]

Summary and Implications: In this analysis of Japanese patients living with metastatic bone pain refractory to opioids and NSAIDs, a medication regimen using 2 drugs (e.g., pregabalin and an antidepressant) led to decreased pain scores when compared to pregabalin alone. While the data were found to be statistically significant, the small sample size limits generalizability and highlights the need for additional studies to validate the findings. When considering combination therapy, appropriate dosing and risks related to polypharmacy should be considered carefully.

CLINICAL CASE: WHO SHOULD BE PRESCRIBED PREGABALIN AND ANTIDEPRESSANTS FOR PAIN? WHAT ARE SOME ADJUVANT PHARMACOLOGIC INTERVENTIONS TO HELP TREAT REFRACTORY METASTATIC BONE PAIN?

Case History

A 57-year-old female with breast carcinoma that has metastasized to the spine is admitted for acute refractory back pain. She receives inpatient intravenous opioid medications, and her acute pain crisis resolves. However, the patient is reporting that her "pain only gets down to a 6 now, when it used to go down to a 3 with my oral medications. They don't seem to have the effect they once did." Prior to this admission, she had only been taking oxycodone and ibuprofen for her pain relief. She is hoping to be discharged soon and does not want to increase the dosage of her opioid medications. She also complains of having no appetite and some difficulty sleeping at night. These symptoms were problematic prior to her pain worsening. Should this patient be started on antiepileptics and antidepressants to help treat her metastatic bone pain?

Suggested Answer

It is reasonable to consider prescribing a trial of combination antiepileptics and antidepressants in this case; however, more research is needed to support this as standard practice. If considering mirtazapine, be aware there is very limited evidence available to support its use specifically for pain. In this case, complaints of anorexia and difficulty sleeping may be helped by mirtazapine and may lower the threshold to consider adding this agent. As always, each patient should be informed of the harm, burden, and benefit related to their treatment plan. If considering combination therapy, monitoring of side effects will be important, and it will be more challenging to identify the cause of the side effects when starting multiple medications at the same time.

References

1. Nishihara M, Arai YC, Yamamoto Y, et al. Combinations of low-dose antidepressants and low-dose pregabalin as useful adjuvants to opioids for intractable, painful bone metastases. *Pain Physician*. 2013 Sep-Oct;16(5):E547–E552. PMID: 24077205.
2. Arai YC, Matsubara T, Shimo K, et al. Low-dose gabapentin as useful adjuvant to opioids for neuropathic cancer pain when combined with low-dose imipramine. *J Anesth*. 2010 Jun;24(3):407–410. doi:10.1007/s00540-010-0913-6. Epub 2010 Mar 10. PMID: 20217150.

3. Berger A, Dukes E, Mercadante S, Oster G. Use of antiepileptics and tricyclic antidepressants in cancer patients with neuropathic pain. *Eur J Cancer Care (Engl)*. 2006 May;15(2):138–145. doi:10.1111/j.1365-2354.2005.00624.x. PMID: 16643261.
4. Derry S, Wiffen PJ, Aldington D, Moore RA. Nortriptyline for neuropathic pain in adults. *Cochrane Database Syst Rev*. 2015;(1):CD011209.
5. Shibata H, Kato S, Sekine I, et al. Diagnosis and treatment of bone metastasis: comprehensive guideline of the Japanese Society of Medical Oncology, Japanese Orthopedic Association, Japanese Urological Association, and Japanese Society for Radiation Oncology. *ESMO Open*. 2016;1(2):e000037–e000037.

8

Intranasal Midazolam Versus Rectal Diazepam for the Home Treatment of Acute Seizures

KIRSTIN L. CAMPBELL

> Given the ease of administration/overall satisfaction, intranasal midazolam via Mucosal Atomization Device may be considered an alternative to rectal diazepam as a rescue medication for the in-home treatment of prolonged seizures.
>
> —Holsti et al.[1]

Research Question: In the home setting, how does intranasal administration of midazolam via use of an atomization device (IN-MMAD) compare with the standard therapy of rectal diazepam (RD)?

Funding: Primary Children's Medical Center Foundation

Year Study Began: 2006

Year Study Published: 2010

Study Location: Primary Children's Medical Center, Salt Lake City, Utah, United States

Who Was Studied: Pediatric patients with any known seizure disorder who were prescribed an antiepileptic rescue medication for use at home.

Who Was Excluded: Patients 18 years of age and older, if their neurologist did not plan to prescribe a rescue medication, or if their prescribed rescue medication was lorazepam.

How Many Patients: 358

Study Overview: This is a randomized controlled trial in which children with epilepsy receiving a prescription for a home seizure rescue medication were randomized to receive IN-MMAD or RD. Physicians, caregivers, and research assistants were blinded to what medication would be received until after consent was obtained. Complete blinding was not possible given differing routes of administration.

Study Intervention: Patients who were randomized to the IN-MMAD group received 0.2 mg/kg (max 10 mg) of midazolam for intranasal administration by atomizer. Patients in the RD group received 0.3–0.5 mg/kg of diazepam for rectal administration. The groups received administration instruction by video for the relevant medication. Both groups received instruction to administer their assigned medication for seizure lasting > 5 minutes and to call 911 for support. Caregivers were provided with a stopwatch and timing sheets to record observations. Requested data included time of seizure onset, time of medication administration, and time to resolution of the seizure. There were no limitations or instructions provided for care at or after the time of emergency medical services (EMS) arrival or for care if patient required transfer to an emergency unit.

Follow-Up: Caregivers were requested to mail in their timing sheet as soon as possible after medication administration. Research assistants would then call participants to gain additional information on ease of administration and satisfaction. Families with no reported use were contacted monthly to inquire if a study medication had been utilized. EMS, emergency department (ED), and hospital records were reviewed, when available, for additional clinical information and investigation of secondary outcomes. Study participation was terminated after the first use of study medication. There was no long-term follow-up.

Endpoints: Primary outcome: Total seizure time after administration of study medication. Secondary outcomes: Time to medication administration, total seizure time, ease of administration, overall medication satisfaction, respiratory complications, EMS support, ED visits, repeat seizure in < 12 hours, and hospitalization rate.

RESULTS

(See Table 8.1.)

Table 8.1 SUMMARY OF STUDY'S KEY FINDINGS

Outcome	RD Group	IN-MMAD	*P* Value
Total received drug (*n*)	42	50	n/a
Time from administration to seizure cessation (min)	4.3	3.0	.09
Total seizure time (min)	12.5	10.5	.25
Outcome	**RD Group**	**IN-MMAD**	**OR**
Repeat seizure within 12 hours (%)	2.4%	2.0%	0.8
Seizure treated in ED (%)	12%	10%	0.8
Outcome	**RD Group**	**IN-MMAD**	***P* Value**
Overall satisfaction (scale 0–10, median)	7.3	9.3	.02
Ease of administration (scale 0–10, median)	9	10	.02

Abbreviations: ED, emergency department; IN-MMAD, intranasal midazolam mucosal atomization; OR, odds ratio; RD, rectal diazepam.

- Time to seizure cessation was 1.3 minutes shorter in the IN-MMAD group, but this finding was not statistically significant.
- Time to administration of the medications did not differ between groups.
- There were no significant differences between groups on secondary clinical outcome measures (repeat seizure, emergency services, ED encounter, or other adverse events).
- Caregivers reported IN-MMAD was easier to give than RD.
- On an 11-point scale (0–10) caregivers reported higher satisfaction in the IN-MMAD group.

Criticisms and Limitations:

- This study could not be fully blinded given the different routes of administration of medications. The authors did not feel that caregivers would want to give both an active drug and a placebo during a seizure event.
- The study was underpowered to detect clinically meaningful differences between IN-MMAD and RD.

Other Relevant Studies and Information:

- Several randomized studies and subsequent review articles assessing different seizure rescue medications, including midazolam, diazepam, and lorazepam in various combinations, have suggested all are effective, but there is insufficient evidence to determine which is best.[2–4]
- A network meta-analysis compared midazolam, lorazepam, and diazepam for status epilepticus in children. Nonintravenous midazolam, intravenous lorazepam, and intravenous diazepam are more successful in achieving seizure cessation compared with nonintravenous diazepam. Among the 3 agents, the highest probability of achieving seizure cessation was with midazolam; however, lorazepam was associated with the greatest safety in regard to respiratory depression. There has been only 1 study comparing lorazepam with midazolam and no direct comparison of intranasal lorazepam with intranasal midazolam.[5]
- The Hann study indicates similar results to the Holsti[1] study in the adult population. No difference in efficacy between IN-MMAD and RD was seen, but both caregivers and patients preferred the intranasal route.[6]
- Two new prefilled intranasal rescue medications have become commercially available since the publication of the Holsti[1] and other studies. They are designed to simplify use in the home setting. Nasal diazepam spray was approved by the Food and Drug Administration in January 2020 for ages 6 and older.[7] Nasal midazolam spray was approved in June 2019 for ages 12 and older.[8]
- The clinical report on rescue medication for epilepsy in education settings lists IN-MMAD as a treatment option.[9]
- Intranasal midazolam is also a recommend option for use in the "Evidence-Based Guideline: Treatment of Convulsive Status Epilepticus in Children and Adults" for patients without available intravenous/intramuscular access.[10]

Summary and Implications: This study failed to prove that IN-MMAD is statistically superior for in-home treatment of acute seizures. The study does show statistical significance for improved ease of administration and caregiver satisfaction in the IN-MMAD group. IN-MMAD should be considered as an option when in-home treatment for acute seizures may be required.

CLINICAL CASE: INTRANASAL MIDAZOLAM VERSUS RECTAL DIAZEPAM FOR SEIZURE RESCUE AT HOME

Case History

A 17-year-old male presents with his parents for follow-up care and discussion of seizure management. This young man is affected by spastic diplegic cerebral palsy resulting in use of a wheelchair, as well as epilepsy. Seizures have been well controlled on daily antiepileptic drugs, but he had a recent breakthrough seizure requiring administration of rectal diazepam. His parents indicate that rectal medication is increasingly difficult to administer given the patient's increased lower extremity tone and his overall size. The patient hates being exposed in a public setting and expresses that this creates more anxiety than the seizure itself. Both parties are interested in discussing alternative options.

Suggested Answer

Many studies have shown that in the prehospital, ED, and inpatient setting the intranasal route of benzodiazepine administration is effective in aborting acute prolonged seizure activity. This study adds evidence that lay caregivers can be successful in administering intranasal midazolam with the use of an atomization device outside of a clinical setting with good response and high user satisfaction. Intranasal midazolam should be discussed with the family and patient as an alternative option for seizure rescue. Discussion should include any concerns related to administration in an educational setting as alternative caregivers may not be familiar with nasal administration. This issue can sometimes be avoided with a prefilled/commercially available option, but such options may include increased cost.

References

1. Holsti M, Dudley N, Schunk J, et al. Intranasal midazolam vs rectal diazepam for the home treatment of acute seizures in pediatric patients with epilepsy. *Arch Pediatr Adolesc Med.* 2010;164(8):747–753.
2. Scott R, Besag F, Neville B. Buccal midazolam and rectal diazepam for treatment of prolonged seizure in childhood and adolescence: a randomized trial. *Lancet.* 1999;353:623–626.
3. Brigo F, Nardone R, Tezzon F, Trinka E. Non-intravenous midazolam versus intravenous or rectal diazepam for the treatment of early status epilepticus. *Epilepsy Behav.* 2015;49:325–336.

4. McTague A, Martland T, Appleton R. Drug management for acute tonic-clonic convulsions including convulsive status epilepticus in children. *Cochrane Database Syst Rev.* 2018;(1):CD001905.
5. Zhao ZY, Wang HY, Wen B, Yang ZB, Feng K, Fan JC. A comparison of midazolam, lorazepam, and diazepam for the treatment of status epilepticus in children: a network meta-analysis. *J Child Neurol.* 2016;31(9):1093–1107.
6. Hann G, Geest P, Doelman G, et al. A comparison of midazolam nasal spray and diazepam rectal solution for the residential treatment of seizure exacerbations. *Epilepsia.* 2010;51(3):478–482.
7. *Valtoco (Diazepam) [prescriber information].* San Diego, CA: Neurelis Inc; Feb 2021.
8. *Nayzilam (Midazolam) [prescribing information].* Plymouth, MN: Proximagen LLC; May 2019.
9. Hartman A, Devore C, Section on Neurology and Council on School Health. Rescue medicine for epilepsy in education settings. *Pediatrics.* 2016;137(1):e20153876.
10. Glauser T, Shinnar S, Gloss D, et al. Evidenced-based guideline: treatment of convulsive status epilepticus in children and adults: report of the Guideline Committee of the American Epilepsy Society. *Epilepsy Curr.* 2016;16(1):48–61.

9

Isopropyl Alcohol Nasal Inhalation for Nausea in the Emergency Department

A Randomized Controlled Trial

ALEX CHOI AND LAURA MORRISON

> Isopropyl alcohol inhalation appears to be a simple and effective short-term therapy for nausea.
>
> — Beadle et al.[1]

Research Question: Given prior studies showing efficacy in patients with post-operative nausea, does nasally inhaled isopropyl alcohol reduce nausea when compared to nasally inhaled normal saline solution in patients presenting to the emergency department (ED) with this symptom?

Funding: None

Year Study Began: Information not provided

Year Study Published: 2016

Study Location: San Antonio Military Medical Center, San Antonio, Texas, United States

Who Was Studied: Adults who presented to the ED with a chief complaint of nausea or vomiting at a level of 3 or greater on a verbal numeric response scale (0–10).

Who Was Excluded: Patients with known allergy to isopropyl alcohol, inability to inhale through the nares, inability to read or write in English, altered mental status, or reported receipt within the past 24 hours of an antiemetic or psychoactive drug or medication known to potentially produce nausea when exposed to alcohol (e.g., disulfiram, metronidazole, cefoperazone).

How Many Patients: 80

Study Overview: This is a randomized, double-blinded, placebo-controlled trial in which 80 adults who presented to the ED with the chief complaint of nausea/vomiting were randomized in a 1:1 ratio to either nasally inhaled isopropyl alcohol or normal saline solution from a saturated pad. To ensure double-blinding, the packaging of individual pads was obscured with tape, instructors opened the pads at arm's length before handing to the patient, and patients were instructed not to describe the pad scent (Figure 9.1).

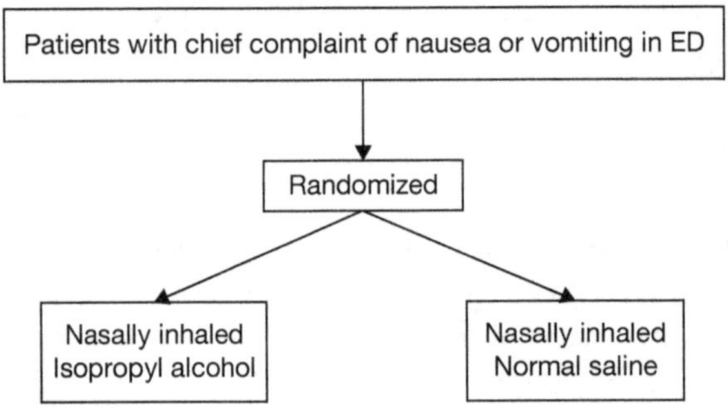

Figure 9.1. Summary of study design.

Study Intervention: The study intervention was completed while patients were in the waiting room or in their ED room before physician arrival. Patients were provided a pad saturated with either alcohol or normal saline solution and instructed to take inhalations at an initial time point and then 2 and 4 minutes later. At each time point, patients were instructed to hold the pad 2.5 cm from their nose and to take no more than 60 seconds of deep inhalations. Verbal nausea and pain scores were recorded by blinded investigators at the study start and at

2, 4, 6, and 10 minutes. At 10 minutes postintervention, they recorded their satisfaction on a 5-point Likert scale. A retrospective review of the paper chart was also performed to collect the frequency of rescue antiemetics given for nausea reported after study completion.

Follow-up: 10 minutes

Endpoints:

Primary outcome: Nausea verbal numeric response scale score at 10 minutes postintervention.

Secondary outcomes: Pain verbal numeric response scale score at 10 minutes postintervention, satisfaction score at 10 minutes postintervention, and receipt of subsequent rescue antiemetics.

RESULTS (TABLE 9.1)

- The isopropyl alcohol group had a lower median nausea score at 10 minutes compared to the placebo group ($P < .001$).
- The isopropyl alcohol group had a higher satisfaction score at 10 minutes compared to the placebo group.
- There was no difference in median pain score at 10 minutes between the 2 groups.
- There was no difference in number of doses dispensed or percentage of antiemetics received postintervention between the 2 groups.

Table 9.1 SUMMARY OF STUDY RESULTS

Outcomes	Placebo (43)	Isopropyl Alcohol(37)	Effect Size (95% CI)
10-minute nausea median VNRS, 0–10	6	3	3 (2–4)
10-minute pain median VNRS, 0–10	6	6	0 (−1 to 2)
10-minute satisfaction score, 1–5	2	4	2 (2–2)
Antiemetic receipt, %	72.1	89.2	17.1 (−0.5 to 34.8)
Antiemetic doses, No.	1.2	1.2	0 (−0.2 to 0.3)

Abbreviation: VNRS, verbal numeric rating scale.

Criticisms and Limitations:

- The study follow-up period was just 10 minutes, and thus this analysis does not offer insights on the long-term outcomes and adverse effects of nasally inhaled isopropyl alcohol.
- The researchers tried to blind patients to their study drug assignment, but because of the scent of isopropyl alcohol, this may not have been effective.
- The mechanism of how isopropyl alcohol alleviates nausea is unclear. Olfactory distraction with other scents (e.g., peppermint) may be effective as well.
- The cause of nausea was documented in < 30% of cases. Nausea is a product of multiple biochemical and physiologic processes. Investigating whether nasally inhaled isopropyl alcohol is more effective in certain disease processes would be worthwhile.

Other Relevant Studies and Information:

- Two subsequent randomized controlled trials[2,3] also support the efficacy of nasally inhaled isopropyl alcohol in treating nausea. In terms of rescue antiemetics given postintervention, 1 study[2] showed no difference after isopropyl alcohol, while the other study[3] showed a significant decrease.
- A 2021 implementation study[4] investigated the consequences of using nasally inhaled isopropyl alcohol as a first-line treatment for nausea in the ED. The results showed an increase in the percentage of patients receiving nausea treatment and a decrease in time to treatment, use of traditional antiemetics, and treatment cost.
- A 2018 Cochrane review[5] analyzing aromatherapy for treating postoperative nausea and vomiting suggested that patients who received isopropyl alcohol showed a shorter time to reach 50% reduction in nausea score and required less rescue antiemetics compared to standard antiemetic treatments. These findings are noted to be based on low-quality evidence.

Summary and Implications: This single-center, double-blinded, randomized controlled trial demonstrates nasally inhaled isopropyl alcohol to be an effective initial treatment for nausea in the ED setting. Although the follow-up time was just 10 minutes, additional studies with longer follow-up have shown improvement in nausea and/or a decrease in subsequent use of traditional antiemetics. These findings suggest that aromatherapy with inhaled isopropyl alcohol may be an effective approach with a low treatment burden for a debilitating symptom.

CLINICAL CASE: WHAT NONINTRAVENOUS, NONORAL INTERVENTION IS THERE FOR NAUSEA IN THE ED?

Case History

A 58-year-old female with stage IV lung cancer presents to the ED with worsening nausea after receiving chemotherapy yesterday. She has been having multiple episodes of emesis and looks dehydrated. Nursing staff state that she is a "hard stick" so they are trying to see if an intensive care unit nurse can come and place an intravenous (IV) line.

What can you do to help with this patient's nausea?

Suggested Answer

The patient in this scenario is suffering from chemotherapy-induced nausea and vomiting. There are multiple antiemetics that could alleviate her nausea. However, she is not able to tolerate any oral medications and lacks IV access for parenteral medications.

The 2016 Beadle trial suggests nasally inhaled isopropyl alcohol to be an effective treatment for nausea in the ED. The study shows nasally inhaled isopropyl alcohol reducing nausea while providing higher satisfaction to patients in 10 minutes compared to nasally inhaled normal saline. Although the 2016 study showed no difference in the number of rescue antiemetics given postintervention, more recent studies[3,4] have shown a decrease in subsequent use of traditional antiemetics. This suggests inhaled isopropyl alcohol as an effective treatment for acute nausea.

In conclusion, the ED staff could provide nasally inhaled isopropyl alcohol as a treatment for the patient's nausea. Nonetheless, they should establish IV access to give traditional antiemetics in case the patient's nausea persists or returns.

References

1. Beadle KL, Helbling AR, Love SL, April MD, Hunter CJ. Isopropyl alcohol nasal inhalation for nausea in the emergency department: a randomized controlled trial. *Ann Emerg Med.* 2016 Jul;68(1):1–9.e1.
2. April MD, Oliver JJ, Davis WT, et al. Aromatherapy versus oral ondansetron for antiemetic therapy among adult emergency department patients: a randomized controlled trial. *Ann Emerg Med.* 2018 Aug;72(2):184–193.
3. Candemir H, Akoglu H, Sanri E, Onur O, Denizbasi A. Isopropyl alcohol nasal inhalation for nausea in the triage of an adult emergency department. *Am J Emerg Med.* 2021 Mar;41:9–13.

4. Veldhuis P, Melse M, Mullaart N. Implementation of isopropyl alcohol (IPA) inhalation as the first-line treatment for nausea in the emergency department: practical advantages and influence on the quality of care. *Int J Emerg Med.* 2021 Feb 24;14(1):15.
5. Hines S, Steels E, Chang A, Gibbons K. Aromatherapy for treatment of postoperative nausea and vomiting. *Cochrane Database Syst Rev.* 2018 Mar 10;3(3):CD007598.

10

Methylphenidate for Cancer-Related Fatigue

DANIEL COGAN

> We observed similar improvements of fatigue and other symptom scores both in the patients receiving methylphenidate and in those receiving placebo.
>
> —BRUERA ET AL.[1]

Research Question: Is methylphenidate superior to placebo in treating cancer-related fatigue?

Funding: US Department of Health and Human Services, National Institutes of Health, Research Project Grant Program (R01)

Year Study Began: 2004

Year Study Published: 2006

Study Location: MD Anderson Cancer Center, Houston, Texas; Lyndon B. Johnson General Hospital, Houston, Texas

Who Was Studied: Adults with cancer reporting moderate or worse chronic fatigue.

Who Was Excluded: Patients with cognitive impairment, recent anemia, uncontrolled hypertension, glaucoma, history of tachycardia, severe anxiety disorders, substance abuse, or use of medications that would interact with methylphenidate.

How Many Patients: 105

Study Overview: This is a randomized, double-blinded, placebo-controlled trial in which patients with cancer and fatigue were randomized to receive either methylphenidate or placebo. The study design is illustrated in Figure 10.1.

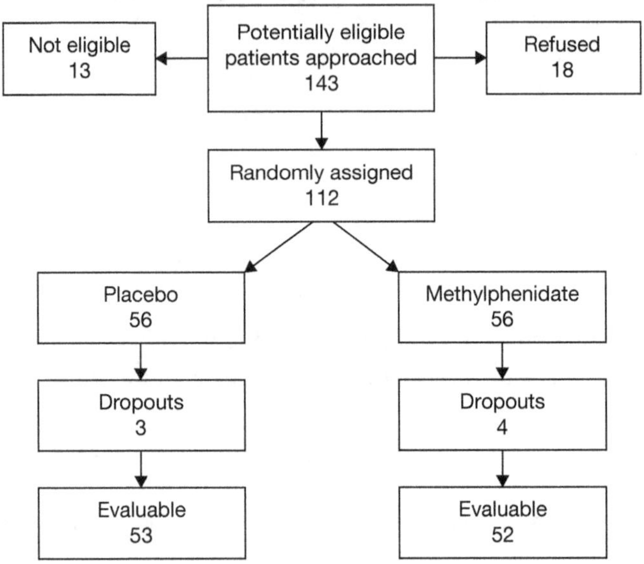

Figure 10.1. Summary of study design.

Study Intervention: Patients were instructed to take a tablet of either 5 mg methylphenidate or placebo every 2 hours as needed for fatigue, with a maximum of 4 doses a day, for 7 days. Patients completed a daily diary recording study drug administration and fatigue intensity. A research nurse conducted daily telephonic assessments of toxicity and fatigue level. After the first 7 days, all patients were offered open-label methylphenidate for 4 weeks. The Functional Assessment of Chronic Illness Therapy—Fatigue (FACIT-F) and Edmonton Symptom Assessment System (ESAS) were assessed at baseline and on days 8, 15, and 36.

Follow-up: 36 days

Endpoints:

Primary outcome: FACIT-F fatigue subscore on day 8.

Secondary outcomes: Fatigue and toxicity scores on days 15 and 36.

RESULTS

- Patients in both the methylphenidate and placebo groups experienced a dramatic and statistically significant reduction in fatigue, but there was no significant difference in fatigue improvement between these 2 groups.
- Incidence and severity of toxicity were also similar between groups (Table 10.1).

Table 10.1 SUMMARY OF STUDY'S KEY FINDINGS. DIFFERENCES IN SCORES FOR SYMPTOM INTENSITY BETWEEN BASELINE AND DAY 8 IN PATIENTS TAKING METHYLPHENIDATE OR A PLACEBO

	Methylphenidate ($n = 52$) **Day 8–Baseline**			**Placebo** ($n = 53$) **Day 8–Baseline**			
Symptom	**Mean**	**SD**	***P***	**Mean**	**SD**	***P***	***P***[a]
FACIT-F							
Physical well-being	4.8	5.6	< .001	3.4	5.8	< .001	.19
Social/family well-being	0.5	3.8	.35	−0.3	4.3	.58	.30
Emotional well-being	1.2	4.1	.04	1.1	3.7	.04	.86
Functional well-being	2.1	5.5	.008	1.3	5.0	.07	.42
Fatigue Subscale	9.6	9.8	< .001	7.5	11.3	< .001	.31
ESAS							
Pain	−1.1	3.0	.01	−1.1	3.0	.01	.95
Fatigue	−2.7	2.6	< .001	−1.9	2.8	< .001	.14
Nausea	−0.7	2.6	.06	−0.2	3.1	.6	.39
Depression	−1.4	2.6	< .001	−1.3	2.9	.002	.77
Anxiety	−1.3	3.0	.004	−1.1	2.7	.006	.70
Drowsiness	−1.4	2.9	< .001	−1.2	2.9	.005	.61
Shortness of breath	−1.4	2.3	< .001	−0.4	3.1	.32	.08
Appetite	−0.4	3.2	.42	−0.7	3.4	.13	.70
Sleep	−0.9	3.1	.04	−1.0	2.9	.02	.95
Feeling of well-being	−1.8	2.7	< .001	−0.7	3.2	.1	.07

Note: There was no significant difference in all of the baseline ESAS and FACIT-F scores between the methylphenidate and placebo group.

Abbreviations: ESAS, Edmonton Symptom Assessment System; FACIT, Functional Assessment for Chronic Illness Therapy—Fatigue; SD, standard deviation.

[a] For day 8 to baseline between methylphenidate and placebo.

Bruera E, Valero V, Driver L, et al. Patient controlled methylphenidate for cancer fatigue: a double-blind, randomized, placebo-controlled trial. *J Clin Oncol.* 2006;24(13):2073–2078.

Criticisms and Limitations:

- The dose of methylphenidate was at the lower end of the dosing range. A higher dose may be superior to placebo.
- The study population was varied in terms of age and type of cancer. Methylphenidate may be beneficial compared to placebo within a more specific subgroup, such as sex,[2] type of cancer, concomitant cancer treatment, age, or other factors.

Other Relevant Studies and Information:

- Despite acknowledging the weakness of evidence, the 2021 National Comprehensive Cancer Network guideline for cancer-related fatigue recommends consideration of methylphenidate.[3]
- Multiple meta-analyses suggest that methylphenidate may have a small but significant benefit compared to placebo.[4–6]
- Nonpharmacologic interventions, exercise and psychological interventions in particular, remain the best-proven intervention for cancer-related fatigue.[3,7]

Summary and Implications: This blinded and randomized study found that methylphenidate was not significantly better than placebo for management of cancer-related fatigue. The design of the study suggests that a daily assessment phone call may be a beneficial intervention for this challenging symptom. Nevertheless, the 2021 National Comprehensive Cancer Network guideline for cancer-related fatigue still recommends consideration of methylphenidate.

CLINICAL CASE: SHOULD YOU PRESCRIBE METHYLPHENIDATE FOR CANCER FATIGUE?

Case History

A 72-year-old man with stage IV cancer of the pancreas complains to you about severe fatigue: "I just don't have any energy." His palliative performance scale score is 80%, and he currently receives gemcitabine. His past medical history includes hyperlipidemia, for which he takes simvastatin. His most recent labs show a normal hemoglobin and hematocrit. He reports sleeping well most nights and feeling occasionally anxious and sad regarding his illness and limited life expectancy but states that he is trying "to live as best I can day to day. I just wish I had more energy."

Should you prescribe methylphenidate to alleviate fatigue for this patient?

Suggested Answer

A common and debilitating problem, the fatigue suffered by those with cancer often frustrates both patient and clinician. Effective treatment is challenging due to the many potential concurrent symptoms and contributing factors. There is surface plausibility for the use of methylphenidate to treat cancer-related fatigue, and some practice guidelines recommend its use. The featured study showed methylphenidate to be no better than placebo for the treatment of cancer-related fatigue and suggests that daily telephonic contact may be a beneficial intervention.

After ruling out any reversible causes for fatigue, it would be appropriate to prescribe a program of modest exercise, as well as frequent telephonic contact with this patient regarding the severity of his fatigue. You should not prescribe methylphenidate for this patient's fatigue.

References

1. Bruera E, Valero V, Driver L, et al. Patient controlled methylphenidate for cancer fatigue: a double-blind, randomized, placebo-controlled trial. *J Clin Oncol.* 2006;24(13):2073–2078.
2. Al Maqbali M, Al Sinani M, Al Naamani Z, Al Badi K, Tanash MI. Prevalence of fatigue in patients with cancer: a systematic review and meta-analysis. *J Pain Symptom Manage.* 2021;61(1):167–189.e114.
3. National Comprehensive Cancer Network. NCCN Clinical Practice Guidelines in Oncology: Cancer-Related Fatigue Version 1.2021. https://www.nccn.org/professionals/physician_gls/pdf/fatigue.pdf. December 1, 2020. Accessed March 1, 2021.
4. Minton O, Richardson A, Sharpe M, Hotpof M, Stone P. Drug therapy for the management of cancer-related fatigue (Review). *Cochrane Database Syst Rev.* 2010;(7):CD006704.
5. Qu D, Zhang Z, Yu X, et al. Psychotropic drugs for the management of cancer-related fatigue: a systematic review and meta-analysis. *Eur J Cancer Care.* 2016;25(6):970–979.
6. Gong S, Sheng P, Jin, et al. Effect of methylphenidate in patients with cancer-related fatigue: a systematic review and meta-analysis. *PLoS One.* 2014;9(1):e84391. doi:10.1371/journal.pone.0084391.
7. Mustian KM, Alfano CM, Heckler C, et al. Comparison of pharmaceutical, psychological, and exercise treatments for cancer-related fatigue: a meta-analysis. *JAMA Oncol.* 2017;3(7):961–968. doi:10.1001/jamaoncol.2016.6914.

11

Duloxetine for the Treatment of Chemotherapy-Induced Peripheral Neuropathy

ALAN PATRICK BALTZ, LAURA ELISABETH GRESSLER, AND RYAN COSTANTINO

> Among patients with painful chemotherapy-induced peripheral neuropathy, the use of duloxetine compared with placebo for 5 weeks resulted in a greater reduction in pain.
>
> —Smith et al.[1]

Research Question: Can duloxetine provide effective pain relief in patients suffering from chemotherapy-induced peripheral neuropathic pain (CIPNP)?

Funding: The study was supported by the National Cancer Institute (NCI) Division of Cancer Prevention, the Alliance Statistics and Data Center, and the Alliance Chairman. The drug and placebo were supplied by Eli Lilly.

Year Study Began: 2008

Year Study Published: 2013

Study Location: 8 NCI-funded cooperative research networks within community and academic settings

Who Was Studied: Patients were eligible if they were 25 years and older, were diagnosed with any cancer at any stage, experienced grade 1 or higher sensory neuropathy according to the NCI Common Terminology Criteria for Adverse

Events (CTCAE), and reported an average chemotherapy-induced pain of at least 4/10 after having received taxanes or oxaliplatin.

Who Was Excluded: Patients with a medical history of known neuropathy due to nerve compression, leptomeningeal carcinomatosis, bipolar disorder, alcohol abuse, severe depression, suicidal ideation, or major eating disorders and patients found to have renal and liver function abnormalities were excluded. In addition, patients with prior or ongoing treatment with other neurotoxic chemotherapeutic agents or concurrent use of other drugs known to influence serotonin levels were excluded.

How Many Patients: 231

Study Overview: This study was a randomized, phase 3, double-blind, placebo-controlled crossover trial in which 231 eligible patients were randomized using a 1:1 ratio. Randomization was further stratified by neurotoxic drug class and CIPNP risk.

Study Intervention: In weeks 1–5, group A received 30 mg of duloxetine for 1 week followed by 60 mg of duloxetine for 4 weeks. Group B received 1 capsule of placebo for 1 week followed by 2 capsules of placebo for 4 weeks. Both groups then underwent a 2-week washout period before crossing over to the other treatment arm. In weeks 8–12, group A received 1 capsule of placebo for 1 week then 2 capsules of placebo for 4 weeks, while group B received 30 mg of duloxetine for 1 week then 60 mg of duloxetine for 4 weeks. Both groups then underwent a second 2-week washout period. This is shown in Figure 11.1.

Follow-Up: 5 weeks for the primary endpoint

Endpoints: The primary endpoint of interest was the change in average pain reported using the Brief Pain Inventory-Short Form (BPI-SF). The primary endpoint was assessed weekly during the initial treatment period, from the start of week 1 to the end of week 5. Change in daily function related to pain was also measured using the BPI-SF. Secondary endpoints of interest were change in CIPNP-related quality of life as measured by the Functional Assessment of Cancer Therapy (FACT)/Gynecologic Oncology Group Neurotoxicity (GOG-NTX) subscale, change in daily function related to pain as measured by the BPI-SF, and adverse effects. The second endpoint related to changes in quality of life was measured on weeks 1, 6, 8, and 13.

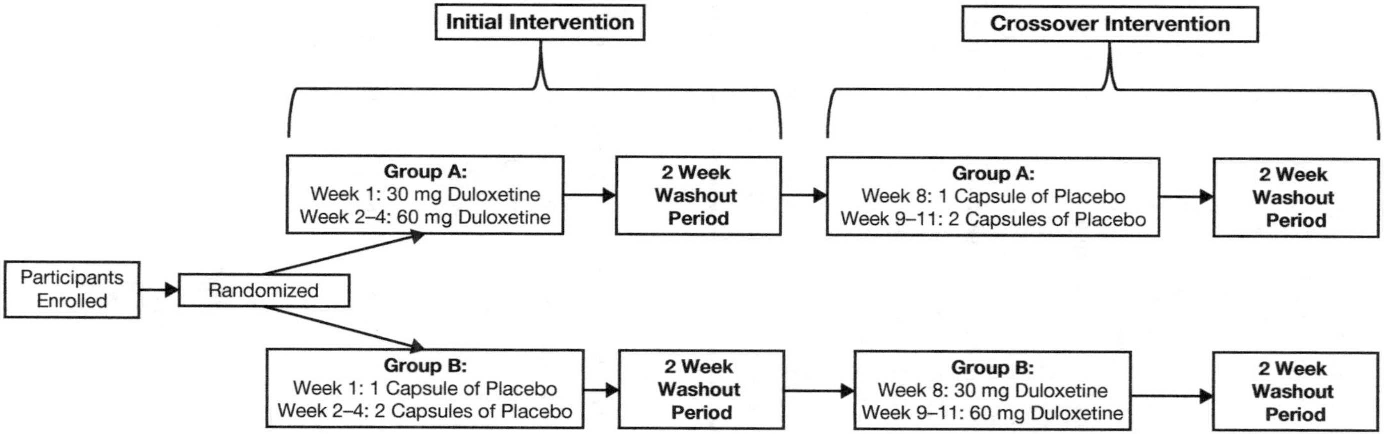

Figure 11.1. Summary of study design and interventions.

RESULTS

- Patients who received duloxetine first in the initial treatment period (group A) reported a statistically significant mean decrease in average pain score compared to the placebo-first initial treatment group (group B) (1.06 vs. 0.34; $P = .003$; Table 11.1).
- The mean difference in average pain score on the BPI-SF between group A and group B was 0.73 (0.60–0.98).
- Patients with CIPNP who had received platinum-based chemotherapy demonstrated greater benefit from duloxetine than those who received taxanes (1.06 vs. 0.19).
- Patients who received duloxetine first reported a greater improvement in quality of life and a greater decrease in pain-related interference in daily function compared to placebo. The mean difference between the 2 groups in mean change scores measuring pain-related interference (4.40, 95% CI: 0.93–7.88) and quality of life (1.58, 95% CI: 0.15–3.00; $P = .03$) was significant.
- The most commonly reported adverse events were fatigue, insomnia, somnolence, nausea, pain, anorexia, and dizziness.

Table 11.1 SUMMARY OF STUDY'S KEY FINDINGS

	Duloxetine-First Group		**Placebo-First Group**		**Mean Difference Between the Groups**	
Sample Size	*n* = 109		*n* = 111		*n* = 220	
	Point Estimate	**95% CI**	**Point Estimate**	**95% CI**	**Point Estimate**	**95% CI**
Mean decrease in average pain score[a]	1.06	0.72–1.40	0.34	0.01–0.66	0.73	0.26–1.20
Decrease in pain interference with daily function[a]	7.9	5.4–10.5	3.5	1.1–5.9	4.40	0.93–7.88
Decrease in chemotherapy-induced peripheral neuropathy–related quality of life[b]	2.44	0.43–4.45	0.87	1.09–2.82	1.58	0.15–3.00

[a] As measured by the Brief Pain Inventory-Short Form (BPI-SF).
[b] As measured by the Functional Assessment of Cancer Therapy (FACT)/Gynecologic Oncology Group Neurotoxicity (GOG-NTX) subscale.

Criticisms and Limitations:

- A higher proportion of patients receiving duloxetine dropped out of the study due to adverse effects versus placebo (11% vs. 1%).
- The exclusion of patients with abnormal liver function testing and kidney disease, which are prevalent in populations with advanced cancer or those receiving chemotherapy, limits the generalizability of the study.
- The limited sample size further limits the generalizability of the study.
- The initial study period including only 5 weeks of treatment did not address the benefits and adverse effects of long-term duloxetine treatment.

Other Relevant Studies and Information:

- Duloxetine has been demonstrated to be a safe and effective treatment for diabetic peripheral neuropathy versus placebo. This shows its utility for a broad array of types of neuropathic pain.[2]
- The study by Farshchian et al. compared the efficacy of duloxetine versus venlafaxine for CIPNP. Duloxetine was more effective than venlafaxine in decreasing motor neuropathy and neuropathic pain grade.[3]

CLINICAL CASE: UTILITY OF DULOXETINE IN A PALLIATIVE CARE SETTING

Case History

A 87-year-old male with a history of stage IV colorectal cancer is status postcolectomy with ileostomy and treatment with oxaliplatin-based chemotherapy. He notes intermittent shooting pain with burning and tingling of his legs that is worse on the left. He notes this pain to be 6/10 in intensity and partially controlled by his current analgesics. Upon the most recent imaging and examination, he is noted to have peritoneal carcinomatosis and enlarging pelvic mass lesions despite chemotherapy. He also reports worsening fatigue, intractable nausea with vomiting, and poor sleep. His functional status is currently very poor due to many factors including his pain, and he has now enrolled in home hospice care.

Would you recommend starting duloxetine to treat CIPNP in this patient?

Suggested Answer

The Smith et al. trial demonstrated an improvement in pain scores, functionality, and quality of life in patients suffering from CIPNP related to oxaliplatin-based chemotherapy. However, this patient's stated pain and symptoms may be multifactorial and related not only to his chemotherapy but also to tumor burden and resulting nerve injury. This study did not evaluate duloxetine's use in the setting of nerve impingement or malignant invasion.

Furthermore, he reports persistent nausea, which is one of the most consistently reported adverse effects reported by patients enrolled in this study. His poor sleep and fatigue may also be further exacerbated as many patients enrolled in the study stopped taking duloxetine after describing these symptoms. This patient would not be an optimal candidate for treatment with duloxetine without further clarification of the presence of true CIPNP and discussion of these known side effects.

Summary and Implications: This study of duloxetine treatment for CIPNP was the first to demonstrate an effective pharmacologic therapy for this condition. It illustrates the importance of exploring novel mechanisms of action in the management of chronic pain syndromes. Duloxetine is now used to treat a variety of types of neuropathic pain.

References

1. Smith EML, Pang H, Cirrincione C, et al. Effect of duloxetine on pain, function, and quality of life among patients with chemotherapy-induced painful peripheral neuropathy: a randomized clinical trial. *JAMA*. 2013;309(13):1359–1367. doi:10.1001/jama.2013.2813
2. Raskin J, Pritchett YL, Wang F, et al. A double-blind, randomized multicenter trial comparing duloxetine with placebo in the management of diabetic peripheral neuropathic pain. *Pain Med*. 2005;6(5):346–356. doi:10.1111/j.1526-4637.2005.00061.x.
3. Farshchian N, Alavi A, Heydarheydari S, Moradian N. Comparative study of the effects of venlafaxine and duloxetine on chemotherapy-induced peripheral neuropathy. *Cancer Chemother Pharmacol*. 2018;82(5):787–793. doi:10.1007/s00280-018-3664-y.

12

Efficacy of Oral Risperidone, Haloperidol, or Placebo for Symptoms of Delirium Among Patients in Palliative Care

A Randomized Clinical Trial

MELLAR P. DAVIS

> Antipsychotic drugs are not useful to reduce symptoms of delirium associated with distress in patients receiving palliative care.
>
> —AGAR ET AL.[1]

Research Question: Is risperidone or haloperidol an effective adjunct for managing symptoms of delirium among patients with distress in the palliative care setting? Both active treatment arms had worse outcomes than placebo

Funding: Australian Government Department of Health

Year Study Began: 2008

Year Study Published: 2017

Study Location: University of Technology Sidney, New South Wales, Australia

Who Was Studied: Adults receiving hospice or palliative care with advanced, progressive disease. Eligible patients were inpatients receiving specialty palliative care within a palliative care unit with delirium based on criteria from the

Diagnostic and Statistical Manual of Mental Disorders (fourth edition).[2] Patients were also required to have a score of 7 or greater on the Memorial Delirium Assessments Scale (MDAS) and a distressful symptom score of 1 or more including inappropriate behavior, inappropriate communication, illusions, and/or hallucinations on the Nursing Delirium Screening Scale (NuDSS).[3–6]

Who Was Excluded: Individuals experiencing substance withdrawal or having a history of neuroleptic malignant syndrome, use of antipsychotics within 48 hours (about 2 days) of admission, previous adverse reactions to antipsychotics, extrapyramidal disorders, prolonged QTc intervals, predicted survival of 7 days or less, a cerebrovascular accident or seizures in the prior 30 days (about 4.5 weeks), pregnancy, or breastfeeding.

How Many Patients: 247 patients: 82 on risperidone, 81 on haloperidol, 84 on placebo

Study Overview: This was a multisite, double-blind, placebo-controlled, randomized trial (Figure 12.1).

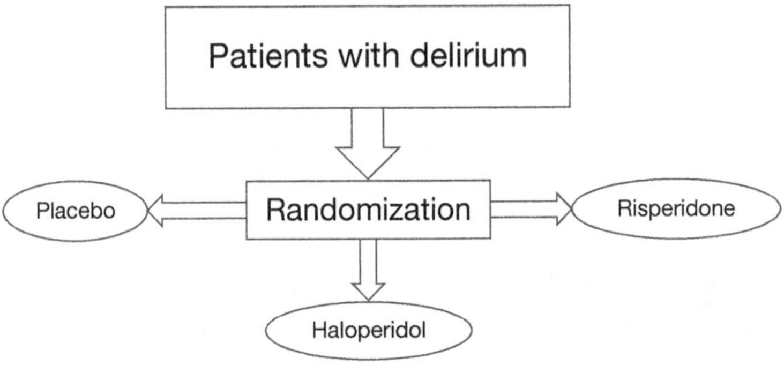

Figure 12.1. Study design.

Study Intervention: Participants 65 years of age or younger received 0.5 mg of haloperidol, 0.5 mg of risperidone, or matching placebo every 12 hours. Doses could be titrated to a maximum of 4 mg/day. Patients over 65 received half of the loading dose and maximum doses compared to younger patients. The study treatment duration was 72 hours (about 3 days). Assessments were done at 8-hour intervals using the MDAS and NuDSS. Midazolam 2.5 mg was available every 2 hours for a NuDSS score of 2 or greater for patients with inappropriate behavior, illusions, and hallucinations.

Follow-up: 72 hours (about 3 days)

Endpoints: The primary outcome was the average of the last 2 delirium symptom scores on day 3 (72 hours) using the average baseline score prior to the first dose of study medication as the baseline. Secondary outcomes included the daily MDAS score, the lowest delirium score, midazolam use, extrapyramidal symptoms (EPSs), sedation by the Richmond Agitation Sedation Scale, toxicity by the Common Terminology Criteria for Adverse Events physician assessment scale, and survival.[7–12]

RESULTS

- At the end of the analysis period, risperidone and haloperidol were associated with greater delirium symptom scores ($P = .02$ and $P = .009$, respectively) than placebo.
- Both risperidone and haloperidol had higher delirium symptom scores per day than placebo.
- Risperidone had higher MDAS scores per day than placebo ($P = .02$).
- Haloperidol had a greater delirium symptom score than placebo ($P = .009$)
- There were no differences between groups in the delirium lowest symptom score.
- There was a higher mean EPS score with haloperidol and risperidone ($P = .01$ and $P = .03$, respectively) than with placebo.
- There were no differences in sedation between treatment arms.
- Deaths were significantly higher with haloperidol than placebo (survival 26 vs. 16 days; $P = .003$; hazard ratio 1.73) but not with risperidone.
- Individuals on antipsychotics had a 1.5 times greater risk of dying.
- Midazolam use was lowest in the placebo arm.

Criticisms and Limitations:

- The outcomes of this trial could have been different had different dosing schedules of risperidone and haloperidol been used.

Other Relevant Studies and Information:

- Since this study was published, a systematic review of haloperidol in the management of delirium in the intensive care unit (ICU) demonstrated no short-term effect on survival, incidence of delirium, ICU length of stay, or delirium- or coma-free days. There were no increased adverse effects but no therapeutic benefit.[13]

- A randomized, placebo-controlled trial of intravenous haloperidol in critically ill patient's failed to demonstrate any effect on the duration of delirium.[14]
- A second systematic review of haloperidol in critically ill patients published in 2020 included 8 randomized trials. There were no benefits to haloperidol in reducing all-cause mortality or delirium severity.[15]
- A Cochrane Database Systematic Review of drug therapy for delirium in terminally ill adults published in 2020 included 4 studies and 399 patients. Haloperidol appeared to worsen delirium at 48 hours. There was no difference between risperidone and haloperidol. There was an increase in EPS adverse effects with haloperidol/risperidone/both haloperidol.[16]
- A systematic review and network meta-analysis published in 2020 found that risperidone appeared to reduce delirium in ICU surgical patients. Neither haloperidol nor risperidone reduced delirium in non-ICU patients.[17]
- A Cochrane Database of Systematic Review of randomized trials involving antipsychotics for treatment of delirium in hospitalized, non-ICU patients was published in 2018. There was no evidence that atypical or typical antipsychotics reduced mortality, altered the duration of delirium, reduced hospital length of stay, improved discharge disposition, or improved health-related quality of life.[18]

Summary and Implications: This rigorous randomized trial failed to demonstrate a benefit—and in fact suggested harm—with the use of haloperidol and risperidone for the management of delirium in patients receiving palliative care. Whether other atypical antipsychotics, such as quetiapine or aripiprazole, are effective requires further research. In the meantime, antipsychotics should be reserved for patients with delirium who are receiving palliative care only when symptoms of agitation cannot be managed using other strategies.

CLINICAL CASE: SHOULD THIS PATIENT BE PLACED ON AN ANTIPSYCHOTIC?

Case History

A 59-year-old man has metastatic lung cancer from the right hilum to the left third and fourth rib in the midaxillary line and left greater trochanter. He has pain in the left hip and left rib. It is continuous and dull. The left hip pain is worse with weight-bearing and the left ribs with deep inspiration. He rates the pain as 8/10 on a numerical rating scale (0 no pain, 10 severe pain). The oncologist starts carboplatin, pemetrexed, and a checkpoint inhibitor. She wished to avoid radiation for the time being since the x-rays of the left hip did not suggest an impending fracture. He was placed on sustained-release morphine 15 mg twice daily with immediate-release morphine 5 mg every 4 hours as needed. The sustained release of morphine was subsequently increased by the oncologist to 30 mg twice daily. He takes 4 "as needed" doses of morphine daily, according to his wife. With this his overall pain is a 4/10.

Socially he is married and works as a machinist. He continues to smoke ½ pack per day. The family history is positive for alcohol abuse in his father, who died in his 50s of cirrhosis. The patient drinks, according to him, 2–3 beers a day, though his wife volunteers that it may in fact be 4–5 beers daily.

He presents to the emergency department with nightmares and some confusion at night associated with visual hallucinations. He had been nauseated for 2 days after his first cycle of chemotherapy and has been able to take his tablets but has been unable to eat or drink. On examination, he is thin with temporal wasting. Pertinent physical findings include dullness in the left lung, diaphoresis, myoclonus, and a right pronator drift. His laboratory studies demonstrated a creatinine of 1.3 mg/mL and blood urea nitrogen of 35 mg/mL. Blood alcohol levels are < 0.1 g%. You are called to the emergency department because he is agitated. The physician on duty asks you if you want to give him quetiapine or haloperidol for his agitation. What would you do?

Suggested Answer

The confusion, visual hallucinations, and myoclonus suggest opioid toxicity; an opioid rotation is a consideration. He also may be withdrawing from alcohol; lorazepam as well as thiamine should be started. The pronator drift suggests that he may have left cerebral metastases close to the motor cortex.

Haloperidol or quetiapine is unlikely to help manage his confusion, myoclonus, agitation, or pronator drift and may reduce seizure thresholds from cerebral metastases or alcohol withdrawal. Morphine was discontinued, followed by rotation to a different opioid, hydromorphone in this case, with a 30%–50 % reduction in equianalgesic dose since the reason for rotation was for opioid toxicity and not uncontrolled pain. Hydromorphone 2 mg every 4 hours by mouth was started. Isopropyl alcohol sniffs controlled his nausea quickly, which allowed for oral administration of oral hydromorphone. Haloperidol, metoclopramide, or olanzapine would have been a reasonable alternative antiemetic for him. A computed tomography scan or brain magnetic resonance imaging was ordered once his agitation improved on lorazepam. It would be important to monitor him for respiratory depression; the combination of a benzodiazepine and opioid increases the risk of respiratory depression, as does the combination of an opioid and alcohol.

References

1. Agar MR, Lawlor PG, Quinn S, et al. Efficacy of oral risperidone, haloperidol, or placebo for symptoms of delirium among patients in palliative care: a randomized clinical trial. *JAMA Intern Med.* 2017;177(1):34–42.
2. Cooper JE. On the publication of the Diagnostic and Statistical Manual of Mental Disorders: Fourth Edition (DSM-IV). *Br J Psychiatry.* 1995;166(1):4–8.
3. Lawlor PG, Nekolaichuk C, Gagnon B, Mancini IL, Pereira JL, Bruera ED. Clinical utility, factor analysis, and further validation of the memorial delirium assessment scale in patients with advanced cancer: assessing delirium in advanced cancer. *Cancer.* 2000;88(12):2859–2867.
4. Breitbart W, Rosenfeld B, Roth A, Smith MJ, Cohen K, Passik S. The Memorial Delirium Assessment Scale. *J Pain Symptom Manage.* 1997;13(3):128–137.
5. Jeong E, Park J, Lee J. Diagnostic test accuracy of the Nursing Delirium Screening Scale: A systematic review and meta-analysis. *J Adv Nurs.* 2020;76(10):2510–2521.
6. Barnes CJ, Webber C, Bush SH, et al. Rating delirium severity using the Nursing Delirium Screening Scale: a validation study in patients in palliative care. *J Pain Symptom Manage.* 2019;58(4):e4–e7.
7. Chouinard G, Margolese HC. Manual for the Extrapyramidal Symptom Rating Scale (ESRS). *Schizophr Res.* 2005;76(2–3):247–265.
8. Bush SH, Grassau PA, Yarmo MN, Zhang T, Zinkie SJ, Pereira JL. The Richmond Agitation-Sedation Scale modified for palliative care inpatients (RASS-PAL): a pilot study exploring validity and feasibility in clinical practice. *BMC Palliat Care.* 2014;13(1):17.
9. Sessler CN, Gosnell MS, Grap MJ, et al. The Richmond Agitation-Sedation Scale: validity and reliability in adult intensive care unit patients. *Am J Respir Crit Care Med.* 2002;166(10):1338–1344.
10. Kluetz PG, Chingos DT, Basch EM, Mitchell SA. Patient-reported outcomes in cancer clinical trials: measuring symptomatic adverse events with the National Cancer Institute's Patient-Reported Outcomes Version of the Common Terminology Criteria for Adverse Events (PRO-CTCAE). *Am Soc Clin Oncol Educ Book.* 2016;35:67–73.
11. Zhong X, Lim EA, Hershman DL, Moinpour CM, Unger J, Lee SM. Identifying severe adverse event clusters using the National Cancer Institute's Common Terminology Criteria for Adverse Events. *J Oncol Pract.* 2016;12(3):e270–280, 245–276.
12. Basch E, Iasonos A, McDonough T, et al. Patient versus clinician symptom reporting using the National Cancer Institute Common Terminology Criteria for Adverse Events: results of a questionnaire-based study. *Lancet Oncol.* 2006;7(11):903–909.
13. Zayed Y, Barbarawi M, Kheiri B, et al. Haloperidol for the management of delirium in adult intensive care unit patients: a systematic review and meta-analysis of randomized controlled trials. *J Crit Care.* 2019;50:280–286.
14. Page VJ, Ely EW, Gates S, et al. Effect of intravenous haloperidol on the duration of delirium and coma in critically ill patients (Hope-ICU): a randomised, double-blind, placebo-controlled trial. *Lancet Respir Med.* 2013;1(7):515–523.

15. Barbateskovic M, Krauss SR, Collet MO, et al. Haloperidol for the treatment of delirium in critically ill patients: a systematic review with meta-analysis and trial sequential analysis. *Acta Anaesthesiol Scand.* 2020;64(2):254–266.
16. Finucane AM, Jones L, Leurent B, et al. Drug therapy for delirium in terminally ill adults. *Cochrane Database Syst Rev.* 2020;1:CD004770.
17. Kim MS, Rhim HC, Park A, et al. Comparative efficacy and acceptability of pharmacological interventions for the treatment and prevention of delirium: a systematic review and network meta-analysis. *J Psychiatr Res.* 2020;125:164–176.
18. Burry L, Mehta S, Perreault MM, et al. Antipsychotics for treatment of delirium in hospitalised non-ICU patients. *Cochrane Database Syst Rev.* 2018;6:CD005594.

13

The Use of Very Low-Dose Methadone for Palliative Pain Control

MELLAR P. DAVIS

> Our method of pain management was quite different from standard palliative care practice and today and appeared to be successful for managing pain without escalation of opiate doses or hyperalgesia.
>
> —SALPETER ET AL.[1]

Research Question: Is methadone, a unique opioid analgesic with high-efficacy opioid receptor stimulation plus an NMDA (N-methyl-D-aspartate) receptor-blocking effect, in very low doses (< 30 mg/day) effective in the long-term management of cancer and noncancer pain?

Funding: Not addressed in the study manuscript

Year Study Began: 2011

Year Study Published: 2013

Who Was Studied: Patients admitted to hospice between July 1, 2011, and April 1, 2012, who were on short-acting or long-acting opioids and had a survival expectation of > 1 week.

Who Was Excluded: Those imminently dying who were on oral or parental opiates and adjuvants as needed.

How Many Patients: 93 of 236 patients were admitted to hospice during the study.

Study Overview: This was a retrospective study of the use of very low-dose methadone in hospice (Figure 13.1).

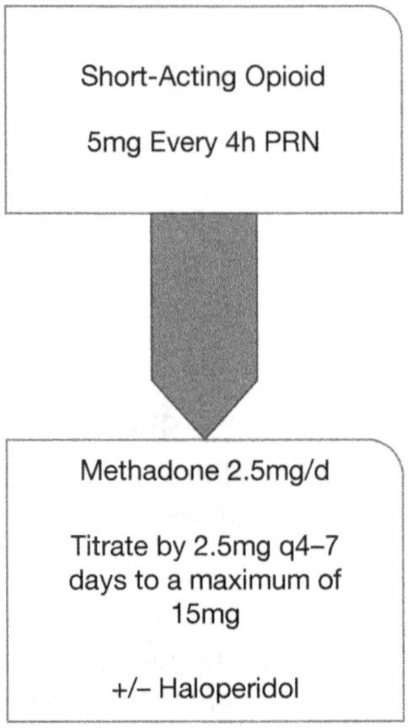

Figure 13.1. Initiating methadone with short-acting opioids as needed.

Study Intervention: Patients on short-acting "as needed" opioids, morphine equivalents of 5 mg, receiving > 2 doses a day were started on methadone 2.5 mg daily with titration by 2.5-mg increments every 4–7 days to a maximum of 15 mg. Patients on sustained-release opioids were offered methadone 2.5–15 mg depending on morphine equivalent daily dose (MEDD). Potent opioids other than methadone were then tapered over several days. The pain was assessed by visiting nurses using a standard numerical rating scale of 0–10 (0 no pain, 10 severe pain). Adjuvant analgesics were used with a preference for haloperidol.

Endpoints: The median and peak pain intensity scores were the primary outcome. Pain scores ≥ 4 were considered a marker of moderate to severe pain.

RESULTS

- The mean age of the patient was 81 years (range 28–105 years).
- 44% of the patients on hospice had a cancer diagnosis.
- 68% died during the study period unrelated to methadone.
- 53% of the methadone-treated subgroup had cancer.
- The median methadone dose was 5 mg. Eighty-one percent received ≤ 7.5 mg daily.
- The median duration of methadone treatment was 34 days (interquartile range 16–59 days).
- Haloperidol was used in 40% of those receiving methadone and in 70% of those converted from long-acting opioids to methadone.
- The median dose of haloperidol was 3 mg (interquartile range 2–6 mg).
- The pain intensity score on admission to the study for cancer was 3 (interquartile range 0 to 4) and for noncancer 2 (interquartile range 0 to 3).
- The median pain intensity score on methadone was 0 (range 0–6) and was similar in cancer and noncancer patients.

Criticisms and Limitations:

- This is a retrospective study and hence patient selection bias is likely to have occurred.
- The frequency of pain assessment in the study was not provided.
- Most patients had mild pain to begin with; therefore, use of this dosing strategy should not be considered in patients with uncontrolled pain on high doses of opioids.

Other Relevant Studies and Information:

- The authors published an additional study 2 years later of 43 patients treated with either full conversion to low-dose methadone or tapered conversion with haloperidol. The average haloperidol dose was 1.5 mg daily. Similar findings were reported for a group of patients with more severe pain (average numerical rating scale pain severity of 5 a week prior to receiving methadone). Interestingly, haloperidol was used for breakthrough pain and was thought to be better than immediate-release opioids in relieving breakthrough pain. The greatest improvement was noted in those with the highest MEDD prior to conversion to low-dose methadone.[2] The rationale for the use of methadone by the author was that it blocked NMDA receptors.

- There have been multiple studies published, mostly retrospective, which have used low-dose methadone as an "add-on" to other potent opioids to improve analgesia.4[3–9]
- In Sprague-Dawley rats on low-dose methadone, as low as 1 ng/g of brain tissue produces antinociception, but this is unlikely to be related to the NMDA receptor (Table 13.1).[10]

Table 13.1 METHADONE AFFINITY FOR THE NMDA RECEPTOR (KI)

Opioid	**Ki Brain (uM)**	**Concentration (ng/mL) Brain**	**Ki Spinal Cord (uM)**	**Concentration (ng/mL) Spinal Cord**
d/l-methadone	8.3	2564	2.5	773
l-methadone	3.4	1050	2.8	865
d-methadone	7.4	2286	2.6	803

Gorman AL, Elliott KJ, Inturrisi CE. The d- and l-isomers of methadone bind to the non-competitive site on the N-methyl-D-aspartate (NMDA) receptor in rat forebrain and spinal cord. *Neurosci Lett.* 1997;223(1):5–8.

- In 35 patients on an average methadone dose of 40 mg (5–80 mg), plasma concentrations were < 80 ng/mL except for 1 patient.[12]
- In a cohort of patients on an average methadone dose of 95 mg/day (30–320), the median d-methadone level was 152 ng/mL, l-methadone level was 144 ng/mL, and d/l-methadone level was 296 ng/mL.[13]
- Cerebrospinal fluid (CSF) methadone levels vary widely, ranging from 2% to 73%, though CSF levels may not reflect brain or spinal cord levels.[14]
- It is very unlikely that methadone, particularly in low doses, interacts and blocks NMDA receptors. The synergy with morphine is independent of NMDA receptors, which was originally proposed by Bolan et al. in 2002.[15]

Summary and Implications: Data from this study suggests that either conversion to low-dose methadone or "add-on" low-dose methadone to potent opioids improves pain and may allow a reduction in MEDD. The mechanism behind the benefits to low-dose methadone are unlikely to be related to NMDA receptors and may be intriguingly associated with binding to a unique set of mu opioid receptor subtypes.[16,17] Randomized trials are needed to confirm these retrospective study results.

CLINICAL CASE: WOULD IT BE REASONABLE TO ROTATE THIS PATIENT TO LOW-DOSE METHADONE?

Case History

A 53-year-old postmenopausal female has breast cancer arising from the left breast with metastasis to the left axilla, L2 vertebral body, right greater trochanter, and right lung. She is experiencing cancer pain in the left axilla and lower back. She rates the pain as a 7/10 (numerical score 0 no pain, 10 severe pain). Her oncologist starts oxycodone 5 mg every 4 hours as needed. She requires 4–5 doses a day. Two weeks later she is placed on sustained-release oxycodone 10 mg twice daily with 5 mg every 4 hours as needed. Her pain diminishes to a 3/10 and she has been able to return to work, which is important in maintaining her insurance. Her breast cancer is estrogen receptor and progesterone receptor positive and HER2 negative. She was placed on letrozole and a CD4/6 inhibitor.

She has diabetes and has some gastroparesis, which leads to intermittent nausea. She receives a letter from her insurance company that states, "Oxycodone and oxycodone sustained release are either not included on our list of covered drugs or are included on a formulary but subject to certain limits. However, the letrozole and CD4/6 inhibitor will be fully covered." The nurse navigator attempts to obtain approval of the oxycodone, but the insurance company is steadfast in its denial. The patient panics and calls you about an alternative treatment for her pain.

Suggested Answer

It is reasonable to start low-dose methadone in a stop-start rotation strategy with this patient. The starting dose would be 2.5 mg once or twice daily. Morphine 5 mg every 4 hours could be used as a breakthrough analgesic as the methadone dose is adjusted to her pain. The cost of methadone 5 mg tablets #60 is $10–$12. Haloperidol may improve her pain and have an added benefit, effectively treating the nausea of gastroparesis related to her diabetes. The evidence for its benefit in treating gastroparesis and associated nausea comes from randomized trials. The dose and frequency of haloperidol for breakthrough pain are not established, and randomized trials are needed, but 1–0.5 mg every 4–6 hours as needed for pain and nausea would be a reasonable starting schedule. Opioids can worsen gastroparesis, and haloperidol is very inexpensive at $16–$25 for 60 of the 1-mg tablets for this purpose. There is a negative trial of haloperidol in the treatment of opioid-related nausea, such that the cause of nausea may determine the efficacy of haloperidol as an antiemetic.

References

1. Salpeter SR, Buckley JS, Bruera E. The use of very-low-dose methadone for palliative pain control and the prevention of opioid hyperalgesia. *J Palliat Med.* 2013;16(6):616–622.
2. Salpeter SR, Buckley JS, Buckley NS, Bruera E. The use of very-low-dose methadone and haloperidol for pain control in the hospital setting: a preliminary report. *J Palliat Med.* 2015;18(2):114–119.
3. Higgins C, Smith BH, Matthews K. Evidence of opioid-induced hyperalgesia in clinical populations after chronic opioid exposure: a systematic review and meta-analysis. *Br J Anaesth.* 2019;122(6):e114–e126.
4. Tognoli E, Proto PL, Motta G, Galeone C, Mariani L, Valenza F. Methadone for postoperative analgesia: contribution of N-methyl-D-aspartate receptor antagonism: a randomised controlled trial. *Eur J Anaesthesiol.* 2020;37(10):934–943.
5. Furst P, Lundstrom S, Strang P. Methadone in Swedish specialized palliative care—is it the magic bullet in complex cancer-related pain? *PLoS One.* 2020;15(4):e0230845.
6. Furst P, Lundstrom S, Klepstad P, Strang P. The use of low-dose methadone as add-on to regular opioid therapy in cancer-related pain at end of life: a national Swedish survey in specialized palliative care. *J Palliat Med.* 2020;23(2):226–232.
7. Furst P, Lundstrom S, Klepstad P, Runesdotter S, Strang P. Improved pain control in terminally ill cancer patients by introducing low-dose oral methadone in addition to ongoing opioid treatment. *J Palliat Med.* 2018;21(2):177–181.
8. Hawley P, Chow L, Fyles G, Shokoohi A, O'Leary MJ, Mittelstadt M. Clinical outcomes of start-low, go-slow methadone initiation for cancer-related pain: what's the hurry? *J Palliat Med.* 2017;20(11):1244–1251.
9. Madden K, Bruera E. Very-low-dose methadone to treat refractory neuropathic pain in children with cancer. *J Palliat Med.* 2017;20(11):1280–1283.
10. Liu SJ, Roerig DL, Wang RI. Brain and plasma levels of methadone and their relationships to analgesic activity of methadone in rats. *Drug Metab Dispos.* 1983;11(4):335–338.
11. Gorman AL, Elliott KJ, Inturrisi CE. The d- and l-isomers of methadone bind to the non-competitive site on the N-methyl-D-aspartate (NMDA) receptor in rat forebrain and spinal cord. *Neurosci Lett.* 1997;223(1):5–8.
12. Rostami-Hodjegan A, Wolff K, Hay AW, Raistrick D, Calvert R, Tucker GT. Population pharmacokinetics of methadone in opiate users: characterization of time-dependent changes. *Br J Clin Pharmacol.* 1999;48(1):43–52.
13. Eap CB, Bertschy G, Baumann P, Finkbeiner T, Gastpar M, Scherbaum N. High interindividual variability of methadone enantiomer blood levels to dose ratios. *Arch Gen Psychiatry.* 1998;55(1):89–90.
14. Rubenstein RB, Kreek MJ, Mbawa N, Wolff WI, Korn R, Gutjahr CL. Human spinal fluid methadone levels. *Drug Alcohol Depend.* 1978;3(2):103–106.
15. Bolan EA, Tallarida RJ, Pasternak GW. Synergy between mu opioid ligands: evidence for functional interactions among mu opioid receptor subtypes. *J Pharmacol Exp Ther.* 2002;303(2):557–562.

16. Fischer BD, Carrigan KA, Dykstra LA. Effects of N-methyl-D-aspartate receptor antagonists on acute morphine-induced and l-methadone-induced antinociception in mice. *J Pain*. 2005;6(7):425–433.
17. Pelissier T, Laurido C, Kramer V, Hernandez A, Paeile C. Antinociceptive interactions of ketamine with morphine or methadone in mononeuropathic rats. *Eur J Pharmacol*. 2003;477(1):23–28.

14

Opioid Therapy for Dyspnea Associated With Chronic Obstructive Lung Disease

Benefits and Harms

MELLAR P. DAVIS

> Among older adults with COPD, incident opioid use and in particular use of the generally more potent opioid-only formulations, regardless of dose, was associated with several significantly increased adverse respiratory outcomes and mortality.
>
> —VOZORIS ET AL.[1]

Research Question: Is there an association of new opioid use with the risk of adverse respiratory outcomes among older adults with chronic obstructive pulmonary disease (COPD)?

Funding: The study was funded by a grant from the Lung Association–Canadian Thoracic National Grant Review/Grant-in-Aid. The Lung Association grant is supported by the Institute of Clinical Evaluative Sciences, funded by an annual grant from the Ontario Ministry of Health and Long-Term Care.

Year Study Began: 2007

Year Study Published: 2016

Study Location: Saint Michael's Hospital, Toronto, Ontario, Canada

Who Was Studied: Community-dwelling older adults and those living in long-term care facilities, 66 years of age or older, with validated physician-diagnosed COPD.

Who Was Excluded: Individuals younger than 66 years and patients receiving palliative care within the year prior to the index date. The index date was the date opioids were started.

How Many Patients: 130 979

Study Overview: This was a population-based retrospective cohort study of Ontario health administrative data from April 1, 2007, to April 1, 2012. Multiple health care administrative databases were linked using unique encoded identifiers. COPD diagnosis was based on an algorithm of 3 or more ambulatory claims of COPD within any 2 years of the study period or 1 or more hospitalizations for COPD. Drug information was derived from the Ontario Drug Benefit Database, which contains all publicly funded outpatient medications dispensed to Ontario residents aged 65 years or older. Oral and transdermal opioid drugs were included, and injectable and rectal administrative opioids were excluded. Opioid agonists-antagonists and methadone were excluded. Opioid drug users were defined by the incidence use of any included opioid. Incidence use was counted only once per individual. Controls were patients with COPD who were dispensed nonopioid medications within the study. The incident use of any included an opioid drug prescribed and subsequently detected on the database. A comparative analysis was done of clinical adverse events between patients receiving opioids and matched controls. Propensity matching between opioid users and nonusers was done through logistic regression for 33 covariates associated with the receipt of opioids in adults with COPD.

Endpoints: Respiratory outcomes occurring within 30 days of the index date (the day opioid therapy was initiated). COPD and pneumonia-related mortality and all-cause mortality were also analyzed.

RESULTS

- Combinations of opioids plus nonopioid COPD therapy reduced outpatient exacerbations and reduced pneumonia and all-cause mortality (Table 14.1).

Table 14.1 OPIOID RELATED RISKS IN OLDER INDIVIDUALS WITH COPD

Event	Hazard Ratio (95% CI)
Outpatient exacerbation	1.27 (1.14–1.41)
Emergency department visits	1.64 (1.35–1.98)
Hospitalizations	1.54 (1.31–1.81)
COPD/pneumonia mortality	4.76 (3.4–6.7)
All-cause mortality	4.01 (3.5–4.6)

- Short-acting opioids were associated with a higher risk for outpatient exacerbation (hazard ratio [HR] 1.37, 95% CI: 1.23–1.53) and emergency department visits (HR 1.70, 95% CI: 1.38–2.09), but sustained-release opioids were not (Table 14.2).

Table 14.2 EVENTS COMPARING SHORT-ACTING AND SUSTAINED OR LONG-ACTING OPIOIDS

Event	Short-Acting: Hazard Ratio (95% CI)	Long-Acting: Hazard Ratio (95% CI)
Hospitalizations	1.5 (1.26–1.79)	1.86 (1.23–2.81)
COPD/pneumonia mortality	4.78 (3.36–6.79)	5.42 (2.53–11.62)
All-cause mortality	3.8 (3.31–4.36)	5.62 (4.46–7.10)

- Combining opioids with nonopioid medications for COPD in patients on ≤ 30 mg of morphine per day did not reduce adverse events.
- Exacerbations that occurred within the year of index opioid use worsened outcomes (Table 14.3).

Table 14.3 MORPHINE EQUIVALENTS PER DAY: LESS THAN OR EQUAL 30 MG VERSUS GREATER THAN 30 MG

Event	Less Than/Equal to 30 mg: Hazard Ratio (95% CI)	Greater Than 30 mg: Hazard Ratio (95% CI)
Hospitalizations	1.93 (1.05–3.54)	1.82 (1.04–3.17)
COPD/pneumonia mortality	6.46 (2.94–14.21)	4.72 (1.24–18.09)
All-cause mortality	6.89 (5.03–9.44)	4.86 (3.47–6.79)

Criticisms and Limitations:

- The diagnosis of COPD was based on physician diagnosis and not pulmonary functions. Physician diagnosis can be inaccurate.
- Associations are not causation in observational studies. Those who received opioids may have more severe COPD, other comorbidities, or greater frailty, which can lead to adverse events.

Other Relevant Studies and Information:

- The benefits of opioids in treating dyspnea associated with COPD are small. In 3 meta-analyses, the standard mean difference (SMD) was less than –0.5, which is considered a small benefit.[2–4]
- One clinical practice guideline made a conditional recommendation suggesting opioid-based therapy be considered for dyspnea management. This statement was made with "very low certainty" due to the supporting studies that were of short duration with small sample sizes, often involving only 30–40 patients.[5]
- In a letter that challenged Vozori's contention that opioids are unsafe in COPD, the evidence presented was a pharmacovigilance study of 85 patients with severe COPD followed for an average of 142 days on low-dose morphine (< 30 mg/day).[6,7] This pharmacovigilance study is inadequately powered for safety.
- Not all opioids are the same. Oral oxycodone in several studies has not been effective in treating dyspnea.[8–10] Although rapid-acting fentanyl modestly reduces dyspnea and prolongs the 6-minute walk time distance in some studies, several of these studies demonstrated that a placebo was just as effective.[11–14] In animal studies, fentanyl had greater risks for respiratory depression than morphine, and it has a narrow utility compared with other opioids.[15–17]
- Several large observational studies have shown increased mortality and morbidity in patients with COPD (including older adults) who are treated with opioids. This adds validity to the findings of this study. A large cohort study of 2000 patients who were oxygen dependent showed increased mortality (HR 1.21, 95% CI: 1.02–1.44) when patients received > 30 mg of morphine daily.[18] A study involving 10 000 Americans with COPD demonstrated an increased risk for hospitalization if patients were treated with opioids (HR 1.73, 95% CI: 1.52–1.97).[19] A case-control observational study of 3000 community-dwelling adults older than 65 demonstrated that opioids within the preceding 6 days increased the risk of pneumonia (odds ratio [OD] 1.38, 95% CI: 1.08–1.76). This was

particularly evident if individuals were treated with sustained-release opioids (OR 3.43, 95% CI: 1.4–8.21). Immunosuppressive opioids such as codeine, morphine, and fentanyl were the most offending agents.[20] A nested case-control study of Americans dispensed opioids demonstrated a significant risk for pneumococcal disease (OR 1.62, 95% CI: 1.36–1.92). This was particularly true for incident users (OR 2.44, 95% CI: 1.49–4.00).[21]

Summary and Implications: This study and others reviewed in this chapter suggest that, contrary to prior guidelines, opioids may worsen respiratory outcomes in older adults with COPD. Opioids are still widely used in this population because while they may not eliminate dyspnea, they might lessen the suffering related to the unpleasantness of dyspnea, providing a benefit that for some outweighs the risks.[22]

CLINICAL CASE: SHOULD MORPHINE BE STARTED ON THIS PATIENT

Case History

A 58-year-old female with COPD Global Initiative for Chronic Obstructive Lung Diseasestage 3, with a body mass index of 35, was previously admitted to the hospital 10 days ago with an exacerbation of her COPD. She had discolored sputum, wheezes, and tachypnea. Her PO_2 on 2 L of oxygen was 92% and her pCO_2 was 43 mmHg. She was placed on bronchodilators, corticosteroids, and antibiotics. She improved and after 5 days in the hospital she was discharged home.

She returns now to the emergency department with increasing dyspnea, mild wheezes, mild lower extremity edema, and chest pain. She is afebrile. Her blood pressure is 110/70 and her respiratory rate is 22, her heart rate is 80 beats per minute, her PO_2 on 2 L of oxygen is 89%, and her pCO_2 is 37 mmHg. A chest x-ray demonstrates mild atelectasis in the right base and normal heart size unchanged from her previous admission. Her white count is 9500/μL, hemoglobin is 11.5 g%, and platelet count is 460 000/μL.

She is treated with multiple bronchodilators without benefit. She is still on corticosteroids from her last admission so the emergency department physician felt that a bolus of corticosteroids would not likely help. The admitting physician consults palliative care to manage her dyspnea. Your fellow has seen the patient in consultation and recommends morphine 5 mg every 4 hours as needed.

Suggested Answer

One of the treatable causes of refractory COPD and repeated exacerbations is pulmonary embolism (PE). The prevalence in a systematic review was 19.9% and in hospitalized patients was as high as 24.7%. Female gender, obesity, and recent hospitalization increase the risks for PE. Some features suggest the diagnosis; a reduced pCO_2 below 40 mmHg, a high platelet count, and hypotension. A D-dimer below 500 ng/mL would effectively exclude the diagnosis, and an elevated D-dimer would bring the diagnosis into consideration. The chest x-ray is often normal or may have a nonspecific infiltrate or atelectasis. A negative lower extremity Doppler scan does not exclude the possibility of a PE if there are other signs suggesting PE. Clinicians should think of the diagnosis particularly when patients are repeatedly admitted at short intervals with refractory COPD symptoms.

References

1. Vozoris NT, Wang X, Fischer HD, et al. Incident opioid drug use and adverse respiratory outcomes among older adults with COPD. *Eur Respir J.* 2016;48(3):683–693.
2. Ekstrom M, Nilsson F, Abernethy AA, Currow DC. Effects of opioids on breathlessness and exercise capacity in chronic obstructive pulmonary disease. A systematic review. *Ann Am Thorac Soc.* 2015;12(7):1079–1092.
3. Jennings AL, Davies AN, Higgins JP, Gibbs JS, Broadley KE. A systematic review of the use of opioids in the management of dyspnoea. *Thorax.* 2002;57(11):939–944.
4. Barnes H, McDonald J, Smallwood N, Manser R. Opioids for the palliation of refractory breathlessness in adults with advanced disease and terminal illness. *Cochrane Database Syst Rev.* 2016;(3):CD011008.
5. Nici L, Mammen MJ, Charbek E, et al. Pharmacologic management of chronic obstructive pulmonary disease. An Official American Thoracic Society clinical practice guideline. *Am J Respir Crit Care Med.* 2020;201(9):e56–e69.
6. Ekstrom M, Bornefalk-Hermansson A, Abernethy A, Currow D. Low-dose opioids should be considered for symptom relief also in advanced chronic obstructive pulmonary disease (COPD). *Evid Based Med.* 2015;20(1):39.
7. Currow DC, McDonald C, Oaten S, et al. Once-daily opioids for chronic dyspnea: a dose increment and pharmacovigilance study. *J Pain Symptom Manage.* 2011;42(3):388–399.
8. Oxberry SG, Torgerson DJ, Bland JM, Clark AL, Cleland JG, Johnson MJ. Short-term opioids for breathlessness in stable chronic heart failure: a randomized controlled trial. *Eur J Heart Fail.* 2011;13(9):1006–1012.
9. Ferreira DH, Louw S, McCloud P, et al. Controlled-release oxycodone vs. placebo in the treatment of chronic breathlessness-a multisite randomized placebo controlled trial. *J Pain Symptom Manage.* 2020;59(3):581–589.

10. Yamaguchi T, Matsuda Y, Matsuoka H, et al. Efficacy of immediate-release oxycodone for dyspnoea in cancer patient: Cancer Dyspnoea Relief (CDR) trial. *Jpn J Clin Oncol.* 2018;48(12):1070–1075.
11. Hui D, Hernandez F, Larsson L, et al. Prophylactic fentanyl sublingual spray for episodic exertional dyspnea in cancer patients: a pilot double-blind randomized controlled trial. *J Pain Symptom Manage.* 2019;58(4):605–613.
12. Hui D, Kilgore K, Frisbee-Hume S, et al. Effect of prophylactic fentanyl buccal tablet on episodic exertional dyspnea: a pilot double-blind randomized controlled trial. *J Pain Symptom Manage.* 2017;54(6):798–805.
13. Hui D, Kilgore K, Park M, Williams J, Liu D, Bruera E. Impact of prophylactic fentanyl pectin nasal spray on exercise-induced episodic dyspnea in cancer patients: a double-blind, randomized controlled trial. *J Pain Symptom Manage.* 2016;52(4):459–468.e451.
14. Pinna MA, Bruera E, Moralo MJ, Correas MA, Vargas RM. A randomized crossover clinical trial to evaluate the efficacy of oral transmucosal fentanyl citrate in the treatment of dyspnea on exertion in patients with advanced cancer. *Am J Hosp Palliat Care.* 2015;32(3):298–304.
15. van Dam CJ, Algera MH, Olofsen E, et al. Opioid utility function: methods and implications. *Ann Palliat Med.* 2020;9(2):528–536.
16. Boom M, Olofsen E, Neukirchen M, et al. Fentanyl utility function: a risk-benefit composite of pain relief and breathing responses. *Anesthesiology.* 2013;119(3):663–674.
17. Hill R, Santhakumar R, Dewey W, Kelly E, Henderson G. Fentanyl depression of respiration: comparison with heroin and morphine. *Br J Pharmacol.* 2020;177(2):254–266.
18. Ekstrom MP, Bornefalk-Hermansson A, Abernethy AP, Currow DC. Safety of benzodiazepines and opioids in very severe respiratory disease: national prospective study. *BMJ.* 2014;348:g445.
19. Baillargeon J, Singh G, Kuo YF, Raji MA, Westra J, Sharma G. Association of opioid and benzodiazepine use with adverse respiratory events in older adults with chronic obstructive pulmonary disease. *Ann Am Thorac Soc.* 2019;16(10):1245–1251.
20. Dublin S, Walker RL, Jackson ML, et al. Use of opioids or benzodiazepines and risk of pneumonia in older adults: a population-based case-control study. *J Am Geriatr Soc.* 2011;59(10):1899–1907.
21. Wiese AD, Griffin MR, Schaffner W, et al. Opioid analgesic use and risk for invasive pneumococcal diseases: a nested case-control study. *Ann Intern Med.* 2018;168(6):396–404.
22. Portenoy RK, Sibirceva U, Smout R, et al. Opioid use and survival at the end of life: a survey of a hospice population. *J Pain Symptom Manage.* 2006;32(6):532–540.

15

Effect of Prophylactic Subcutaneous Scopolamine Butylbromide on Death Rattle in Patients at the End of Life

MELLAR P. DAVIS

Study Nickname: The SILENCE Randomized Clinical Trial, *JAMA*. 2021 Oct 5;326(13):1268–1276

This multicenter RCT found that the occurrence of the death rattle was significantly reduced by prophylactic subcutaneously administered scopolamine butylbromide. The prespecified adverse events were not substantially different between the 2 groups.

Research Question: Are antimuscarinic antisecretory drugs more effective when given prophylactically in someone actively dying than at the onset of the death rattle?

Funding: Palliative Care Research Programme Palliatie from the Netherlands Organization for Health Research and Development

Year Study Began: 2017

Year Study Published: 2021

Study Location: Erasmus Medical Center, Rotterdam, the Netherlands

Who Was Studied? Adults admitted to hospice with a life expectancy of at least 3 days with expected hospitalization until death and the ability to understand the information given to them about the study.

Who Was Excluded? Patients with tracheostomies or tracheal cannulas, patients using anticholinergics or octreotide, patients with active respiratory infection.

How Many Patients? 157

Study Overview: This was a multicenter, randomized, double-blind trial of scopolamine butylbromide or placebo administered subcutaneously 4 times daily. Treatment was started when patients stopped eating, could only take sips of water, could no longer swallow, and were semicomatose. The medications were continued until death or grade 2 terminal secretions (audible at the foot of the bed by the Back scale[1]) measured at 2 consecutive time points 4 hours apart.

Study Intervention: Scopolamine butylbromide 20 mg subcutaneously 4 times daily or placebo.

Follow-up: Median observation time on placebo was 33 hours (interquartile range [IQR] 13.8–63.4); median observation time on scopolamine butylbromide was 45.8 hours (IQR 20.9–92.0).

Endpoints:

Primary endpoint: The occurrence of a grade 2 or higher death rattle based on the Back scale (grade 0—no rattle, grade 1—rattle heard when next to the patient, grade 2—rattle heard at the foot of the bed, grade 3—rattle heard at the door) on 2 consecutive time points, 4 hours apart.

Secondary endpoints: (1) The time between recognition of the dying phase and the occurrence of the death rattle in hours. (2) Prespecified adverse events potentially related to the use of an anticholinergic drug.

Exploratory endpoint: The time between the recognition of the dying phase and death in hours.

Power calculations: In a previous study of 400 patients, 39% had a death rattle grade 2 or higher. Investigators considered a 50% relative reduction to be clinically relevant (reducing death rattle occurrence to 19%). For a 2-sided significance of 0.05 and 80% power, 180 patients are needed.

Secondary outcomes: There were no differences in adverse outcomes or other symptoms such as pain, nausea, dyspnea, or vomiting.

Table 15.1 STUDY RESULTS

Outcomes	**Scopolamine ($n = 79$)**	**Placebo ($n = 78$)**	***P* Value**	**Hazard Ratio**
Death rattle at 2 timepoints	10 (13%)	21 (27%)	.02	N/A
Death rattle at 1 timepoint, no improvement	15 (19%)	29 (37%)	.01	N/A
Time from dying phase to death rattle	48 hours, 8%	48 hours, 17%	.03	0.44
Time from dying phase to death rattle, 1 timepoint without improvement	48 hours, 8%	48 hours, 22 %	.006	0.40

Exploratory outcome: The dying phase was longer with scopolamine butylbromide at 42.8 hours than placebo at 29.5 hours (median); hazard ratio 0.71, $P = .04$.

Criticisms and Limitations:

- The accrual did not reach its goal at 180 patients.
- Only 10% of admitted patients participated in the study.
- "Dying phase" criteria were based on a Dutch guideline previously published in 2010.
- There are other alternatives such as a scopolamine transdermal patch or scopolamine (hyoscine) hydrobromide sublingual that would not require a subcutaneous line. However, the scopolamine patch contains scopolamine hydrobromide, which crosses the blood–brain barrier and may contribute to increased sedation and delirium.
- Glycopyrrolate, which is also a quaternary amine antimuscarinic antisecretory drug, may be an alternative in countries like the United States where scopolamine butylbromide is not available.

Other Relevant Studies and Information:

- An earlier study conducted by Mercadante and colleagues randomized patients who were actively dying with a Richmond Agitation Sedation Scale (RASS) of ≤ 3 and without death rattle.[2]
- Randomization was between scopolamine butylbromide 20 mg every 8 hours subcutaneously or as a subcutaneous infusion prophylactically or treatment of using the same at the onset of the death rattle (grade 1 by the Back scale).

- Eighty-one patients were treated at the onset of the death rattle and 51 were treated prophylactically.
- Similar to the present study, there was improvement in and prevention of the death rattle with prophylactic use of scopolamine butylbromide. The death rattle occurred in 49 of 81 patients treated at the onset of the death rattle and 3 of 51 treated prophylactically ($P = .001$).
- The onset of the death rattle from the "dying phase" was 12 hours for those in the control group and 36 hours for those treated prophylactically ($P = .0001$).
- Response to scopolamine butylbromide when the death rattle occurred was 20%.
- Survival in those who were treated prophylactically was 45.26 hours and for those treated with the onset of the death rattle was 41.1 hours with a P value of .05.

Summary and Implications: Grade 2 death rattle occurs in 39%–60% of patients who are actively dying. This and a prior study have demonstrated that the prophylactic use of quaternary scopolamine significantly reduces the death rattle. What is apparent from both studies is that once terminal secretions are present, the response to antimuscarinics is likely not to occur. As a result, antimuscarinics should be given prophylactically, that is, prior to the onset of the death rattle and around the clock rather than with the onset of the death rattle and "as needed." This requires timing the initiation of antimuscarinics with the projected time of death, which may be difficult to do.

CLINICAL CASE

Case History

MS is a 57-year-old male with advanced lung cancer who received palliative carboplatin plus pemetrexed and second-line pembrolizumab. On his fourth cycle of pembrolizumab, he developed pneumonitis and was placed on corticosteroids assuming the pneumonitis was related to the checkpoint inhibitor. A computed tomography scan demonstrated multiple ground-glass infiltrates in his lung. He elected not to pursue further anticancer therapy and decided to enroll in home hospice. However, he developed a fever of 38.3° C and was admitted to the inpatient hospice unit from home with weakness, anorexia, cough, and confusion with mild stupor. The family wanted him to be comfortable and did not want him to "drown" in his own secretions since he was short of breath at baseline. On examination, there were crackles in both lungs, and he had some discolored sputum according to the nurse. His respiratory rate was 30 breaths per minute, and he had some retractions of accessory muscles. What would be the best initial treatment option?

1. Empirically treat him as if he had pneumonia with antibiotics in hopes of reducing his secretions and respiratory distress.
2. Start morphine infusion at 1 mg/hour and titrate based on a respiratory rate above 24 breaths per minute.
3. Increase the steroid dose using dexamethasone 4 mg every 8 hours.
4. Start glycopyrrolate 0.2–0.4 mg intravenously or subcutaneously every 8 hours given the family's concern about "drowning" in his secretions.

Suggested Answer

The patient wanted comfort only and so antibiotics would be inappropriate for the most part. Antibiotics may reduce shortness of breath and secretions arising from the lung, but this is not a well-established practice. Further studies would be needed to clarify the benefits and detriments of antibiotics at the end of life. Antimuscarinics are great for oral secretions but may be detrimental if secretions are arising from the lungs. Desiccation of pulmonary mucus may lead to mucus plugging and increase dyspnea. One study recently found that corticosteroids may help terminal dyspnea but are unlikely to help if dyspnea is caused by pneumonia.

References

1. Back IN, Jenkins K, Blower A, Beckhelling J. A study comparing hyoscine hydrobromide and glycopyrrolate in the treatment of death rattle. *Palliat Med.* 2001;15(4):329–336.
2. Mercadante S, Marinangeli F, Masedu F, et al. Hyoscine butylbromide for the management of death rattle: sooner rather than later. *J Pain Symptom Manage.* 2018;56(6):902–907.

16

Palmitoylethanolamide (PEA) as Adjunctive Therapy May Offer Benefit to Patients With Major Depressive Disorder (MDD)

SUSAN DESANTO-MADEYA AND CONSTANCE DAHLIN

> [Palmitoylethanolamide (PEA) was] revealed to be a safe and well tolerated adjuvant to citalopram in patients (predominantly male) with major depressive disorder (MDD). Male patients in the PEA group demonstrated rapid onset and significantly greater improvements in depressive symptom scores from week 2 compared to the placebo group.
>
> —Ghazizadeh-Hashemi et al.[1]

Research Question: What are the efficacy and tolerability of palmitoylethanolamide (PEA) as an adjunct to citalopram versus placebo and citalopram in patients with major depressive disorders (MDD)?

Funding: The study was supported by a grant from Tehran University of Medical Sciences to Professor Shahin Akhondzadeh (Grant No. 33136).

Year Study Began: 2017

Year Study Published: 2018

Study Location: This study was conducted as a 2-center, double-blind, parallel-group randomized controlled trial at the outpatient clinic of Iran Hospital and Tehran Psychiatric Institute.

Who Was Studied: Men and women 18–50 years of age with a diagnosis of MDD according to the *Diagnostic and Statistical Manual of Mental Disorders*, fifth edition, with a score of ≥ 19 on the 17-item Hamilton Depression Rating Scale (HAM-D) and with a score of at least 2 on item 1 of the HAM-D.

Who Was Excluded: Exclusion criteria were the receipt of any antidepressant medication and psychotherapy treatments in the previous month; receipt of electroconvulsive therapy (ECT) in the last 2 months, presence of psychosis or diagnosis of other mental disorders, alcohol or substance use or dependence within 1 year, risk of suicide or suicidal ideations, and uncontrolled medical problems (i.e., cardiovascular disease, hypertension, thyroid disorders, or pregnancy).

How Many Patients: 58 patients were randomized (29 patients in each group), and 54 patients (27 patients in each group) completed the trial; 85 patients were screened for eligibility, and 27 were excluded due to not meeting inclusion criteria or declined participation.

Study Overview: A randomized double-blind and placebo-controlled study (Figure 16.1).

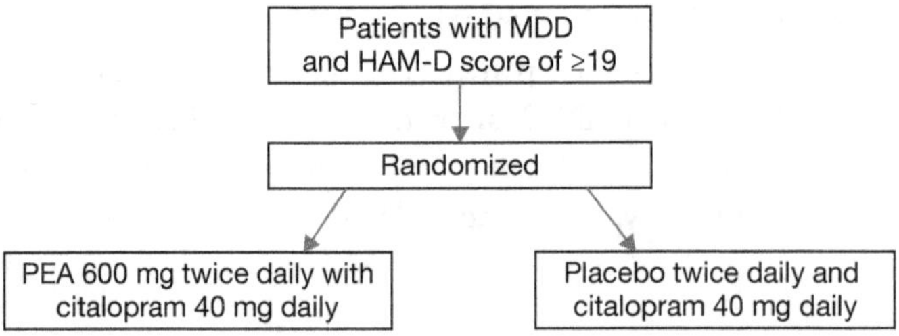

Figure 16.1. Flow diagram representing case selection.

Study Intervention: Patients were randomly assigned to receive PEA 600 mg twice daily with citalopram 40 mg daily or a placebo with citalopram 40 mg daily. Citalopram was administered at half dose in the first week. Patients were not treated with any other psychiatric or nonpsychiatric medication during the trial period.

Follow-Up: 6 weeks

Endpoints: The primary outcome was to evaluate PEA in improving depression using the HAM-D score compared with placebo at weeks 2, 4, and 6 postintervention.

RESULTS

- Fifty-four patients completed the trial (27 per group).
- The PEA group demonstrated significantly greater reduction in HAM-D scores compared to the placebo group at week 2 (Table 16.1).
- Throughout the trial period, the PEA group had significantly greater improvement in depressive symptoms compared to the placebo group.
- There were no differences in baseline characteristics and side effects between the 2 groups (Table 16.2).

Table 16.1 COMPARISON OF HAM-D SCORE CHANGE FROM BASELINE

Week	PEA + Citalopram Group[a]	Placebo + Citalopram Group	Mean Difference	*P* Value
2	8.30 ± 2.41	5.1 ± 3.57	2.48 (0.81–4.15)	.004
4	12.52 ± 2.69	10.89 ± 3.69	1.63 (−0.14 to 30.07)	.070
6	16.30 ± 2.38	14.40 ± 4.15	1.89 (0.03–3.75)	.047

Abbreviation: PEA, palmitoylethanolamide. 95% CI: 95% confidence interval.

Table 16.2 COMPARISON OF RESPONSE TO TREATMENT AND REMISSION RATES

HAM-D	PEA Arm (*n* = 27)	Placebo Arm (*n* = 27)	*P* Value	Relative Risk
Week 2				
n (%) with response to treatment	0	0	1.00	n/a
Week 4				
n (%) with response to treatment	14 (51.8%)	10 (37%)	.27	1.4
Week 6				
n (%) with response to treatment	27 (100%)	20 (74%)	.01	1.35
Week 2				
n (%) with remissions	0	0	1.00	n/a
Week 4				
n (%) with remissions	1 (3.7%)	0	1.00	n/a
Week 6				
n (%) with remissions	6 (22.2%)	3 (11.1%)	.46	1.92

Abbreviations: HAM-D, Hamilton Depression Rating Scale; PEA, palmitoylethanolamide
[a] Reported by Fischer's exact test.

Criticisms and Limitations: The sample size was small, and the study was underpowered to identify clinically important differences. Male and female populations were not equal; females were underrepresented (35%). The duration of treatment and observation was relatively short.

Other Relevant Studies and Information:

- In another clinical study, the response of 14 patients with major depressive episodes to PEA was followed over 20–50 weeks. The antidepressant response was maintained in 12 of the 14 patients. Effective dosage did not change with time and no apparent side effects were experienced. PEA produced sustained relief of depression in a significant number of patients, including some unresponsive to the standard treatments.[2]
- A study by Kawamura and colleagues found that the circulating palmitoylethanolamide levels inversely correlated with the severity of major depression, with an area under the receiver-operator curve of 0.92 and a sensitivity/specificity > 88% at a cutoff level of 1.46 μM. These results suggest that plasma PEA level could be a candidate biomarker of MDD in the clinical setting as well as a therapeutic target.[3]

Summary and Implications: This study suggests that PEA may be effective as an adjunct treatment to citalopram for patients with MDD. The use of PEA with citalopram was well tolerated with rapid improvement in depressive symptoms within 2 weeks and continued through 6 weeks. Because this was a small study, the findings are preliminary and further research is needed before PEA can be recommended for the treatment of MDD.

CLINICAL CASE: PATIENT WITH CANCER AND DEPRESSION

Case History

A 50-year-old man with stage II colon cancer, otherwise healthy, is noted to have a HAM-D score of 22. He is feeling guilty about not feeling present with his family—a spouse and 2 teenage daughters. He is struggling to make decisions about treatment. Moreover, he is anxious to participate in family activities and complete financial and advance care planning documents but feels too depressed and tired to do so. He has not had any prior treatment for his depression. He does not want to use a stimulant as he has seen the negative side of their use on his children's school. How should the patient be treated?

Suggested Answer

Initiating PEA and citalopram has been found to be effective for male patients with MDD over a short time interval. Given that the patient has cancer, he will probably need long-term treatment for depression. The patient could have a trial of PEA 600 mg twice a day with citalopram 40 mg once a day for rapid decline in depressive symptoms. He would experience few side effects and would most likely experience a better quality of life.

References

1. Ghazizadeh-Hashemi M, Ghajar A, Shalbafan MR, et al. Palmitoylethanolamide as adjunctive therapy in major depressive *J Affect Disord*. 2018;232:127–133. doi:10.1016/j.jad.2018.02.057. Epub 2018 Feb 21. PMID: 29486338.
2. Sabelli H, Fink P, Fawcett J, Tom C. Sustained antidepressant effect of PEA replacement. *J Neuropsychiatry Clin Neurosci*. 1996;8(2):168–171. doi:10.1176/jnp.8.2.168.
3. Kawamura N, Shinoda K, Sato H, et al. Plasma metabolome analysis of patients with major depressive disorder. *Psychiatry Clin Neurosci*. 2018;72(5):349–361.

17

Haloperidol as an Adjunct Therapy for Pain and Nausea in Acute Gastroparesis

SANDRA DISCALA AND CHRISTINE M. VARTAN

> Haloperidol was superior to placebo in reducing nausea and pain, and our findings suggest that the addition of haloperidol to conventional therapy was better than conventional therapy alone. And therefore our study suggests that haloperidol is an effective first-line agent in combination with standard analgesic and antiemetic agents for the treatment of gastroparesis in the ED.
>
> —Roldan et al.[1]

Research Question: Is the addition of haloperidol to conventional therapy superior to conventional therapy for treating nausea and abdominal pain in patients with gastroparesis?

Funding: The authors had no relevant financial information or potential conflicts to disclose in preparation of this study.

Year Study Began: 2013

Year Study Published: 2017

Study Location: 2 academic urban hospital emergency departments (EDs) (1 private and 1 county hospital) located in Texas, United States

Who Was Studied: Adults with a history of gastroparesis who were seen in the EDs for nausea, vomiting, and abdominal pain related to gastroparesis diagnosis.

Who Was Excluded: Age < 18 years, QT prolongation (past or current), hypotension (defined as systolic blood pressure < 90 mmHg), other acute abdominal conditions, allergy to haloperidol, pregnancy, those who were incarcerated, or patients who were not able to provide informed consent.

How Many Patients: 33

Study Overview: This study was a randomized, double-blind, placebo-controlled trial at the ED of 2 urban hospitals. A total of 33 patients were randomized in a 1:1 ratio to different treatment arms (Figure 17.1).

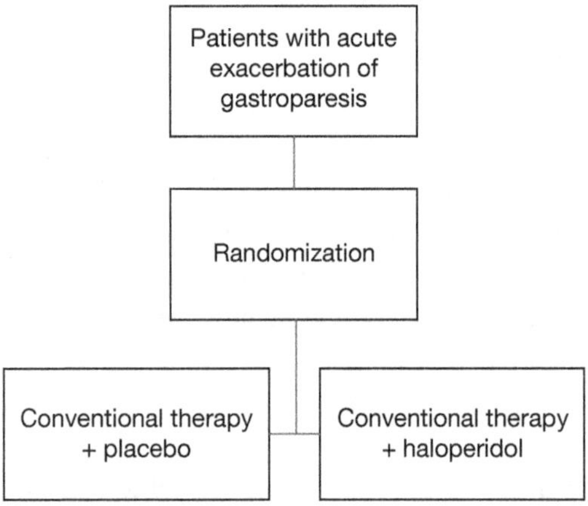

Figure 17.1. Overview of study design.

Study Intervention: Patients enrolled in this study received a blinded prepackaged study medication that was either haloperidol 5 mg intravenously or an equivalent volume of a placebo. Patients received conventional treatment, which was determined by the physician. Conventional treatments such as hydromorphone, morphine, metoclopramide, ondansetron, promethazine, pantoprazole, famotidine, erythromycin, diphenhydramine, magnesium hydroxide, haloperidol, and lorazepam were administered before and/or after blinded intervention. Abdominal pain using a 10-point visual analog scale and nausea using a 5-point visual analog scale were measured at randomization and in 15-minute increments for 1 hour. Additional monitoring parameters were cardiac activity, pulse oximetry, and blood pressure along with any adverse effects. After the 1-hour interval, patients were given additional symptomatic treatment as needed.

Follow-Up: 1 hour

Endpoints: Primary outcome: Change in symptoms of abdominal pain and nausea assessed by a 10-point and 5-point visual analog scale, respectively. Secondary outcomes: Disposition such as discharge or hospital admission, length of stay (LOS) in ED, and resolution of nausea at 1 hour determined by request for further nausea medications.

RESULTS

- After 1 hour, mean pain scores had decreased by 5.37 points in the haloperidol group with a *P* value of ≤ .001 versus 1.11 points in the placebo group with a *P* value of .11 (Table 17.1). The *n* = 15 in the haloperidol group did not meet the a priori specification for a sample size of at least 18 subjects in each group.

Table 17.1 PAIN AND NAUSEA SCORES PRE- AND POSTINTERVENTION

Time from Intervention	**Haloperidol Group (*n* = 15) Mean Pain Score (± SD)**[1]	**Placebo Group (*n* = 18) Mean Pain Score (± SD)**[1]
Pretreatment	8.5 (± 1.82)	8.28 (± 1.77)
30 minutes posttreatment	4.67 (± 3.59)	8.06 (± 1.86)
60 minutes posttreatment	3.13 (± 3.6); *P* value ≤ .001	7.17 (± 2.81); *P* value .11
Time from Intervention	**Mean Nausea Score (± SD)**	**Mean Nausea Score (± SD)**
Pretreatment	4.53 (± 0.83)	4.11 (± 0.96)
30 minutes posttreatment	2.20 (± 1.96)	3.67 (± 1.37)
60 minutes posttreatment	1.83 (± 1.92)	3.39 (± 1.68)

[1] Pain scores are based on the visual analog scale ranging from 0 to 10.
Roldan CJ, Chambers KA, Paniagua L, Patel S, Cardenas-Turanzas M, Chathampally Y. Randomized controlled double-blind trial comparing haloperidol combined with conventional therapy to conventional therapy alone in patients with symptomatic gastroparesis. *Acad Emerg Med.* 2017;24(11):1307–1314.

- After 1 hour, mean nausea scores had decreased by 2.7 points in the haloperidol group with a *P* value of ≤ .001 versus 0.72 points in the placebo group with a *P* value of .05 (Table 17.1). The *n* = 15 in the haloperidol group did not meet the a priori specification for a sample size of at least 18 subjects in each group.

- In those who did not receive opioids ($n = 21$), the 1-hour postintervention reduction in mean pain score was 5 points in those receiving haloperidol ($n = 9$, $P \leq .001$) versus 1.31 in those receiving placebo ($n = 13$, $P = .14$); results for nausea were 2.61 reduction in haloperidol ($P \leq .01$) versus 0.77 in the placebo group ($P = .13$).
- The secondary outcome favored the haloperidol group as hospitalizations in the haloperidol group were $n = 4$ (26.7%) versus in the placebo group $n = 13$ (72.2%) ($P = .009$).
- The secondary outcome favored the haloperidol group as ED median LOS was 4.8 hours in the haloperidol group and 9 hours in the placebo group ($P = .77$).

Criticisms and Limitations:

- Due to the small sample size, the primary outcome did not meet the expected sample size required to meet the a priori power calculation. Therefore, the study did not reach statistical significance, but the outcomes did favor a trend in the haloperidol intervention arm compared to placebo.
- Conventional therapy varied widely as there was no specific protocol.

Other Relevant Studies and Information:

- Ramirez et al. retrospectively reviewed 52 patients with diabetic gastroparesis who were treated in the ED with haloperidol and compared their outcomes to outcomes during their own previous ED visits for gastroparesis when haloperidol was not given.[2] The use of haloperidol was found to decrease rates of hospital admission (5 vs. 14; $P = .02$) and morphine-equivalent analgesic use (median 6.75 vs. 10.75; $P = .009$) but not ED or hospital LOS.[2]
- In a retrospective chart review of patients with diabetic gastroparesis who received haloperidol ($n = 22$) versus those who did not ($n = 99$), the haloperidol group had a median ED LOS of 8.5 hours versus 6 hours in those who did not ($P < .011$), but lower rates of hospitalization (45.5% vs. 70.7%, $P < .024$).[3]
- Despite the results of this analysis, the 2021 American Diabetes Association standards of care discuss the use of metoclopramide,

domperidone (only available outside the United States) and erythromycin, but not haloperidol, for the treatment of diabetic gastroparesis.[4] These guidelines have not yet been updated to include the results of this analysis, however.

Summary and Implications: This small double-blind randomized controlled trial showed promise for the use of haloperidol as adjunct pharmacotherapy in reducing pain and nausea associated with acute gastroparesis presenting in the ED. Larger randomized controlled trials are needed to further assess haloperidol for this challenging condition for which there are few effective therapies.

CLINICAL CASE: WHERE DOES HALOPERIDOL FIT IN THE TREATMENT OF SYMPTOMATIC GASTROPARESIS?

Case History

A 47-year-old Hispanic female with symptomatic diabetic gastroparesis presents to the ED. She has been having issues with nausea and difficulty eating at home over the past 2 days and is concerned with using insulin without eating. She now reports abdominal pain that is 8 out of 10 on the visual analog scale and nausea that is 5 out of 5 on the visual analog scale. Blood pressure is 141/90 mmHg, QTc interval is 400 ms, and pregnancy test is negative. She does not have any medication allergies or any significant cardiac disease. She was provided metoclopramide and ondansetron without relief. No abnormal movements have been observed.

Should this patient be offered haloperidol as adjunct treatment of gastroparesis?

Suggested Answer

The Roldan trial utilized haloperidol as adjunct therapy in adults with acute symptomatic gastroparesis in the ED. The mean severity of pain and nausea intensity were both severe at baseline in the trial, with improvements to mild pain intensity and minimal nausea in the haloperidol treatment arm in comparison to placebo.

The patient in this case meets similar inclusion criteria of the Roldan et al. trial in that adults presenting to the ED with abdominal pain and nausea attributed to their gastroparesis were included. This patient has high symptom burden and is not deriving benefit from the current standard of care. Ondansetron is well known for its constipating effects and therefore would limit its further utility here. Haloperidol and metoclopramide increase antidopaminergic effects and require close monitoring with use.

The patient is not pregnant and QTc is normal; therefore, it would be reasonable to offer haloperidol 5 mg intravenously once. Continue to monitor cardiac and clinical status along with improvement in pain and nausea over the next hour after haloperidol administration.

References

1. Roldan CJ, Chambers KA, Paniagua L, Patel S, Cardenas-Turanzas M, Chathampally Y. Randomized controlled double-blind trial comparing haloperidol combined with conventional therapy to conventional therapy alone in patients with symptomatic gastroparesis. *Acad Emerg Med.* 2017;24(11):1307–1314.
2. Ramirez R, Stalcup P, Croft B, Darracq MA. Haloperidol undermining gastroparesis symptoms (HUGS) in the emergency department. *Am J Emerg Med.* 2017;35(8):1118–1120.
3. Heuser W, Carp S, Fuehrer J, et al. Haloperidol in lieu of conventional therapy in the treatment of diabetic related gastroparesis in the emergency department. *Clin Pharmacol Toxicol Res.* 2019;2(1):1–5.
4. American Diabetes Association. Microvascular complications and foot care: standards of medical care in diabetes—2021. *Diabetes Care.* 2021;44(Suppl 1):S151–S167.

18

Neuroleptic Strategies for Terminal Agitation in Patients With Cancer and Delirium at an Acute Palliative Care Unit

A Single-Center, Double-Blind, Parallel-Group, Randomized Trial

ALLISON E. JORDAN AND ALEXANDER GAMBLE

> Our data provide preliminary evidence that the three strategies of neuroleptics might reduce agitation in patients with terminal agitation. These findings are in the context of the single-centre design, small sample size, and lack of a placebo-only group.
>
> —Hui et al.[1]

Research Question: What is the most effective neuroleptic strategy in the treatment of refractory agitation in cancer patients with terminal delirium?

Funding: National Institute of Nursing Research

Year Study Began: 2017

Year Study Published: 2020

Study Location: Palliative and Supportive Care Unit, University of Texas MD Anderson Cancer Center Houston, Texas, United States

Who Was Studied: Patients over the age of 18 with advanced cancer admitted to the palliative and supportive care unit with refractory agitation despite low-dose haloperidol.

Who Was Excluded: Patients with Parkinson disease, Alzheimer disease, myasthenia gravis, acute narrow-angle glaucoma, neuroleptic malignant syndrome, active seizure disorder, documented QTc prolongation, or hypersensitivity or who were already on scheduled chlorpromazine within the past 48 hours of study enrollment.

How Many Patients: 68

Study Overview: See Figure 18.1.

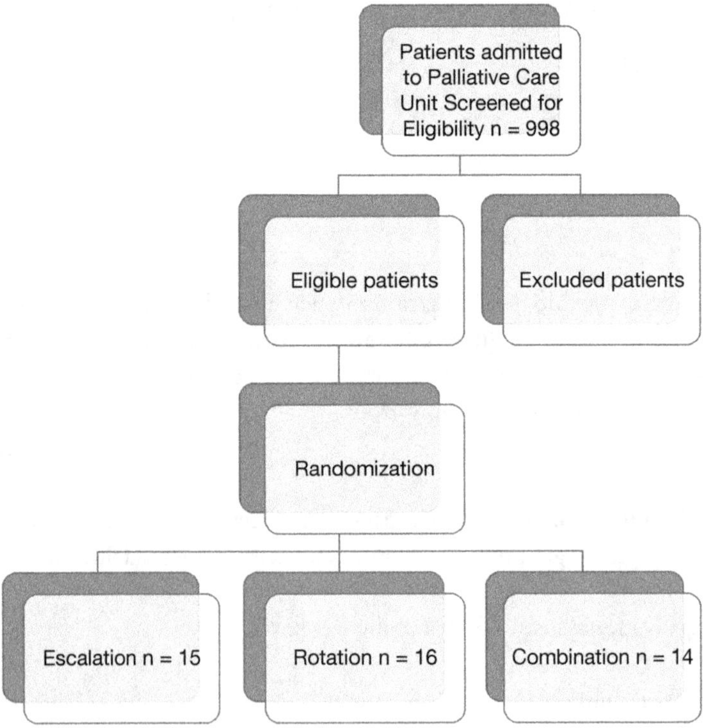

Figure 18.1. Summary of study design.

Study Intervention: Immediately after enrollment into the study, the neuroleptic regimen was standardized to intravenous open-label haloperidol 2 mg every 6 hours and 2 mg every hour as needed. The Richmond Agitation Sedation Scale (RASS) score was monitored every 2 hours. When the RASS score was 1 or greater, the masked medication regimen was started.

The masked study medication regimen consisted of a scheduled dose intravenously every 4 hours and a rescue dose every hour as needed. At the initiation of the masked study medication, the patients received their scheduled dose and a rescue dose. The study used a double-dummy design. The starting schedule and rescue dose for the escalation group was 2 mg haloperidol, 25 mg chlorpromazine for the rotation group, and 1 mg haloperidol and 12.5 mg chlorpromazine for the combination group. The bedside nurse assessed the RASS score at fixed intervals. Scheduled and as-needed medication doses were increased by 1 dose level if a patient had a RASS score of 2 or more at any time or required 3 or more rescue doses within a 4-hour period.

Follow-Up: Death, discharge, or withdrawal

Endpoints:

Primary outcome: Change in RASS from initiation of study to 24 hours later.

Secondary outcomes: Proportion of patients with a target RASS of –2 to 0 within the first 24 hours; the need for rescue neuroleptics or benzodiazepines and the need for dose-level increase during the first 24 hours; perceived level of comfort and agitation by caregivers and nurses.

RESULTS

- RASS scores decreased in all 3 groups after administration of masked treatment (Figure 18.2).
- The rotation group had fewer patients who required a dose-level increase within the first 24 hours.
- The combination group was significantly more likely to require rescue benzodiazepines.
- 60%–75% of patients were perceived by caregivers and nurses to be more comfortable the day after treatment when compared to the day before.
- Hypotension was the most common severe adverse event.
- No patients had worsening of any of the 8 neuroleptic symptoms listed in the UKU questionnaire between days 0 and 3.
- There were no treatment-related deaths.

Criticisms and Limitations:

- The study did not have a placebo-only control group; thus, it is not possible to know how the various treatment strategies compared to a placebo treatment.

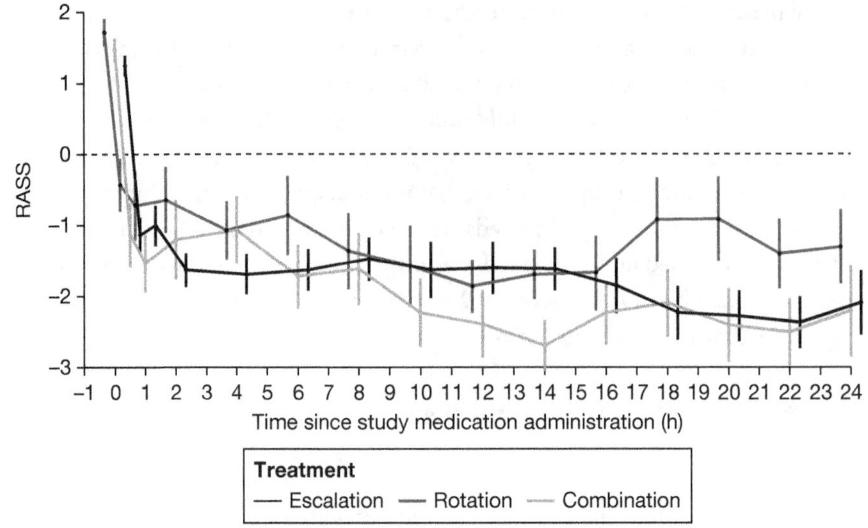

Figure 18.2. Change in RASS score over the first 24 h after study medication administration.
The mean RASS scores (data markers) are plotted for each study group starting at time 0 (i.e., immediately before masked study medication administration) over the next 24 h, with error bars indicating standard error.

RASS, Richmond Agitation Sedation Scale.

- While increased sedation may be perceived as increased comfort, for some families this may not be desirable because they may not be able to communicate with the patient.
- The sample size in each group was small, thus limiting the power of the analysis for identifying significant results.

Other Relevant Studies and Information:

- The Breitbart and Asadollahi trials (see Chapters 1 and 47 respectively) demonstrated the potential benefit of neuroleptics in managing symptoms of delirium in the hospital and emergency settings.[2,3]
- An earlier study by Hui (Chapter 21) showed superior reduction in delirious agitation with addition of lorazepam to haloperidol compared to haloperidol alone.[4]
- The Agar trial (Chapter 12) found that individualized management of delirium precipitants and supportive strategies alone result in better reductions in distressing symptoms as compared to treatment with neuroleptics.[5]

- A 2018 *New England Journal of Medicine* study by Girard et al. concluded that neuroleptics did not alter the duration, severity, or symptoms of delirium, nor the length of hospital stay for patients with delirium in the intensive care unit.[6] Importantly, that study did not look specifically at management of agitation in delirium, with most patients enrolled experiencing a hypoactive delirium.

Summary and Implications: Prior studies have offered seemingly contradictory findings with respect to the role of neuroleptics in delirium management; however, these prior studies did not focus on symptoms of agitation, a primary reason medications are considered for patients experiencing delirium in clinical practice. This analysis suggests that neuroleptics may have a role as an adjunct to nonpharmacologic approaches for controlling delirium-related agitation among patients with cancer in palliative care settings.

CLINICAL CASE: HOW BEST TO ADDRESS TERMINAL AGITATION IN DELIRIUM?

Case History

A 78-year-old woman with known metastatic breast cancer is admitted to the hospital with complaint of altered mental status gradually worsening over the prior several days. Urinalysis suggested urinary tract infection (UTI), but the rest of her workup, including computed tomography of the head, is negative for significant findings. She is treated with appropriate antibiotic therapy, but mentation does not improve over the initial days of treatment, including the best nonpharmacologic approaches to delirium. On the third hospital day a brain magnetic resonance image is obtained and shows numerous new lesions concerning for metastatic disease.

Her family indicates that given advancing disease, the patient would want to transition to comfort-focused care and return home with hospice services if possible. They express concern that her agitation has become severe and has not improved despite being started on 1 mg of haloperidol intravenously every 4 hours as needed for agitation over the past day.

Suggested Answer

The Hui trial highlights the potential for neuroleptics to both decrease agitation and improve patient comfort in the setting of terminal agitation, as well as the importance of titration and potential for rotation.

The patient in this case scenario may have a terminal delirium driven by the progression of her underlying malignancy with new brain metastases, but it is also possible that this may represent a reversible delirium driven by her acute UTI in addition to the new metastatic disease.

While a case could be made to target her agitation by addition of lorazepam, we would suggest consideration for the dose escalation, rotation, or combination approaches of the current study. This would hopefully avoid potentially prolonging the underlying delirium by addition of benzodiazepines such that, should her delirium prove reversible with further treatment of the UTI, she may have the opportunity for meaningful connection with her family, as well as potential to return home with hospice services.

References

1. Hui D, De La Rosa A, Wilson A, et al. Neuroleptic strategies for terminal agitation in patients with cancer and delirium at an acute palliative care unit: a single-centre, double-blind, parallel-group, randomised trial. *Lancet Oncol.* 2020;21(7):989–998.
2. Breitbart W, Marotta R, Platt MM, et al. A double-blind trial of haloperidol, chlorpromazine, and lorazepam in the treatment of delirium in hospitalized AIDS patients. *Am J Psychiatry.* 1996;153:231–237.
3. Asadollahi S, Heidari K, Hatamabadi H, et al. Efficacy and safety of valproic acid versus haloperidol in patients with acute agitation: results of a randomized, double-blind, parallel-group trial. *Int Clin Psychopharmacol.* 2015;30(3):142–150.
4. Hui D, Frisbee-Hume S, Wilson A, et al. Effect of lorazepam with haloperidol vs haloperidol alone on agitated delirium in patients with advanced cancer receiving palliative care: a randomized clinical trial. *JAMA.* 2017;318(11):1047.
5. Agar MR, Lawlor PG, Quinn S, et al. Efficacy of oral risperidone, haloperidol, or placebo for symptoms of delirium among patients in palliative care: a randomized clinical trial. *JAMA Intern Med.* 2017;177(1):34–42.
6. Girard TD, Exline MC, Carson SS, et al. Haloperidol and ziprasidone for treatment of delirium in critical illness. *N Engl J Med.* 2018;379(26):2506–2516.

19

Methadone Versus Morphine as a First-Line Strong Opioid for Cancer Pain

JENNIFER ALLEN AND BRIAN GANS

> Our results suggest that methadone deserves additional study as a first-line strong opioid for cancer pain.
>
> —BRUERA ET AL.

Research Question: To compare the effectiveness and side effects of methadone and morphine as first-line treatment with opioids for cancer pain

Funding: Supported in part by the Brown Foundation, Houston, Texas, and the Tobacco

Settlement Foundation. One of the authors is supported by a grant from Swiss Cancer Research (BIL grant KFS 950-09-1999).

Year Study Began: 2000

Year Study Published: 2004

Study Location: This double-blind parallel trial was conducted by 7 international palliative care groups (Table 19.1): Argentina, Yugoslavia, Brazil, Columbia, Chile, Australia, and Spain. The Department of Palliative Care and Rehabilitation Medicine at the University of Texas MD Anderson Cancer Center (Houston, Texas) coordinated the study but did not enroll patients.

Table 19.1 DAY 29 OUTCOMES BY INTENTION-TO-TREAT ANALYSIS (N = 49 METHADONE, 54 MORPHINE)

Parameter	No. of Responders	% of Responders	95% CI (%)	*P*
Pain response of 20% or greater				
Methadone	24	49	34–64	.50
Morphine	30	56	41–70	
Composite toxicity worse by 20% or more				
Methadone	33	67	53–82	.94
Morphine	36	67	53–80	
Pain response with stable composite opioid toxicity (obvious benefit)				
Methadone	12	24	11–38	.56
Morphine	16	30	16–43	
Patient-reported global benefit (at least moderate)				
Methadone	26	53	38–68	.41
Morphine	33	61	47–75	

Who Was Studied: Patients with poor control of pain caused by advanced cancer. To be eligible, patients were also required to have normal renal function, life expectancy of at least 4 weeks, and normal cognition as defined by the Mini-Mental State Examination.

Who Was Excluded: Patients were not eligible if they were already receiving strong opioids, radiation therapy for pain control, or antineoplastic therapy expected to produce an analgesic response.

How Many Patients: A total of 103 patients were randomly assigned to treatment (49 in the methadone group and 54 in the morphine group). Of those, only 66 completed the study.

Study Overview: This is a randomized double-blind trial of patients with uncontrolled advanced cancer pain that necessitated the use of strong opioids. The patients were randomized to receive either oral methadone or oral morphine (Figure 19.1).

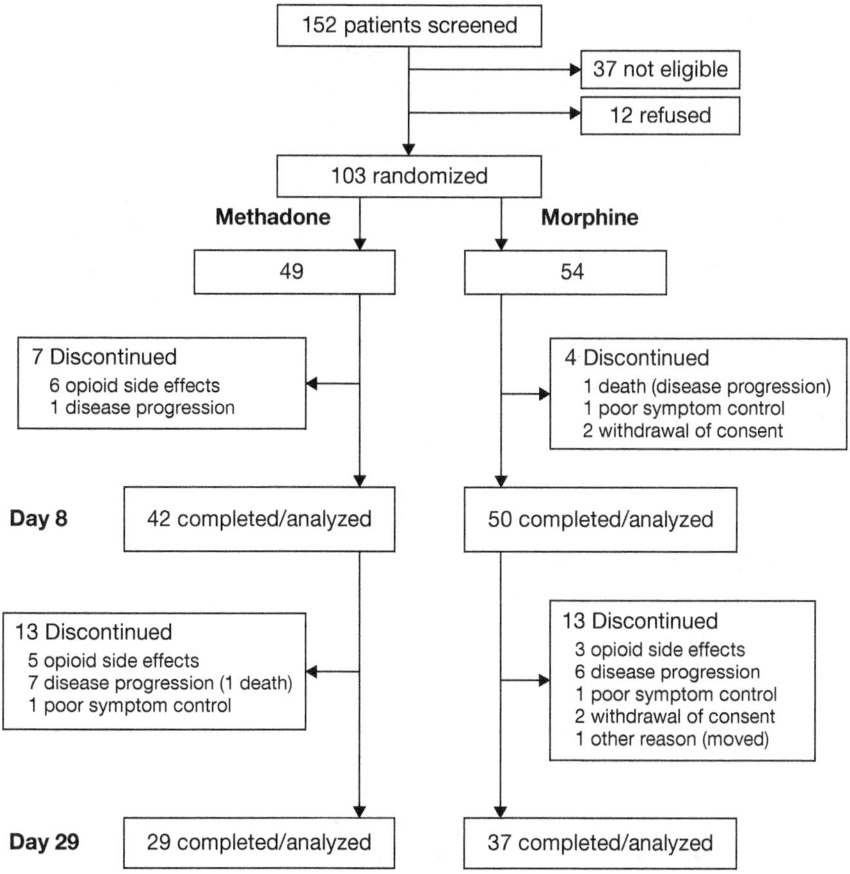

Figure 19.1. Patient flow chart.

Reprinted with permission from Bruera E, Palmer JL, Bosnjak S, et al. Methadone versus morphine as a first-line strong opioid for cancer pain: a randomized, double-blind study. J Clin Oncol. 2004;22(1):185–192.

Study Intervention: For a period of 4 weeks, patients received either methadone 7.5 mg every 12 hours and methadone 5 mg every 4 hours as needed for breakthrough pain or long-acting morphine 15 mg twice daily and immediate-release morphine 5 mg every 4 hours. All nonopioid analgesic drugs were discontinued on admission to the study. The dose of the study drug was increased if patients received more than 2 breakthrough doses a day and was decreased if patients reported sedation.

- For the first 8 days of the study patients were monitored by office visits or phone calls. In-person assessments occurred on days 8, 15, 22, and

29 of treatment. During the first 8 days, assessments of pain (using the Edmonton Staging System for Cancer Pain), sedation, confusion, nausea, and constipation were conducted. For the weekly assessment, cognitive function and global assessment of overall benefit were completed by the patient and the investigator. Patients were removed from the study if pain became intractable, if they developed a new severely painful site, or if they developed a complication from their cancer or cancer treatment.

- On days 14 and 28, the percent increase of morphine or methadone compared to the starting dose was calculated as the opioid escalation index [total dose on day (14 or 28) / total dose on day 1 × 100]

Follow-Up: 28 days

Endpoints:

Primary outcome: Pain intensity at 4 weeks
Secondary outcomes: Medication adverse effects, including sedation, nausea, confusion, and constipation

RESULTS

- The proportion of patients with a 20% or more improvement in pain expression at day 8 was similar for both groups (methadone and morphine).
- The development of sedation in the methadone group showed a distinct pattern, with a more delayed onset of symptom severity than in the morphine group.
- The opioid dose escalation index for the methadone group was a median of 12.5 and 18.3 on days 14 and 28, respectively, versus 16.7 and 16.7 for the morphine group.
- The quantity of bowel movements did not differ at baseline between the 2 groups, nor was there a different number of bowel movements compared with baseline between the groups during the study.

Criticisms and Limitations:

- The higher dropout rate due to sedation in the methadone group may be secondary to the high methadone-to-morphine dose ratio of 0.5 (7.5:15). A lower ratio may have revealed superior efficacy in the methadone group.

- The study did not meet the accrual goal of 100 assessable patients, thus limiting its power. While 103 patients were randomly assigned to treatment, only 66 patients completed the study and were analyzed.
- The use of a 20% reduction in pain intensity is not the standard measure of response, which has usually been defined as a 30% or 50% reduction in pain intensity or a 2-point reduction in a numerical rating scale.[9,10]

Other Relevant Studies and Information: A study from Argentina used a methadone dose titration strategy in opioid-naïve patients with cancer and severe pain.[11] Controlled pain was considered when there was an improvement of ≥ 30% or ≥ 2 points in the numerical pain score. Pain control was achieved in 50/62 patients (81%). Adult Cancer Pain Clinical Practice Guidelines from the National Comprehensive Cancer network indicate that appropriately titrated methadone may have superior tolerability compared to other opioids in patients experiencing chronic pain.

[(Notes BG) I took the above straight from the "Adult Cancer Pain" NCCN guidelines also "Pain-G 15 of 18" as I did below]

Summary and Implications: This double-blind trial found that twice-daily methadone at a total dose of 15 mg/day provided similar analgesia for the treatment of cancer versus sustained-release morphine at a dose of 30 mg/day. There were no differences in toxicity outcomes at 4 weeks, but the dropout rate because of opioid side effects was higher for the methadone group at days 8 and 29. Based on this and other studies, methadone can be considered even as a first-line treatment for cancer-related pain.

CLINICAL CASE: SHOULD WE START METHADONE IN THIS PATIENT?

Case History

A 57-year-old woman with a new diagnosis of metastatic non–small cell lung carcinoma to the spine, bilateral femurs, and pelvis presents to your palliative care outpatient practice. Her primary complaint is pain, which she notes is 9/10, that is diffuse and at times lancinating, limiting her functioning and quality of life. Previous interventions include acetaminophen, tramadol, and ibuprofen with very little effect. The patient has no medical insurance and is very worried about how she is going to pay for her medications. She tells you that it is very important to her to be able to be fully present with her family and to not be "knocked out."

Suggested Answer

The Bruera study found that methadone did not produce superior analgesic efficacy over morphine at a ratio of 0.5. However, the methadone was well tolerated, and more than 75% of patients did have significant improvement in their cancer-related pain. Also, more patients in the methadone group at this ratio noted significant sedation.

In this patient scenario where she is suffering from disabling levels of cancer-related pain that has some neuropathic qualities and she is concerned about how she is going to pay for her medication, it would be very reasonable to start a trial of methadone. To prevent sedation, a starting dose of 2.5 mg every 12 hours could be used. She could continue to use acetaminophen or ibuprofen for breakthrough pain while the methadone is reaching steady state. A decision about titration could be made at 5–7 days after starting the medication.

Methadone would also be a good choice in terms of her concern about cost, as GoodRx quotes prices of methadone as low as $10 for 90 tablets of 10 mg.

References

1. Nicholson AB, Watson GR, Derry S, Wiffen PJ. Methadone for cancer pain. *Cochrane Database Syst Rev.* 2017;(2):CD003971.
2. Mercadante S, Casuccio A, Agnello A, Serretta R, Calderone L, Barresi L. Morphine versus methadone in the pain treatment of advanced-cancer patients followed up at home. *J Clin Oncol.* 1998;16(11):3656–3661.
3. Bruera E, Palmer JL, Bosnjak S, et al. Methadone versus morphine as a first-line strong opioid for cancer pain: a randomized, double-blind study. *J Clin Oncol.* 2004;22(1):185–192.
4. Swarm RA, Paice JA, Anghelescu DL, et al. Adult Cancer Pain, version 3.2019, NCCN Clinical Practice Guidelines in Oncology. *J Natl Compr Canc Netw.* 2019;17(8):977–1007.
5. McPherson ML, Walker KA, Davis MP, et al. Safe and appropriate use of methadone in hospice and palliative care: expert consensus white paper. *J Pain Symptom Manage.* 2019;57(3):635–645.e4.
6. Bruera E, Sweeney C. Methadone use in cancer patients with pain: a review. *J Palliat Med.* 2002;5:127–138.
7. Hanna V, Senderovich H. Methadone in pain management: a systematic review. *J Pain.* Epub 2021; 22(3): 233–245.
8. Mercadante S, Bruera E. Methadone as a first-line opioid in cancer pain management: a systemic review. *J Pain Symptom Manage.* 2018 Mar;55(3):998–1003.
9. Farrar JT, Berlin JA, Strom BL. Clinically important changes in acute pain outcome measures: a validation study. *J Pain Symptom Manage.* 2003;25(5):406–411.
10. Farrar JT. What is clinically meaningful: outcome measures in pain clinical trials. *Clin J Pain.* 2000;16(2 Suppl):S106–S112.
11. Mammana G, Bertolino M, Bruera E, et al. First-line methadone for cancer pain: titration time analysis. *Support Care Cancer.* 2021;29(11):6335–6341.

20

Methylnaltrexone for Opioid-Induced Constipation

ELIZABETH HIGGINS, JOAN CAIN, AND DWIGHT BLAIR

> This trial shows that methylnaltrexone rapidly induces laxation (defecation) without compromising analgesia in patients with advanced illness and [opioid-induced constipation].
>
> —THOMAS ET AL.[1]

Research Question: Does methylnaltrexone improve laxation in patients with opioid-induced constipation (OIC) who have advanced illness, and is it safe?

Funding: The study was supported by Progenics Pharmaceuticals, which also designed the protocol and collected and analyzed the data. A consultant who was paid by the sponsor participated in the writing and editing of the manuscript.

Year Study Began: 2004

Year Study Published: 2008

Study Location: 27 US and Canadian nursing homes, hospice sites, and palliative care centers

Who Was Studied: Patients 18 years of age and older with incurable cancer or other end-stage disease with a life expectancy of 1 month or more and who had received opioids for 2 weeks or more and had OIC (< 3 laxations during preceding week) and were taking laxatives.

Who Was Excluded: Patients who had a positive pregnancy test were excluded. Patients were also excluded if they had constipation that was not primarily caused by opioids. Patients with mechanical obstruction, fecal impaction, or fecal ostomy were also excluded.

How Many Patients: 133

Study Overview: This study was a randomized, double-blind, placebo-controlled phase 3 trial with a subsequent 3-month open-label extension phase (Figure 20.1).

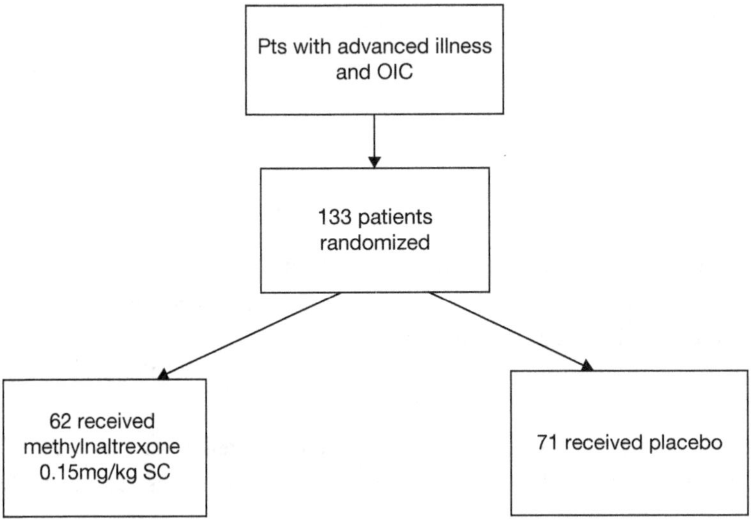

Figure 20.1. Summary of study design.

Study Intervention: Patients who were randomized to get methylnaltrexone received 0.15 mg/kg of the drug subcutaneously on alternating days of the week for 2 weeks. They were allowed to continue their baseline laxative regimen as well as their current rescue laxatives as long as they were not used within 4 hours before or after receiving a dose of the study drug. By day 8, if patients had < 3 rescue-free laxations, the initial volume of the study drug could be doubled to 0.30 mg/kg. Patients on the placebo arm received an equivalent volume of saline.

Follow-Up: 3 months

Endpoints: Primary outcomes were laxation within 4 hours after the first dose of the study drug and laxation within 4 hours after 2 or more of the first 4 doses. Secondary outcomes were consistency and difficulty of bowel movements and adverse events (National Cancer Center Institute's Common Toxicity Criteria version 2.0).

RESULTS

- Please see summary of findings in Table 20.1.
- Patients in the methylnaltrexone group were more likely to have laxation within 4 hours after the study group than patients in the placebo group.
- Patients who received methylnaltrexone were more likely to have laxation without the use of a rescue laxative after 2 or more of the first 4 doses compared to patients in the placebo group.
- Treatment with methylnaltrexone did not appear to affect patients' perceptions of pain or precipitate opioid withdrawal.
- Patients in the methylnaltrexone groups suffered similar adverse effects compared to patients in the placebo group.
- Serious adverse events that were thought to be due to the study drug were muscle spasm (1 patient) and abdominal pain (1 patient).

Table 20.1 SUMMARY OF FINDINGS

Outcome	**Methylnaltrexone Group (*n* = 62)**	**Placebo Group (*n* = 71)**	***P* Value**
Laxation within 4 hours (after first dose)	30	11	.001
Laxation within 4 hours (after first 4 doses)	32	6	.001
Rescue-free laxation within 4 hours in 13-day period	24	4	.001
Any adverse event	57	51	NS
Abdominal pain	9	11	NS
Flatulence	5	8	NS

Criticisms and Limitations:

- The clinical response rate with methylnaltrexone was greater than with the placebo, but overall low.
- Approximately 14% of patients dropped out of the study by the end of 7 days (the duration of primary outcome measurement), but 1 in 4 dropped out by 13 days (the end of the study period), raising the possibility of attrition bias.

- The population studied was not racially diverse, as 94% of subjects were White. This could potentially limit generalizability.

Other Relevant Studies and Information:

- Brenner et al.[2] found that both naloxegol and polyethylene glycol (PEG) 3350 were effective options for OIC, with similar proportions of patients reporting a strong preference for either treatment.
- Naldemedine was approved by the Food and Drug Administration based on 2 industry-sponsored, large multinational, phase 3, randomized, double-blind, placebo-controlled clinical trials.[3] Compared to the placebo, naldemedine resulted in statistically more people having spontaneous bowel movements (SBMs), although absolute efficacy rates were low. Compared to the placebo, about 14%–22% of patients had at least 3 SBMs per week or an increase of at least 1 SBM above baseline, translating into needing to treat about 5–7 patients for one to meet these endpoints. The overall efficacy is similar to that found for methylnaltrexone.
- An observational study by Dols et al.[4] suggested efficacy of naloxegol on symptoms and quality of life related to OIC in patients with cancer.
- In a meta-analysis of 8 randomized trials comparing methylnaltrexone to placebo, there was a significantly increased rate of rescue-free bowel movements within 4 hours with the first dose of methylnaltrexone relative to placebo (relative risk [RR] 3.74), rescue-free bowel movements within 24 hours (RR 1.98), and rescue-free bowel movements > 3 times weekly (RR 1.33).[8] There was an overall reduction in the need for rescue laxatives (RR 0.73). The only adverse effect that was greater than placebo was abdominal pain (RR 2.3).
- The American Gastroenterological Association has issued a clinical guideline on OIC, incorporating several trials on peripherally acting μ-receptor opioid receptor antagonists (PAMORAs). The guidelines recommend traditional laxatives (osmotic laxatives, lubricants, and stimulants) as first-line therapy, with PAMORAs (naldemedine, naloxegol, and methylnaltrexone) as next-line treatment for "laxative-refractory OIC," with naldemedine having the strongest recommendation in this class.[5]

Summary and Implications: This multicenter, randomized, double-blind, placebo-controlled trial was the first published study of a selective peripherally acting opioid receptor blocker. It suggested that methylnaltrexone is a safe treatment for OIC. However, due to low overall efficacy as well as high cost, methylnaltrexone is generally reserved for patients with persistent symptoms despite aggressive use of traditional bowel regimens.

CLINICAL CASE: WHO SOULD RECEIVE METHYLNALTREXONE FOR OPIOID-INDUCED CONSTIPATION

Case History

A 55-year-old female with diagnosed stage IV breast cancer has been requiring opioids over the past month for chest and back pain. She reports taking 150 opioid morphine equivalents (OME) per day with no bowel movement for the past 4 days even with the use of PEG 3350 (MiraLAX) daily and senna (2 pills) twice per day for 3 days. She reports no history of constipation until starting opioids. She reports flatulence without laxation during this timeframe.

Should this patient receive methylnaltrexone?

Suggested Answer

The Thomas et al. manuscript describes the double-blind placebo-controlled study of patients randomized to receive methylnaltrexone (at a dose of 0.15 mg/kg) or equal volume of a placebo administered subcutaneously on alternate days for 2 weeks. Patients were allowed to continue a baseline laxative regimen throughout the study and take rescue laxatives as needed. Compared to the placebo, the study found that 33% of the patients had rescue-free laxation without changes in pain scores or evidence of withdrawal.

The patient in this scenario would qualify for the use of methylnaltrexone for her OIC. She is in need of the opioids for the pain related to her stage IV breast cancer and her constipation is caused by the opioid use, as she shows no signs/symptoms of other primary causes.

An additional positive outcome of the study, which will benefit the patient in this case, is that no changes in pain score or symptoms of opioid withdrawal were noted as the medication does not affect the central nervous system in humans. She should receive the methylnaltrexone at the standard dose of 0.15 mg/kg. She may continue with her baseline regimen as noted above and should hold off on taking any rescue laxative (suppository or enema) 4 hours before or after the administration of methylnaltrexone.

References

1. Thomas J, Karver S, Cooney GA, et al. Methylnaltrexone for opioid-induced constipation in advanced illness. http://dx.doi.org/10.1056/NEJMoa0707377. doi:10.1056/NEJMoa0707377
2. Brenner DM, Hu Y, Datto C, Creanga D, Camilleri M. A randomized, multicenter, prospective, crossover, open-label study of factors associated with patient preferences for naloxegol or PEG 3350 for opioid-induced constipation. *Am J Gastroenterol.* 2019;114(6):954–963. doi:10.14309/ajg.0000000000000229.
3. Hale M, Wild J, Reddy J, Yamada T, Arjona Ferreira JC. Naldemedine versus placebo for opioid-induced constipation (COMPOSE-1 and COMPOSE-2): two multicentre, phase 3, double-blind, randomised, parallel-group trials. *Lancet Gastroenterol Hepatol.* 2017;2(8):555–564. doi:10.1016/S2468-1253(17)30105-X.
4. Dols MC, Zambrano CB, Gutiérrez LC, et al. Efficacy of naloxegol on symptoms and quality of life related to opioid-induced constipation in patients with cancer: a 3-month follow-up analysis. *BMJ Support Palliat Care.* 2021;11(1):25–31. doi:10.1136/bmjspcare-2020-002249.
5. Crockett SD. American Gastroenterological Association Institute guideline on the medical management of opioid-induced constipation. 2019;156(1):9.
6. Nalamachu SR, Pergolizzi J, Taylor R Jr, et al. Efficacy and tolerability of subcutaneous methylnaltrexone in patients with advanced illness and opioid-induced constipation: a responder analysis of 2 randomized, placebo-controlled trials. *Pain Pract.* 2015;15(6):564–571.
7. Chamberlain BH, Rhiner M, Slatkin NE, Stambler N, Israel RJ. Subcutaneous methylnaltrexone for treatment of opioid-induced constipation in cancer versus noncancer patients: an analysis of efficacy and safety variables from two studies. *J Pain Res.* 2021;14:2687–2697.
8. Zhang YY, Zhou R, Gu WJ. Efficacy and safety of methylnaltrexone for the treatment of opioid-induced constipation: a meta-analysis of randomized controlled trials. *Pain Ther.* 2021;10(1):165–179.
9. Liao SS, Slatkin NE, Stambler N. The influence of age on central effects of methylnaltrexone in patients with opioid-induced constipation. *Drugs Aging.* 2021;38(6):503–511.
10. Lin AJ, Costandi AJ, Kim E, et al. Improved bowel function with oral methylnaltrexone following posterior spinal fusion for adolescent idiopathic scoliosis. *J Pediatr Orthop.* 2021.
11. Chamie K, Golla V, Lenis AT, Lec PM, Rahman S, Viscusi ER. Peripherally acting mu-opioid receptor antagonists in the management of postoperative ileus: a clinical review. *J Gastrointest Surg.* 2021;25(1):293–302.
12. Beavers J, Orton L, Atchison L, et al. The efficacy and safety of methylnaltrexone for the treatment of postoperative ileus. *Am Surg.* 2021:31348211048825.
13. Yu CS, Chun HK, Stambler N, et al. Safety and efficacy of methylnaltrexone in shortening the duration of postoperative ileus following segmental colectomy: results of two randomized, placebo-controlled phase 3 trials. *Dis Colon Rectum.* 2011;54(5):570–578.

14. Gifford CS, McGahan BG, Miracle SD, et al. Perioperative subcutaneous methylnaltrexone does not enhance gastrointestinal recovery after posterior short-segment spinal arthrodesis surgery: a randomized controlled trial. *Spine J.* 2021.
15. Franke AJ, Iqbal A, Starr JS, Nair RM, George TJ Jr. Management of malignant bowel obstruction associated with GI cancers. *J Oncol Pract.* 2017;13(7):426–434.
16. Liu X, Yang J, Yang C, et al. Morphine promotes the malignant biological behavior of non-small cell lung cancer cells through the MOR/Src/mTOR pathway. *Cancer Cell Int.* 2021;21(1):622.
17. Janku F, Johnson LK, Karp DD, Atkins JT, Singleton PA, Moss J. Treatment with methylnaltrexone is associated with increased survival in patients with advanced cancer. *Ann Oncol.* 2018;29(4):1076.

21

Lorazepam and Haloperidol Versus Haloperidol Monotherapy for the Treatment of Agitated Delirium

KATHERINE M. JUBA AND JEFFERSON S. SVENGSOUK

> In this preliminary trial of hospitalized patients with agitated delirium in the setting of advanced cancer, the addition of lorazepam to haloperidol compared with haloperidol alone resulted in a significantly greater reduction in agitation at 8 hours.
>
> —Hui et al.[1]

Research Question: Does the combination of lorazepam and haloperidol provide superior treatment of agitation compared to haloperidol alone in patients with advanced cancer and delirium?

Funding: National Cancer Institute, National Institutes of Health, American Cancer Society, Andrew Sabin Family Foundation

Year Study Began: 2014

Year Study Published: 2017

Study Location: MD Anderson Cancer Center, Houston, Texas

Who Was Studied: Adults with advanced cancer in the inpatient palliative care unit who had a diagnosis of delirium and Richmond Agitation-Sedation Scale

(RASS) score ≥ 2 (later revised to ≥ 1) in the previous 24 hours despite use of scheduled haloperidol (1–8 mg/day).

Who Was Excluded: Patients with dementia, use of scheduled benzodiazepines or chlorpromazine within previous 48 hours, uncontrolled seizures, contraindications to benzodiazepines and/or neuroleptics, or concurrent heart failure exacerbation.

How Many Patients: 90 patients were randomized and 52 patients completed the study.

Study Overview: This study was a randomized, double-blind, placebo-controlled, parallel-group trial. Palliative care patients with advanced cancer and hyperactive or mixed delirium were randomized in a 1:1 ratio to receive a single dose of 3 mg intravenous (IV) lorazepam or placebo for the treatment of agitation in addition to scheduled and as-needed IV haloperidol (Figure 20.1).

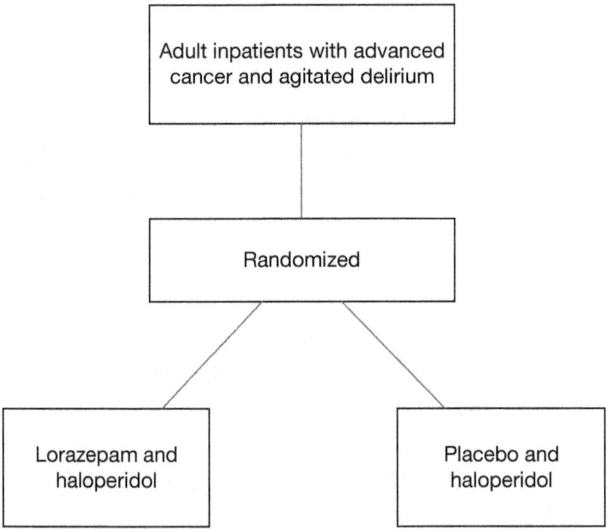

Figure 21.1. Study overview.

Study Intervention: Patients in the lorazepam and placebo arms received haloperidol 2 mg IV every 4 hours and haloperidol 2 mg IV every 1 hour as needed for agitation upon enrollment. Each patient had their RASS[2] score monitored every 2 hours until they had a score of ≥ 2, later changed to ≥ 1, and required administration of an as-needed haloperidol dose. Patients then received the study medication as either a single dose of 3 mg IV lorazepam or placebo, and 2 mg IV haloperidol once. RASS scores were obtained at baseline and 0.5, 1, 1.5, 2, 3, 4, 5, 6, 7, and 8 hours.

Follow-Up: Duration of each patient's stay in the inpatient palliative unit (mean of 6 days)

Endpoints: Primary endpoints: Change in and severity of agitation (RASS) at 8 hours. Secondary endpoints: Severity of delirium (Memorial Delirium Assessment Scale [MDAS]); use of as-needed antipsychotic medications; study medication–related adverse effects (Udvalg for Kliniske Undersoøgelser [UKU]); length of stay; overall survival; patient symptom burden (Edmonton Symptom Assessment Scale [ESAS]).

RESULTS

- The lorazepam + haloperidol group experienced a greater reduction in agitation and a deeper state of sedation at 8 hours compared with the placebo + haloperidol group (Table 21.1).
- The lorazepam + haloperidol group also had a greater reduction in agitation at 30 minutes of treatment compared with haloperidol alone. Both groups experienced reductions in agitation within 30 minutes that was maintained at 8 hours (Table 21.1).
- In the lorazepam + haloperidol group there was a smaller proportion of patients with hyperactivity and a larger proportion with sedation compared with the placebo + haloperidol group.
- The researchers noted that individual patients' agitation scores showed rapid reductions when treated with lorazepam + haloperidol and variable response when treated with placebo + haloperidol.
- The lorazepam + haloperidol group required lower doses and fewer numbers of rescue neuroleptics and lower total neuroleptics (Table 21.1).
- The lorazepam + haloperidol group experienced greater drowsiness as assessed by caregivers and appeared to be in greater comfort as assessed by both caregivers and nurses (Table 21.1).
- There were otherwise no significant differences between groups in ESAS symptoms, severity of delirium, delirium recall, communication capacity, respiratory rate, discharge outcomes, or overall survival.
- The most common adverse effects seen in both groups were hypokinesia and akathisia.

Table 21.1 SUMMARY OF KEY FINDINGS

	Lorazepam + Haloperidol	Placebo + Haloperidol	*P* Value
RASS score change by 8 hours	−4.1 (−4.8 to −3.4)	−2.3 (−2.9 to −1.6)	< .01
RASS score at 8 hours	−2.5 (−3.2 to −1.9)	−0.7 (−1.3 to −0.1)	< .01
RASS score change by 30 minutes	−3.6 (−4.3 to −2.9)	−1.6 (−2.2 to −1.0)	< .01
Rescue neuroleptic use within 8 hours, HEDD, median	2.0 (2.0–2.0)	4.0 (2.0–5.0)	.009
Rescue neuroleptic use within 8 hours, No. of doses, median	1.0 (1.0–1.0)	2.0 (1.0–2.0)	.008
Overall survival, median hours	68 (49–130)	73 (38–106)	.56
Patients with improvement in comfort on day 1, caregiver assessment	16 (84%)	7 (37%)	.007
Patients with improvement in comfort on day 1, nurse assessment	17 (77%)	6 (30%)	.005

Abbreviations: HEDD, haloperidol equivalent daily dose; RASS, Richmond Agitation-Sedation Scale.

Criticisms and Limitations:

- Study findings are not generalizable to patients with hypoactive delirium, noncancer diagnosis, early-stage cancer, and those cared for outside of an inpatient palliative care setting.
- Since only a single dose of lorazepam 3 mg was used, these findings may not apply to lorazepam given at different doses or according to alternative dosing schedules.

Other Relevant Studies and Information:

- Breitbart et al. conducted a double-blind, randomized controlled trial comparing the efficacy and adverse effects of haloperidol, chlorpromazine, and lorazepam in hospitalized patients with acquired immunodeficiency syndrome and delirium.[3] Use of haloperidol or chlorpromazine resulted in improved delirium symptoms. Patients who received lorazepam had treatment-limiting adverse effects without an improvement in their delirium symptoms.
- Four randomized controlled trials assessing the effectiveness of pharmacotherapy in patients with advanced illness and delirium were included in a 2020 Cochrane Database Review.[4] The trials by Hui et al. and

Breitbart et al. were included among the studies.[1,3] The authors concluded that low-quality evidence suggests that these medications may increase delirium symptoms in patients with mild to moderate delirium and advanced illness.

Summary and Implications: This preliminary study of the treatment of persistent agitated delirium in patients with advanced cancer suggests that the addition of 3 mg IV lorazepam to IV haloperidol versus haloperidol alone resulted in a significantly greater reduction in agitation at 30 minutes and at 8 hours with a lower risk of hyperactivity. Lorazepam treatment was associated with a higher rate of caretaker-reported sedation. Further research is needed to confirm these findings and determine the optimal dose and schedule.

CLINICAL CASE: WHAT PATIENT IS APPROPRIATE TO RECEIVE IV LORAZEPAM IN ADDITION TO HALOPERIDOL FOR AGITATED DELIRIUM?

Case History

The patient is a 66-year-old male in the inpatient palliative care unit with metastatic pancreatic cancer and a life expectancy of days to weeks. The patient has become increasingly agitated over the past day despite use of scheduled and rescue IV haloperidol, nonpharmacologic interventions, aggressive symptom management, and workup for potentially reversible etiologies of delirium. He repeatedly attempts to climb out of bed and strikes the nurses and patient care technicians when they are providing care (RASS: +2 to +3). The patient's family and interdisciplinary team are concerned about the patient's level of distress and safety.

Is this patient appropriate to receive a dose of IV lorazepam in addition to his current haloperidol regimen?

Suggested Answer

The patient described in the case fits the enrollment criteria in the study by Hui et al. and is appropriate to receive a dose of IV lorazepam.[1] He continues to experience agitated delirium (RASS: +2 to +3) with concurrent use of an antipsychotic regimen, nonpharmacologic treatments, assessment for treatable causes of delirium, and symptom management. The benefit of decreased patient agitation and optimizing the safety of the patient and staff with the use of a dose of lorazepam outweighs the risk of sedation.

References

1. Hui D, Frisbee-Hume S, Wilson A, et al. Effect of lorazepam with haloperidol vs haloperidol alone on agitated delirium in patients with advanced cancer receiving palliative care: a randomized clinical trial. *JAMA*. 2017 Sept 19;318(11):1047–1056.
2. Sessler CN, Gosnell MS, Grap MJ, et al. The Richmond Agitation-Sedation Scale: validity and reliability in adult intensive care unit patients. *Am J Respir Crit Care Med*. 2002 Nov 15;166(10):1338–1344.
3. Breitbart W, Marotta R, Platt MM, et al. A double-blind trial of haloperidol, chlorpromazine, and lorazepam in the treatment of delirium in hospitalized AIDS patients. *Am J Psychiatry*. 1996 Feb 15;3(2):231–237.
4. Finucane AM, Jones L, Leurent B, Sampson EL, Stone P, Tookman A, Candy B. Drug therapy for delirium in terminally ill adults. *Cochrane Database of Syst Rev*. 2020;(1):CD004770.

22

Treatment of Cancer-Related Fatigue With Dexamethasone

LYDIA MIS AND ARIF KAMAL

> Our data suggest that dexamethasone acts rapidly in relieving cancer-related fatigue. This rapid response is of interest because patients with advanced cancer usually have moderate to severe levels of fatigue at the time of initial assessment by a palliative care team.
>
> —YENNURAJALINGAM ET AL.[1]

Research Question: Does the short-term use of dexamethasone in patients with advanced cancer improve cancer-related fatigue (CRF) and other disease-related symptoms?

Funding: Mentored Research Scholar Grant No. MRSG-07-001-01-CCE01 from the American Cancer Society; Clinical Trial Information: NCT009489307

Year Study Began: 2006

Year Study Published: 2013

Study Locations: MD Anderson Cancer Center and Lyndon B. Johnson General Hospital, Houston, Texas; Four Seasons Hospice, Flat Rock, North Carolina

Who Was Studied: Patients aged 18 or older with advanced cancer and 3 or more symptoms during the previous 24 hours (e.g., pain, fatigue, chronic nausea and anorexia/cachexia, sleep problems, depression, or poor appetite) of moderate to severe intensity.

Who Was Excluded: Patients currently receiving corticosteroid therapy and those with impaired cognition, active infection, anemia, neutropenia, history of diabetes or human immunodeficiency virus infection, surgery within 2 weeks prior to enrollment in the study, and life expectancy < 4 weeks.

How Many Patients: 132

Study Overview: See Figure 22.1.

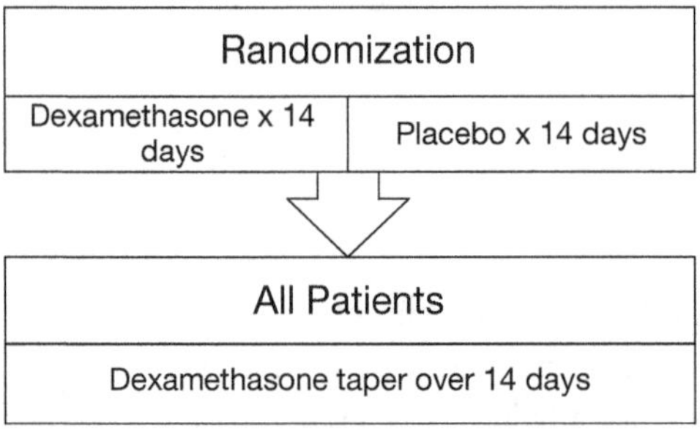

Figure 22.1. Summary of study design.

Study Intervention: Patients were randomized to dexamethasone 4 mg orally or placebo twice daily (with food). On day 15, all patients began a 2-week taper, receiving dexamethasone 4 mg orally twice daily for 7 days followed by 2 mg orally twice daily for 7 days (not included in the published study). Patients completed a validated quality-of-life instrument on days 8 and 15 for the assessment of CRF and symptom-specific questionnaires to measure anorexia/cachexia, depression and anxiety, and additional symptoms commonly seen in cancer patients (pain, fatigue, nausea, drowsiness, dyspnea, and feeling of well-being). If the patient was able to return to the clinic, bloodwork to assess protein levels and anemia was drawn. Adverse events were assessed in accordance with the National Cancer Institute Common Toxicity Criteria (version 3.0).

Follow-Up: Patients were evaluated at days 8 and day 15 (end of study) and followed for up to 43 days for safety and toxicity assessments.

Endpoints: Primary outcome was change in CRF using the Functional Assessment of Chronic Illness Therapy-Fatigue (FACIT-F) subscale from baseline to day 15 in patients randomized to dexamethasone or placebo. Secondary outcomes included changes in the Hospital Anxiety and Depression Scale (HADS), Functional Assessment of Cancer Therapy-Anorexia-Cachexia (FAACT) scale, and Edmonton Symptom Assessment Scale (ESAS).

RESULTS

- There were no differences in baseline characteristics between the dexamethasone and placebo groups except that the dexamethasone group had more females.
- Moderate to severe fatigue was present at baseline in 58 (93.5%) of 62 patients randomized to dexamethasone and 56 (97%) of 58 patients randomized to placebo.
- The FACIT-F total (quality-of-life) score is the sum of physical, social, emotional, and functional distress scores plus the fatigue subscore. At days 8 and 15, as shown in Table 22.1, dexamethasone improved the FACIT-F and physical distress subscales, and at day 15, there was improvement in the FACIT-F total score.

Table 22.1 SIGNIFICANT CHANGES IN SYMPTOM SCORES AT DAY 8 AND DAY 15

	Day 8			Day 15		
	Dexamethasone *N* = 43	Placebo *N* = 41	***P***	Dexamethasone *N* = 43	Placebo *N* = 41	***P***
FACIT-F subscale	8.01	3.06	.005	9	3.1	.008
FACIT physical	4.37	1.34	.007	5.25	1.32	.002
FACIT-F total score	13.37	7.5	NS	18.16	7.87	.030
ESAS pain	−1.77	−0.13	.014	−1.35	−0.17	NS
ESAS physical	-9.10	-3.42	.009	−10.86	−4.78	.013
FAACT	4.78	1.49	NS	6.82	1.95	.013
HADS depression	−1.23	−0.43	NS	−1.39	−0.31	NS

Abbreviations: ESAS, Edmonton Symptom Assessment Scale; FAACT, Functional Assessment of Cancer Therapy-Anorexia-Cachexia; FACIT-F, Functional Assessment of Chronic Illness Therapy-Fatigue; HADS, Hospital Anxiety Depression Scale; NS, no significant improvement.

- Dexamethasone improved the ESAS for pain only at day 8 but improved the physical distress scores at both day 8 and day 15, as shown in Table 22.1.
- There was no difference between dexamethasone and placebo as measured by the ESAS scores for the following: fatigue, nausea, depression, anxiety, drowsiness, shortness of breath, appetite, sleep, feeling of well-being, psychological distress, and symptom distress.
- Dexamethasone did not improve depression or anxiety as measured by the HADS at either 8 or 15 days, as shown in Table 22.1.
- Dexamethasone improved the FAACT score only at day 15, as shown in Table 22.1.

Criticisms and Limitations: The major criticism of this trial was the small sample size and a dropout rate of approximately 28%, which reduced the power to potentially detect a difference in certain outcomes. Limitations of this study include the short study period of 15 days and allocation bias in that more patients randomized to placebo were reporting moderate to severe fatigue at baseline than patients randomized to dexamethasone.

Other Relevant Studies and Information:

- The short-term use of methylprednisolone (MP) in patients with advanced cancer has shown variable effects on cancer-related symptoms.[2–4]
- Bruera and colleagues showed that MP 32 mg orally daily (16 mg twice daily) for 20 days improved pain, depression, appetite, and food consumption, whereas anxiety and performance status did not show improvement.[2] Change in fatigue was not an endpoint of this study.
- Paulsen and colleagues did not show an improvement in pain after MP 32 mg daily for 7 days; however, their analysis did show improvements in fatigue, appetite loss, and patient satisfaction.[3] A similar trend in improved quality of life was seen in a study by Eguchi and colleagues; however, the sample size was too small to show a similar trend in fatigue reduction due to inadequate patient recruitment.[4]

Summary and Implications: Dexamethasone is widely used in patients with advanced and terminal cancer to alleviate fatigue, pain, anorexia, and cachexia and to improve appetite and well-being despite the lack of randomized, double-blinded, controlled trials that demonstrate long-term benefit. This short-term randomized, double-blinded, controlled trial showed benefits of dexamethasone with respect to quality of life at 8 and 15 days but failed to show benefit in pain past 8 days. There were also favorable effects on appetite and cachexia after 15 days. More research is needed to better assess the long-term benefits and risks.

CLINICAL CASE: DEXAMETHASONE FOR FATIGUE IN CANCER PATIENT WITH ADVANCED DISEASE

Case History

A 74-year-old woman with metastatic non–small cell lung cancer (received 3 of 4 planned cycles of chemotherapy) was admitted for extreme fatigue and inability to care for herself. She had a cough and a new oxygen requirement. Chest x-ray showed no consolidation suggestive of pneumonia, and computed tomography scan was negative for pulmonary embolism but revealed progressive disease. The patient is considering further therapy with pembrolizumab as an alternative to further chemotherapy. The team does not want to start methylphenidate or modafinil for fatigue based on history of rate-controlled atrial fibrillation on metoprolol. The palliative care team recommends dexamethasone 4 mg by mouth twice daily for fatigue, but the team is unclear how long to continue treatment with this dose.

Suggested Answer

The Yennurajalingam trial showed that dexamethasone was effective for the treatment of fatigue given for 2 weeks at 4 mg by mouth twice daily. The original clinical trial schema described a 2-week taper off dexamethasone after the initial 2 weeks. It is important to note that patients should not be continued long term on this dose of dexamethasone as it can lead to corticosteroid-induced side effects. Additionally, it is recommended that patients be on no more than 10 mg of prednisone equivalents per day prior to the (re)start of checkpoint inhibitors such as pembrolizumab as doses higher than 10 mg daily may be associated with poorer outcomes.

References

1. Yennurajalingam S, Frisbee-Hume S, Palmer JL, et al. Reduction of cancer-related fatigue with dexamethasone: a double-blind, randomized, placebo-controlled trial in patients with advanced cancer. *J Clin Oncol.* 2013;31(25):3076–3082. doi:10.1200/JCO.2012.44.4661.
2. Bruera E, Roca E, Cedaro L, et al. Action of oral methylprednisolone in terminal cancer patients: a prospective randomized double-blind study. *Can Treat Rep.* 1985;69(7–8):751–754.

3. Paulsen O, Klepstad P, Rosland JH, et al. Efficacy of methylprednisolone on pain, fatigue, and appetite loss in patients with advanced cancer using opioids: a randomized, placebo-controlled, double-blind study. *J Clin Oncol.* 2014;32(29):3221–3228. doi:10.1200/JCO.2013.54.3926.
4. Eguchi K, Honda M, Kataoka T, et al. Efficacy of corticosteroids for cancer-related fatigue: a pilot randomized placebo-controlled trial of advanced cancer patients. *Palliat Support Care.* 2016;13:1301–1308. doi:10.1017/S1478951514001254.

23

Octreotide in Malignant Bowel Obstruction

NATALIE M. LATUGA, DEBRA L. LUCZKIEWICZ,
AND MELLAR P. DAVIS

> This study does not support the routine use of octreotide in addition to ranitidine and dexamethasone for the symptomatic treatment of inoperable malignant bowel obstruction.
>
> —CURROW ET AL.[1]

Research Question: What is the net effect of adding octreotide to standardized therapies in the setting of inoperable malignant bowel obstruction on the number of days free of vomiting?

Funding: Australian Government's Department of Health under the National Palliative Care Strategy

Year Study Began: 2008

Year Study Published: 2015

Study Location: 12 palliative care service networks across Australia

Who Was Studied: Adults with advanced cancer presenting with vomiting secondary to bowel obstruction where surgery or anticancer therapies were not immediately indicated.

Who Was Excluded: Patients with poor functional status, severe renal impairment (creatinine clearance < 10 mL/min), severe liver cirrhosis, or preexisting venting gastrostomy or jejunostomy.

How Many Patients: 87

Study Overview: This is a double-blind, placebo-controlled, randomized study in which 87 patients with advanced cancer were randomized to receive either octreotide 600 mcg per 24 hours infused or placebo if they presented with bowel obstruction and vomiting. Patients were randomized in blocks of 4 by site in a 1:1 ratio (Figure 23.1).

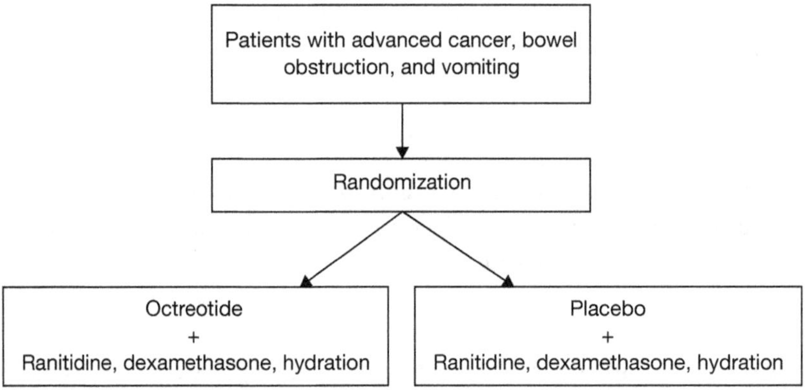

Figure 23.1. Summary of study design.

Study Intervention: All patients received standardized supportive therapy of ranitidine, dexamethasone, and hydration. "As needed" symptom management medications were also standardized to include parenteral opioids for pain, hyoscine butylbromide for colicky pain, and haloperidol for nausea. 5-HT_3 antagonists could be considered for use. Metoclopramide was only allowed if part of a local protocol for the site and under close supervision of the site investigator.

In addition to this treatment, patients in the octreotide arm received a subcutaneous infusion of octreotide 600 mcg per 24 hours. Bowel obstructions were diagnosed clinically by 2 independent medical practitioners. Patients were asked to complete a quality-of-life measure (Global Impression of Change [GIC]) and report episodes of vomiting.

Follow-up: 72 hours

Endpoints: Primary endpoint: Number of days free of vomiting measured at 72 hours. Secondary endpoints: GIC, number of episodes of vomiting, survival, nausea, the Brief Pain Inventory (BPI), functional status, "as needed" symptom control medication use, treatment failure, toxicity, and clinical/demographic factors that predict response.

RESULTS

- For the primary endpoint, there was no statistically significant difference between groups for number of days free of vomiting, total number of people free of vomiting for all 72 hours, and mean number of days free of vomiting (Table 23.1).
- Between baseline and day 1, both groups showed a significant drop in the mean unadjusted number of vomiting episodes, with no significant difference over the course of the study. However, the octreotide group showed a statistically significant reduced incidence of vomiting over the duration of the study following an adjusted multivariate regression analysis.
- Both groups were likely to report a positive daily change in outlook (GIC), but there was no difference between groups.
- There was no difference between groups for secondary outcomes of nausea, pain, survival, treatment failure, or toxicity. No clinical/demographic features were identified that predicted response.
- The octreotide group had better control of vomiting ($P = .019$) but was more likely to be administered hyoscine butylbromide for colicky pain.

Table 23.1 SUMMARY OF STUDY'S KEY FINDINGS

Primary Outcomes	**Octreotide Group**	**Placebo Group**	***P* Value**
Number of days free of vomiting			.41
0 days	11	13	
1 day	9	12	
2 days	12	11	
3 days	17	14	
Total number of people free of vomiting for all 72 hours	17	14	.67
Mean (SD) number of days free of vomiting in each group	1.87 (1.10)	1.69 (1.15)	.47

Primary Outcomes	Octreotide Group	Placebo Group	P Value
Secondary Outcomes[a]			
Adjusted incidence of vomiting	IRR = 0.4; 95% CI: 0.19–0.86		.019
GIC > 0	74%	84%	> .75
Presence of nausea	Postintervention values not reported		.37
Intensity of nausea	Postintervention values not reported		> .36
BPI score, mean	5.7	5.7	Not reported
Baseline change	−0.25	−0.25	
Survival	HR = 1.24; 95% CI: 0.81–1.92		.33
"As needed" medication use	OR = 3.24; 95% CI: 1.06–9.96		.041
Hyoscine butylbromide			

Abbreviations: BPI, Brief Pain Inventory; GIC, Global Impression of Change; HR, hazard ratio; IRR, incidence rate ratio; OR, odds ratio; SD; standard deviation.
[a] Outcomes reported as ratios are octreotide:placebo.

Criticisms and Limitations:

- Study duration was 72 hours, which may not have been enough time to see effects.
- The octreotide dose was not titrated, which would be more typical of clinical practice.
- Ranitidine is known to increase the endogenous release of somatostatin,[2–5] which may have masked the response to octreotide.

Other Relevant Studies and Information:

- These results are similar to those of 2 other randomized, double-blind controlled trials. Mariani et al.[6] evaluated lanreotide versus placebo in 80 patients and found no difference in the percentage of responders. Laval et al.[7] evaluated octreotide immediate release and octreotide LAR in 64 patients, but the study was underpowered.
- Several smaller studies comparing octreotide to anticholinergics show benefit.[8–10]
- There are no long-term studies that provide evidence of sustained benefits to ranitidine or octreotide.
- Obita et al.[11] conducted a systematic review of somatostatin analogues compared to placebo or other agents. Seven trials met the inclusion criteria. The Currow study had the lowest risk of bias. Four randomized trials found that somatostatins were more effective than hyoscine butylbromide in reducing vomiting.

- Despite a low level of evidence and acknowledgment of this negative trial, somatostatin analogues are recommended in the National Comprehensive Cancer Network (NCCN) Palliative Care Version 1.2021 guidelines[12] and the 2016 Multinational Association of Supportive Care in Cancer/European Society of Medical Oncology (MASCC/ESMO) consensus recommendations for the management of nausea and vomiting in advanced cancer.[13]
- The 2021 MASCC guideline update for medical management of malignant bowel obstruction indicates that octreotide should be considered first-line treatment based on systematic review and the possibility that the negative results of this trial may be related to the use of ranitidine in both study arms.[14]

Summary and Implications: This double-blind, randomized, placebo-controlled trial involving patients with malignant bowel obstruction did not demonstrate benefit of adding octreotide to standardized supportive therapy of ranitidine, dexamethasone, and hydration and showed that it may have increased symptom burden as shown by the increased need for hyoscine butylbromide in the octreotide arm. Certain subpopulations may benefit, although which and how much is not yet clear. These findings argue against routine use of octreotide in addition to ranitidine and dexamethasone.

CLINICAL CASE: SHOULD OCTREOTIDE BE USED FOR MALIGNANT BOWEL OBSTRUCTION?

Case History

A 64-year-old female with stage IV ovarian cancer and peritoneal carcinomatosis presents to the hospice inpatient unit with intractable vomiting lasting 3 days. She complains of severe abdominal cramping as well. Complete bowel obstruction is confirmed radiographically. Should this patient be started on octreotide?

Suggested Answer

The results of the study by Currow et al. did not demonstrate benefit when adding octreotide to a regimen of dexamethasone, ranitidine, and hydration. Because of the potential to worsen colicky pain and the uncertain benefit for the reduction of vomiting episodes, one could argue to avoid octreotide for this patient and add supportive measures such as anticholinergics/antiemetics/

opioids as needed. However, current NCCN and MASCC/ESMO guidelines continue to advocate for the early use of octreotide to manage vomiting, particularly in the setting of complete bowel obstruction, where maintenance of gut function is not possible. If the decision was made to initiate octreotide for this patient, she would need to be closely monitored for benefits, such as reduced episodes of vomiting, versus adverse effects, particularly worsening of colicky pain.

References

1. Currow DC, Quinn S, Agar M, et al. Double-blind, placebo-controlled, randomized trial of octreotide in malignant bowel obstruction. *J Pain Symptom Manage.* 2015;49(5). doi:10.1016/j.jpainsymman.2014.09.013.
2. Itoh H. [Clinicopharmacological study of gastrointestinal drugs from the viewpoint of postmarketing development]. *Yakugaku Zasshi.* 2006;126(9):767–778.
3. Yang H, Lou D, Zou Y. [Effect of ranitidine on the gastric acid, plasma endothelin, and calcitonin gene-related peptide in patients undergoing the brain operation]. *Zhong Nan Da Xue Xue Bao Yi Xue Ban.* 2007;32(2):295–298.
4. Ren J, Dunn S, Tang Y, et al. Effects of calcitonin gene-related peptide on somatostatin and gastrin gene expression in rat antrum. *Regul Pept.* 1998;73(2):75–82.
5. Ren J, Young R, Lassiter D, Rings M, Harty R. Calcitonin gene-related peptide: mechanisms of modulation of antral endocrine cells and cholinergic neurons. *Am J Physiol.* 1992;262(4 Pt 1):G732–G739.
6. Mariani P, Blumberg J, Landau A, et al. Symptomatic treatment with lanreotide microparticles in inoperable bowel obstruction resulting from peritoneal carcinomatosis: a randomized, double-blind, placebo-controlled phase III study. *J Clin Oncol.* 2012;30(35). doi:10.1200/JCO.2011.40.5712.
7. Laval G, Rousselot H, Toussaint-Martel S, et al. SALTO: a randomized, multicenter study assessing octreotide LAR in inoperable bowel obstruction. *Bull Cancer.* 2012;99(2). doi:10.1684/bdc.2011.1535.
8. Mercadante S, Ripamonti C, Casuccio A, Zecca E, Groff L. Comparison of octreotide and hyoscine butylbromide in controlling gastrointestinal symptoms due to malignant inoperable bowel obstruction. *Support Care Cancer.* 2000;8(3). doi:10.1007/s005200050283.
9. Murakami H, Matsumoto H, Nakamura M, Hirai T, Yamaguchi Y. Octreotide acetate-steroid combination therapy for malignant gastrointestinal obstruction. *Anticancer Res.* 2013;33(12).
10. Ripamonti C, Panzeri C, Groff L, Galeazzi G, Boffi R. The role of somatostatin and octreotide in bowel obstruction: pre-clinical and clinical results. *Tumori.* 2001;87(1). doi:10.1177/030089160108700101.
11. Obita GP, Boland EG, Currow DC, Johnson MJ, Boland JW. Somatostatin analogues compared with placebo and other pharmacologic agents in the management of

symptoms of inoperable malignant bowel obstruction: a systematic review. *J Pain Symptom Manage.* 2016;52(6). doi:10.1016/j.jpainsymman.2016.05.032.

12. National Comprehensive Cancer Network. Palliative Care (Version 1.2021). https://www.nccn.org/professionals/physician_gls/pdf/palliative.pdf. Accessed January 20, 2021.
13. Walsh D, Davis M, Ripamonti C, Bruera E, Davies A, Molassiotis A. 2016 Updated MASCC/ESMO consensus recommendations: management of nausea and vomiting in advanced cancer. *Support Care Cancer.* 2017;25(1). doi:10.1007/s00520-016-3371-3.
14. Davis M, Hui D, Davies A, et al. Medical management of malignant bowel obstruction in patients with advanced cancer: 2021 MASCC guideline update. *Support Care Cancer.* 2021;29(12). doi:10.1007/s00520-021-06438-9.

24

Efficacy of Levetiracetam, Fosphenytoin, and Valproate for Established Status Epilepticus by Age Group (ESETT)

A Double-Blind, Responsive-Adaptive, Randomized Controlled Trial

ANGELA YEH AND EMILY J. MARTIN

> Any of the three drugs can be considered as a potential first-choice, second-line drug for benzodiazepine-refractory status epilepticus.
>
> —Chamberlain et al.[1]

Research Question: What is the efficacy and safety of levetiracetam, fosphenytoin, and valproate in benzodiazepine-refractory status epilepticus?

Funding: National Institute of Neurological Disorders and Stroke, National Institute of Health

Year Study Began: 2015

Year Study Published: 2020

Study Location: 58 hospital emergency departments across the United States

Who Was Studied: Patients aged 1 year or older with persistent or recurrent convulsions of at least 5 minutes duration who had received adequate doses of benzodiazepines with the last dose of benzodiazepine administered within 30 minutes.

Who Was Excluded: Prisoners, pregnant patients, postanoxic patients, and those with seizures precipitated by trauma, hypoglycemia, or hyperglycemia were excluded. Those with allergies or contraindications to the study drugs and those already treated for this episode of status epilepticus with nonbenzodiazepine anticonvulsants were also excluded.

How Many Patients: In total, 462 patients were enrolled, including 225 children (aged 1–17 years), 186 adults (aged 18–65 years), and 51 older adults (aged over 65 years).

Study Overview: This is a multicenter, double-blind, randomized controlled trial evaluating the comparative effectiveness of levetiracetam, fosphenytoin, and valproate in treating patients with benzodiazepine-refractory status epilepticus in emergency departments across the United States. Patients with established status epilepticus were randomly assigned to receive levetiracetam, fosphenytoin, or valproate. Randomization was response adaptive and stratified by age group (younger than 18 years, 18–65 years, and older than 65 years). The initial 300 patients underwent equal allocation (1:1:1). Afterward, the target allocation ratio was updated every 100 patients, and the response-adaptive randomization was used primarily to allocate more patients to the treatment group likely to be the most effective. Allocation was concealed. All investigators, patients, clinical and study teams, and pharmacists were masked to study drug allocation (Figure 24.1).

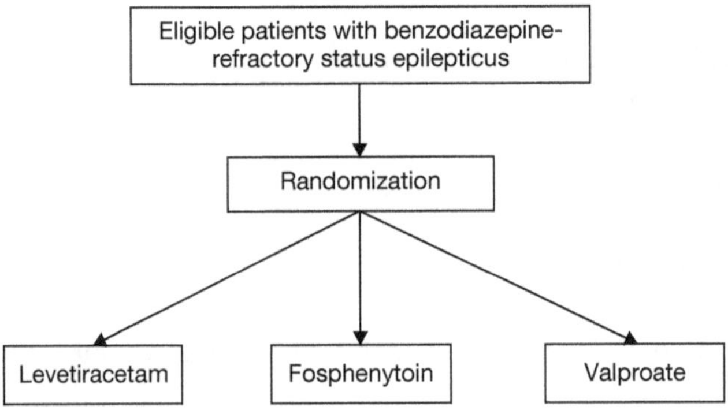

Figure 24.1. Summary of study design.

Study Intervention: Patients with persistent status epilepticus after having received a minimal adequate cumulative dose of benzodiazepines were randomly assigned to receive levetiracetam, fosphenytoin, or valproate. Minimal adequate cumulative doses of benzodiazepines were defined as diazepam 10 mg intravenously (IV), lorazepam 4 mg IV, or midazolam 10 mg IV or intramuscularly (IM) for all adults and children with body weight of ≥ 32 kg, and diazepam 0–3 mg/kg IV, lorazepam 0–1 mg/kg IV, or midazolam 0–3 mg/kg IM or 0–2 mg/kg IV for children with body weight of < 32kg. Weight-based infusion rates provided treatment doses of levetiracetam 60 mg/kg (maximum 4500 mg), fosphenytoin 20 mg PE per kg (maximum 1500 mg PE), or valproate 40 mg/kg (maximum 3000 mg) infused over 10 minutes.

Follow-Up: Patients were followed until hospital discharge or for 30 days, whichever occurred first.

Endpoints: The primary outcome was the absence of clinically apparent seizure activity with improving responsiveness at 60 minutes after the start of the study drug infusion, without additional anticonvulsant medication, including medications required for endotracheal intubation. Secondary outcomes included admission to intensive care unit (ICU), length of ICU stay, length of hospital stay, life-threatening hypotension or cardiac arrhythmia or intubation within 60 minutes of starting the study drug infusion, acute respiratory depression, acute seizure recurrence 1–12 hours after start of the study drug infusion, and death.

RESULTS

- Baseline characteristics were balanced across treatment groups within age groups.
- No difference was found in the primary outcome between treatment groups within each age group (Table 24.1).
- Life-threatening hypotension or life-threatening cardiac arrhythmia was rare and did not differ by treatment group in any age group.
- Endotracheal intubation of children occurred more frequently in the fosphenytoin group but did not differ by treatment group in either adult age group.
- No other differences in safety outcomes were detected.

Table 24.1 SUMMARY OF KEY FINDINGS

	Children (1–18 years) n = 225			**Adults (18–65 years) n = 186**			**Older adults (>65 years) n = 51**		
	Levetiracetam	**Fosphenytoin**	**Valproate**	**Levetiracetam**	**Fosphenytoin**	**Valproate**	**Levetiracetam**	**Fosphenytoin**	**Valproate**
Treatment Efficacy	44 (52%)	35 (49%)	36 (52%)	31 (44%)	25 (46%)	28 (46%)	7 (37%)	6 (35%)	7 (47%)
Admission to ICU	53 (62%)	45 (63%)	43 (62%)	38 (54%)	26 (48%)	34 (56%)	15 (79%)	13 (76%)	8 (53%)
Length of ICU stay, days	1 (0–2)	1 (0–2)	1 (0–2)	1 (0–3)	0 (0–3)	1 (0–3)	3 (1–6)	2 (1–7)	2 (0–6)
Length of hospital stay, days	2 (1–3)	2 (1–3)	2 (1–4)	3 (1–6)	3 (1–7)	2 (1–6)	7 (5–12)	5 (3–16)	5 (3–16)
Safety Population	86	73	70	74	58	64	20	18	15
Life-threatening hypotension	0	2 (3%)	3 (4%)	0	2 (3%)	0	1 (5%)	1 (6%)	0
Life-threatening cardiac arrhythmia	0	0	0	1 (1%)	0	0	0	0	0
Endotracheal intubation	7 (8%)	24 (33%)	8 (11%)	19 (26%)	13 (22%)	14 (22%)	7 (35%)	5 (28%)	2 (13%)
Acute respiratory depression	5 (6%)	13 (18%)	7 (10%)	10 (14%)	6 (10%)	5 (8%)	0	2 (11%)	0
Acute seizure recurrence within 1-12 hours	8 (9%)	11 (15%)	6 (9%)	5 (7%)	3 (5%)	5 (8%)	4 (20%)	4 (22%)	3 (20%)
Death	1 (1%)	0	1 (1%)	2 (3%)	2 (3%)	1 (2%)	4 (20%)	1 (6%)	0

Data are n, n (%), or median (IQR).

Criticisms and Limitations:

- The primary outcome in this study was the absence of clinically apparent seizure activity and increased responsiveness. The investigators did not confirm the presence or absence of seizures with electroencephalograms.
- Given that fewer older adults were enrolled in this study, meaningful inferences about the older adult age group are limited.

Other Relevant Studies and Information:

- The Established Status Epilepticus Treatment Trial (ESETT)[2] was a double-blinded trial of fosphenytoin, levetiracetam, and valproate in adults and children with established status epilepticus. While the trial did not find differences in overall outcomes, it did not determine if efficacy was modulated by age. This trial is an extension of ESETT and shows that a lack of difference in outcomes between drugs is similar across age groups.
- Prior to ESETT, the Emergency Treatment with Levetiracetam or Phenytoin in Convulsive Status Epilepticus in Children (EcLiPSE)[3] and the Levetiracetam Versus Phenytoin for Second-Line Treatment of Convulsive Status Epilepticus in Children (ConSEPT)[4] trials showed no difference in outcomes between those treated with fosphenytoin or levetiracetam. Both EcLiPSE and ConSEPT were open-label randomized trials in children with established status epilepticus.
- Together with data from EcLiPSE, ConSEPT, and the original ESETT, this study indicates that any of the 3 anticonvulsants—fosphenytoin, levetiracetam, or valproate—can be considered as a reasonable and appropriate second-line medication in the treatment of children and adults with established, benzodiazepine-refractory status epilepticus.

Summary and Implications: This large, randomized controlled trial showed that approximately half of patients across 3 age groups (children, adults, and older adults) with established status epilepticus respond to high doses of levetiracetam, fosphenytoin, or valproate. Any of these 3 drugs can be considered an equally effective, second-line medication for benzodiazepine-refractory status epilepticus.

CLINICAL CASE: MANAGEMENT OF BENZODIAZEPINE-REFRACTORY STATUS EPILEPTICUS IN A PEDIATRIC PATIENT

Case History

A 2-year-old boy with congenital epilepsy presents to the emergency department with altered mental status and tonic-clonic movement of his right arm with right-sided eye deviation. There is no history of trauma and his blood glucose is within normal range. He shows no signs of clinical improvement after receiving 4 doses of lorazepam 0.1 mg/kg administered IV. His last dose of lorazepam was administered 10 minutes ago. What medication should be administered next?

Suggested Answer

Based on the results of ESETT, levetiracetam, fosphenytoin, and valproate are equally effective and safe in treating benzodiazepine-refractory status epilepticus in children and adults. If there are no allergies or contraindications to these medications, each can be considered an appropriate first-choice, second-line therapy.

References

1. Chamberlain JM, Kapur J, Shinnar S, et al.; Neurological Emergencies Treatment Trials; Pediatric Emergency Care Applied Research Network investigators. Efficacy of levetiracetam, fosphenytoin, and valproate for established status epilepticus by age group (ESETT): a double-blind, responsive-adaptive, randomised controlled trial. *Lancet.* 2020 Apr 11;395(10231):1217–1224. doi:10.1016/S0140-6736(20)30611-5. Epub 2020 Mar 20. PMID: 32203691; PMCID: PMC7241415.
2. Kapur J, Elm J, Chamberlain JM, et al.; NETT and PECARN Investigators. Randomized trial of three anticonvulsant medications for status epilepticus. *N Engl J Med.* 2019 Nov 28;381(22):2103–2113. doi:10.1056/NEJMoa1905795. PMID: 31774955; PMCID: PMC7098487.
3. Lyttle MD, Rainford NEA, Gamble C, et al.; Paediatric Emergency Research in the United Kingdom & Ireland (PERUKI) collaborative. Levetiracetam versus phenytoin for second-line treatment of paediatric convulsive status epilepticus (EcLiPSE): a multicentre, open-label, randomised trial. *Lancet.* 2019 May 25;393(10186):2125–2134. doi:10.1016/S0140-6736(19)30724-X. Epub 2019 Apr 17. PMID: 31005385; PMCID: PMC6551349.
4. Dalziel SR, Furyk J, Bonisch M, et al.; PREDICT research network. A multicentre randomised controlled trial of levetiracetam versus phenytoin for convulsive status epilepticus in children (protocol): Convulsive Status Epilepticus Paediatric Trial (ConSEPT)—a PREDICT study. *BMC Pediatr.* 2017 Jun 22;17(1):152. doi:10.1186/s12887-017-0887-8. PMID: 28641582; PMCID: PMC5480418.

25

Donepezil and Memantine for Moderate-to-Severe Alzheimer Disease

When Is It Appropriate to Discontinue Therapy?

KRISTINA MARCHAND AND KEVIN MCGEHRIN

> **Study Nickname:** DOMINOAlthough the cognitive benefit associated with donepezil therapy exceeded a distribution-based minimum clinically important difference, the cognitive benefits associated with memantine treatment were smaller and did not reach the minimum clinically important difference.
>
> —*HOWARD ET AL.*[1]

Research Question: Do patients with moderate-to-severe Alzheimer disease already receiving donepezil benefit from the addition of memantine?

Funding: United Kingdom Medical Research Council, Alzheimer's Society

Year Study Began: 2008

Year Study Published: 2012

Study Location: Multicenter study across the United Kingdom

Who Was Studied: Community-dwelling patients with moderate-to-severe Alzheimer disease (Standardized Mini-Mental Status Examination [SMMSE] score 5–13) already being treated with donepezil 10 mg daily for at least 3 months.

Who Was Excluded: Patients with other severe medical conditions, already treated with memantine, or determined unable to comply with treatment.

How Many Patients: 295

Study Overview: In this double-blinded, placebo-controlled clinical trial, subjects were randomly assigned to 1 of 4 possible treatment groups (Figure 25.1).

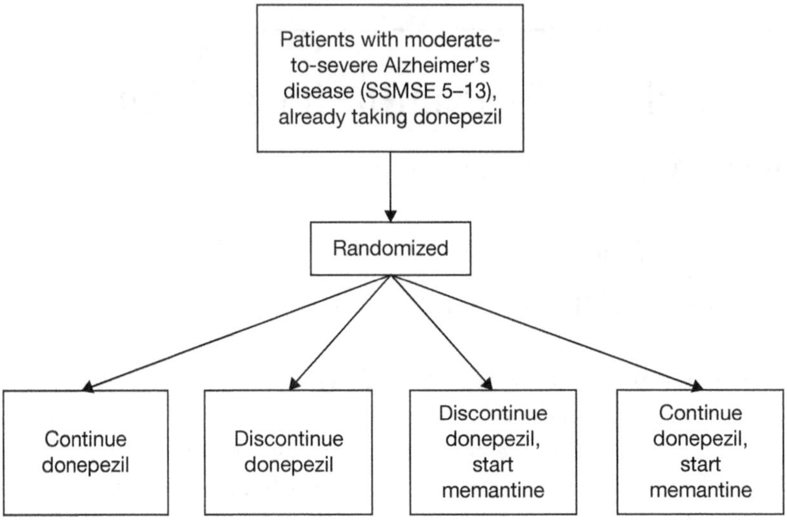

Figure 25.1. Summary of study design.

Study Intervention: Participants spent weeks 1–4 undergoing dose tapers and placebo additions, with final dosing during weeks 5–52. Utilizing a 2×2 factorial design, differences in cognition and function were compared between 3 potential therapy changes: continuation versus discontinuation of donepezil, addition versus no addition of memantine, and combination of donepezil and memantine.

Follow-Up: Assessed at enrollment, then at 6, 18, 30, and 52 weeks

Endpoints:

Primary:

- SMMSE scores—cognitive function on a scale of 0 (severe impairment) to 30 (no impairment). Minimal clinically important difference was 1.4 points when comparing 2 groups.
- Bristol Activities of Daily Living Scale (BADLS) scores—functional ability on a scale of 0 (no impairment) to 60 (severe impairment). Minimal clinically important difference was 3.5 points when comparing 2 groups.

Secondary: Neuropsychiatric Inventory (NPI) scale, Dementia Quality of Life (DEMQOL-Proxy) scale, and caregiver General Health Questionnaire (GHQ-12) scale.

RESULTS (TABLE 25.1)

Table 25.1 Estimate of Treatment Differences in Cognitive and Functional Outcomes

	Cognitive Impairment			**Functional Impairment**		
	Δ SMMSE Score*	**95% CI**	***P* Value**	**Δ BADLS Score****	**95% CI**	***P* Value**
Continue vs. discontinue donepezil	1.9	1.3 to 2.5	<0.001	−3.0	−4.3 to −1.8	<0.001
Active vs placebo memantine	1.2	0.6 to 1.8	<0.001	−1.5	−2.8 to −0.3	0.02
Combination therapy (donepezil + memantine)	0.8	−0.1 to 1.6	0.07	−0.5	−2.2 to 1.2	0.57

*MCID defined as ≥ 1.4.
**MCID defined as ≥ −3.5.

- All groups showed continued cognitive and functional decline during the study (none improved). Results were reported as between-group differences, since some groups declined further than others.
- There was a statistically significant benefit between SMMSE scores (1.9 points higher) for patients who continued donepezil, which exceeded the study's definition for a minimum clinically important difference (MCID) of 1.4 points.
- There was a difference in SMMSE response in the group that continued donepezil, depending on the severity of dementia at the start of the trial. For patients with an SMMSE score of 10–13, there was a 2.6-point improvement in the SMMSE score between those who continued and those who discontinued memantine. However, for patients with a baseline SMMSE score of 5–9, the difference between these 2 groups was 1.3 points (failing to meet the predetermined "clinically important" mark of 1.4).

- Combined treatment (addition of memantine to donepezil) was not superior to treatment with donepezil alone and did not meet the MCID in SMMSE or BADLS.
- There were no significant differences in secondary outcomes.
- There were no unexpected serious adverse reactions reported. Some of the most commonly reported side effects were gastrointestinal side effects, falls, and infections.

Criticisms and Limitations:

- Recruitment was smaller than called for by study design.
- Dropout rates were high and differed between treatment groups (higher dropout in discontinuation of donepezil and placebo memantine groups), raising concerns that the analysis may have underestimated the benefits of medication continuation.
- The authors separately published their justification for determining the MCID[2] utilizing a distribution-based definition derived from their own data set. Their MCID (1.4 SMMSE points) was substantially smaller than the MCID defined in similar dementia drug trial models (3.72 SMMSE points) determined using expert opinion.[3]
- Preservation of cognition and function has greater value for patients with mild-to-moderate disease. Difficult behaviors, which were not impacted as secondary outcomes, become more meaningful in the severe disease stage when treatment focus is more likely to be palliative.[4]

Other Relevant Studies and Information:

- Tapered discontinuation of donepezil is well tolerated and safe.[5]
- Two systematic reviews of related studies showed modest statistically significant benefits in outcomes when combining cholinesterase inhibitors and memantine, but the authors of those reviews concluded the clinical relevance of these findings was uncertain.[6,7]
- A 2018 review recommended that discontinuation of donepezil be considered periodically if no cognitive or functional benefits are observed by caregivers.[8]
- Xu and colleagues evaluated the long-term effects of cholinesterase inhibitors on cognitive decline and mortality over a 5-year period. Their results showed that cholinesterase inhibitor use results in higher SMMSE scores annually and showed a 27% lower risk of death compared to

nonusers. Only galantamine was associated with a lower risk of death and severe dementia.[9]

- This study influenced a change in guidelines published in 2018 by the United Kingdom's National Institute for Health and Care Excellence (NICE), which now recommends that clinicians not stop donepezil based on disease severity alone and that adding memantine be considered in moderate-to-severe disease.[10]

Summary and Implications: This trial is widely cited as justification for continuing donepezil or adding memantine in late-stage Alzheimer disease. However, only continued therapy with donepezil reduced decline in cognitive score and did not significantly change functional scores. The small cognitive benefit reflected only a fractional reduction in the scope of overall decline. Some of the most commonly reported side effects were gastrointestinal side effects, falls, and infections. The discerning palliative care clinician will wonder whether such small changes in SMMSE scores translate to meaningful benefit for patients living with late-stage Alzheimer disease.

CLINICAL CASE: WILL MORE MEDICATIONS HELP MS. SMITH'S WORSENING DEMENTIA?

Case History

Ms. Smith is a 77-year-old woman with Alzheimer disease who lives at home with her daughter. Her family is considering hospice enrollment after noticing a steady decline over the past 3 years. She now requires assistance with all activities of daily living and has mild dysphagia. Ms. Smith has lost 11 pounds and speaks only in short sentences. Her most recent SMMSE score was 6/30. She has been taking donepezil 10 mg daily for over a year, but her family is unsure if this is providing benefit. Should donepezil be continued? Should memantine be added?

Suggested Answer

Based on this study, for patients like Ms. Smith in the moderate-to-severe stages of Alzheimer disease, we should not expect to see observable improvements in cognitive or functional status by adding or changing to memantine, so we should not recommend it. Although there might be a small change in her SMMSE scores if we continue donepezil, this improvement would be minimal compared to the overall continuation of decline over time. However, in the DOMINO trial, patients with an SMMSE score below 10 did not achieve their "clinically important" endpoint of a difference of 1.4 points or greater. It would be sensible to weigh the potential cognitive benefits against the burdens of continuing donepezil. Common side effects of this drug class include gastrointestinal upset, appetite loss, and malaise. Continuing therapy also adds to polypharmacy and pill burden in a patient with dysphagia. Our most helpful intervention is to thoughtfully discuss what we expect for the natural course of her condition over time and identify potential pros and cons for continuing versus discontinuing donepezil.

References

1. Howard R, McShane R, Lindesay J, et al. Donepezil and memantine for moderate-to-severe Alzheimer's disease. *N Engl J Med.* 2012;366(10):893–903.
2. Howard R, Phillips P, Johnson T, et al. Determining the minimum clinically important differences for outcomes in the DOMINO trial. *Int J Geriatr Psychiatry.* 2011;26(8):812–817.
3. Burback D, Molnar FJ, St. John P, Man-Son-Hing M. Key methodological features of randomized controlled trials of Alzheimer's disease therapy: minimal clinically important difference, sample size and trial duration. *Dement Geriatr Cogn Disord.* 1999;10(6):534–540.
4. Raina P, Santaguida P, Ismaila A, et al. Effectiveness of cholinesterase inhibitors and memantine for treating dementia: evidence review for a clinical practice guideline. *Ann Intern Med.* 2008;148(5):379–397.
5. Herrmann N, O'Regan J, Ruthirakuhan M, et al. A randomized placebo-controlled discontinuation study of cholinesterase inhibitors in institutionalized patients with moderate-to-severe Alzheimer disease. *J Am Med Dir Assoc.* 2016;17(2):142–147.
6. Farrimond L, Roberts E, McShane R. Memantine and cholinesterase inhibitor combination therapy for Alzheimer's disease: a systematic review. *BMJ Open.* 2012;2(3):e000917.
7. Muayqil T, Camicioli R. Systematic review and meta-analysis of combination therapy with cholinesterase inhibitors and memantine in Alzheimer's disease and other dementias. *Dement Geriatr Cogn Disord Extra.* 2012;2:546–572.
8. Kim L, Factora R. Alzheimer dementia: starting, stopping drug therapy. *Cleve Clin J Med.* 2018;85(3):209–214.
9. Xu H, Garcia-Ptacek S, Jonsson L, et al. Long-term effects of cholinesterase inhibitors on cognitive decline and mortality. *Neurology.* 2021;96:e2220–e2230.
10. National Institute for Health and Care Excellence. *Dementia: Assessment, Management and Support for People Living With Dementia and Their Carer.* London: National Institute for Health and Care Excellence; 2018.

26

Use of Mirtazapine for Cancer-Associated Anorexia and Cachexia

ALEXANDRA L. MCPHERSON

> Based on the results of the current trial and those previously reported, it would be advisable not to use mirtazapine as an appetite stimulant in non-depressed advanced cancer patients with [cancer-associated anorexia-cachexia syndrome].
>
> —HUNTER ET AL.[1]

Research Question: Does mirtazapine improve appetite and other cachexia measurements in patients with incurable cancer and with cancer-associated anorexia and cachexia (CAC)?

Funding: Cairo University Research Support Program, Friends of Patients of Kasr Al-Ainy Oncology Center Association

Year Study Began: 2018

Year Study Published: 2021

Study Location: Kasr Al-Ainy Center of Clinical Oncology and Nuclear Medicine, Kasr Al-Ainy School of Medicine, Cairo University, Cairo, Egypt

Who Was Studied: Adults with incurable solid tumor, predicted prognosis > 3 months, cachexia (defined as unintentional loss of > 5% body weight over the past 6 months or loss of > 2% body weight over the past 6 months plus body mass index < 20), loss of appetite score ≥ 4 on the Edmonton Symptom Assessment System (ESAS), Eastern Cooperative Oncology Group performance of 0–2, normal renal and hepatic function, ability to take oral medications, not dependent on tube feeding, and ability to understand and communicate in Arabic.

Who Was Excluded: Weight gain for a known cause, score ≥ 4 on a single-item 7-point Likert scale assessing depression, cognitive impairment, uncontrolled symptoms and/or comorbidities that may affect appetite, treatment with antipsychotic agents for 30 days prior to or during protocol therapy, supplement or medication use that may stimulate appetite, and positive pregnancy test in premenopausal women.

How Many Patients: 120

Study Overview: This is a parallel-group, placebo-controlled, double-blind, randomized phase 3 trial in which 120 patients were randomized to either mirtazapine 15 mg at night or placebo in a 1:1 ratio. The patients, recruiter, providers, and outcome assessor were blinded to treatment allocation (Figure 26.1).

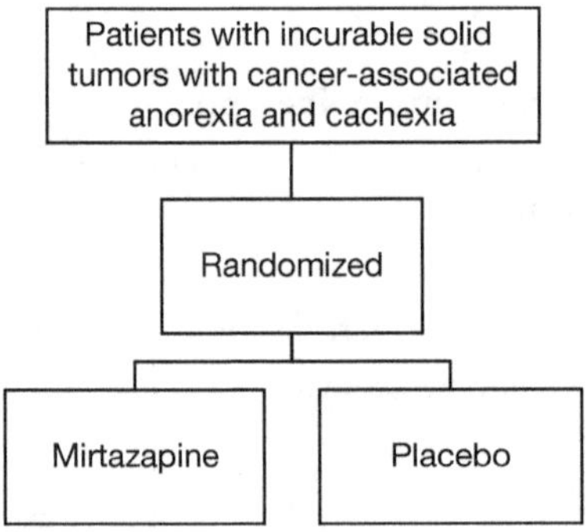

Figure 26.1. Summary of study design.

Study Intervention: Patients in the intervention arm received oral mirtazapine 15 mg (half tablet of Remeron 30 mg), while those in the control arm received a half tablet of placebo. Both were administered once daily at bedtime for 28 days with the option to continue for another 28 days.

Follow-Up: 28 days, with an optional additional 28-day period

Endpoints:

Primary outcome: Change in appetite score from baseline to day 28, measured by a 0–10 appetite scale, where 0 indicates no appetite at all and 10 the best appetite possible.

Secondary outcomes: Change in appetite score from baseline to day 56 (measured using the same 0–10 scale), change in quality of life from baseline to days 28 and 56 (measured by Functional Assessment of Anorexia/Cachexia Therapy [FAACT] questionnaire), change in fatigue from baseline to days 28 and 56 (assessed by the ESAS-revised), change in depressive symptoms from baseline to days 28 and 56 (assessed by the Hospital Anxiety and Depression Scale [HADS-D]), change in body weight and lean body mass from baseline to days 28 and 56, change in handgrip strength from baseline to days 28 and 56, overall survival, and changes in inflammatory markers from baseline to day 56.

RESULTS

- In general, there were no significant differences between mirtazapine or placebo regarding change in appetite score (primary endpoint) or any of the other outcome measures from baseline to days 28 and 56, except for the HADS-depression score, which was significantly higher in the placebo arm at days 28 and 56. A higher HADS-depression score is indicative of more depression (Table 26.1).
- Less than half (48%) of patients in the mirtazapine arm completed 56 days of treatment, compared to 75% of those in the placebo arm.
- Patients in the mirtazapine arm reported more somnolence and hallucinations, which contributed to treatment discontinuation.
- Patients in the mirtazapine arm had significantly less progression of depression.
- There was no difference in survival between the mirtazapine and placebo arms.

Table 26.1 SUMMARY OF STUDY'S KEY FINDINGS

Outcome		**Mirtazapine 28 Days**	**Placebo 28 Days**	***P* Value**		**Mirtazapine 56 Days**	**Placebo 56 Days**	***P* Value**
Appetite score	Median	2	2	.472	Median	2.5	1.5	.326
	IQR	0–2	0–2		IQR	1–3	0-3	
Body weight (kg)	Median	−0.8	−0.6	.948	Mean	−0.64	−1.58	.264
	IQR	−1.5 to 0.75	−1.4 to 0.1		SD	4.2	2.85	
Lean body mass (kg)	Median	−0.16	−0.37	.411	Mean	−0.05	−0.64	.349
	IQR	−1.1 to 1	−1 to 0.32		SD	2.56	2.56	
Handgrip strength (kg)	Median	−0.76	0	.31	Median	−0.76	−0.15	.166
	IQR	−1.51 to 0.76	−0.91 to 0.76		IQR	−5.3 to 1.3	−1.7 to 1.1	
HADS-Depression	Median	1	2	.018	Median	2	3	.006
	IQR	0–2	1–2		IQR	1–3	2–4	
FAACT Total	Mean	2.17	0.62	.286	Mean	−0.09	−3.7	.153
	SD	7.58	6.86		SD	9.6	10.77	
Tiredness (ESAS-r)	Median	0	0.5	.098	Median	1	1	.119
	IQR	0–1	0–1		IQR	−0.5 to 1	0–2	

Abbreviations: ESAS-r: Edmonton Symptom Assessment System-Revised; FAACT, Functional Assessment of Anorexia/Cachexia Therapy; HADS, Hospital Anxiety and Depression Scale; IQR, interquartile range; SD, standard deviation.

Criticisms and Limitations:

- This is a single-center study, which may limit its broader generalizability.
- This study was limited to patients with an ECOG performance score of 0–2, indicating decent functional status, and may not be generalizable to other patients.

Other Relevant Studies and Information:

- Theobald et al. conducted a pilot open-label, crossover trial of mirtazapine (15 and 30 mg at night) in 20 advanced cancer patients. No difference was observed in the numeric rating scale measuring appetite; however, the single Zung items measuring appetite and weight exhibited significant improvement at week 8.[2]
- Riechelmann et al. conducted an open-label phase 2 study of mirtazapine (15–30 mg daily) in 17 nondepressed patients with CAC. Mirtazapine improved appetite in 24% of patients at week 4.[3]
- Cankurtaran et al. conducted a study designed to compare the effectiveness of mirtazapine, imipramine, or placebo for symptom management in 53 cancer patients with psychological morbidity. No significant difference was observed between groups for appetite loss. The mirtazapine group had improvements in insomnia, anxiety, and depression.[4]
- Davis et al. treated 57 patients with either 15 or 30 mg of mirtazapine daily. Quality of life, the primary outcome, improved in 5 of 57 (9%).[5] Insomnia and anxiety met the target response rate of 33% improvement in the intention-to-treat analysis. No further symptom response was seen with dose escalation. Secondary outcomes based on the presence of the symptom at baseline occurred within the first week and did not improve thereafter. A 1-point improvement (on a 1–4 scale) was shown for insomnia (19/43, 44%), nausea (12/31, 38%), and anxiety (19/50, 38%). Patient-perceived toxicity and intolerance to mirtazapine were significant, with only 40% completing 2 weeks of mirtazapine.
- The 2020 American Society of Clinical Oncology (ASCO) Clinical Practice Guideline for the Management of Cancer Cachexia mentions the lack of data surrounding the use of mirtazapine and, as a result, does not recommend its use. These guidelines do not reflect the findings from this study, which were published in 2021.[6]

Summary and Implications: This parallel-group, placebo-controlled, double-blind, randomized phase 3 trial found that, compared to placebo, mirtazapine 15 mg once daily at bedtime did not improve appetite, body weight, handgrip strength, or quality of life in patients with advanced cancer and anorexia and cachexia. Based on these results, mirtazapine should not be routinely recommended for cancer-associated cachexia. Mirtazapine may have more utility in clinically depressed patients with CAC; however, more research needs to be done.

CLINICAL CASE: SHOULD MIRTAZAPINE BE USED FOR APPETITE STIMULATION IN CANCER PATIENTS?

Case History

A 62-year-old woman with an unremarkable past medical history was recently diagnosed with metastatic ovarian cancer and presents to the outpatient palliative care clinic for symptom management. Her pain is well controlled on her current analgesic regimen, and she is happy to share that she's been able to go out for evening walks with her husband and dog. Her most bothersome symptoms at present are fatigue and lack of appetite with resulting weight loss. She states that she has lost 22 pounds over the past 6 months (she was 143 pounds and is now 121 pounds). She is planning to start cancer-directed therapy in the next few weeks and is worried this is going to make her appetite even worse. She does not have a history of depression, anxiety, or insomnia. Her estimated prognosis is 6–12 months. She states her friend takes mirtazapine for depression and gained weight while taking it. After doing some research, she saw that mirtazapine may also be used as an appetite stimulant, and she wonders whether this might be a potential option for her.

Should mirtazapine be prescribed for appetite stimulation in this patient?

Suggested Answer

While several prior studies examined the effects of mirtazapine on appetite, the Hunter study was the first placebo-controlled randomized controlled trial conducted in advanced cancer patients with CAC. As stated above, the 2020 ASCO Clinical Practice Guideline does not provide a recommendation regarding use of mirtazapine for CAC due to lack of available data.

Based on her 22-pound weight loss over the past 6 months (15.4%), this patient meets criteria for cachexia. A trial of corticosteroids or megestrol acetate could be considered. It is also important to regularly assess for and ensure adequate control of nausea/vomiting, as it can have a detrimental effect on appetite. It may be beneficial to have the patient follow up with an oncology-trained nutritionist to discuss strategies for weight gain.

References

1. Hunter C, Abdel-Aal H, Elsherief W, et al. Mirtazapine in cancer-associated anorexia and cachexia: a double-blind placebo-controlled randomized trial. *J Pain Symptom Manage.* 2021;62(6):1207–1215.
2. Theobald DE, Kirsh KL, Holtsclaw E, Donaghy K, Passik SD. An open-label, crossover trial of mirtazapine (15 and 30 mg) in cancer patients with pain and other distressing symptoms. *J Pain Symptom Manage.* 2002;23:442–447.
3. Riechelmann RP, Burman D, Tannock IF, Rodin G, Zimmermann C. Phase II trial of mirtazapine for cancer-related cachexia and anorexia. *Am J Hosp Palliat Care.* 2010;27:106–110.
4. Cankurtaran ES, Ozalp E, Soygur H, Akbiyik DI, Turhan L, Alkis N. Mirtazapine improves sleep and lowers anxiety and depression in cancer patients: superiority over imipramine. *Support Care Cancer.* 2008;16:1291–1298.
5. Davis MP, Kirkova J, Lagman R, Walsh D, Karafa M. Intolerance to mirtazapine in advanced cancer. *J Pain Symptom Manage.* 2011;42(3):e4–e7.
6. Roeland EJ, Bohlke K, Baracos VE, et al. Management of cancer cachexia: ASCO guideline. *J Clin Oncol.* 2020;38:2438–2453.

27

Epidemiology of Amyotrophic Lateral Sclerosis and Effect of Riluzole on Disease Course

RYAN C. COSTANTINO

> A reasonable interpretation of the data could be that, at least on a population level, riluzole's effect on survival diminishes over time and is lost approximately 6 months after starting treatment.
>
> —CETIN ET AL.[1]

Research Question: What is the incidence and prevalence of amyotrophic lateral sclerosis (ALS) and how does a person's age, gender, and duration of riluzole treatment impact survival?

Funding: No external funding was obtained for this study.

Year Study Began: January 1, 2008, to June 30, 2012

Year Study Published: 2015

Study Location: Austria

Who Was Studied: Patients 20 years or older discharged from a hospital during the study period with a primary diagnosis of ALS or who were prescribed riluzole.

Who Was Excluded: Individuals younger than 20.

How Many Patients: 911

Study Overview: This was an observational study that leveraged hospital discharge and prescription records within databases containing information from 9 regional sickness funds in the country of Austria. Together the data within registries capture approximately 77.7% of the population aged 20 or older.

Study Intervention: Not applicable

Follow-Up: Not applicable

Endpoints: Incidence, prevalence, patients' survival based on age and gender, and riluzole treatment.

RESULTS

- The median time from ALS diagnosis to death was 676 days (95% CI: 591–761).
- Riluzole had a favorable effect on survival, but only for approximately 6 months after diagnosis, with survival curves crossing between the groups at 540 days (~18 months); beyond this time period, those patients not taking riluzole had a better prognosis.
- Overall, the group that received riluzole had 15% higher survival compared to the group that did not receive riluzole at 6 months. However, at 48 months the group that received riluzole had a 14% lower survival compared to the group that did not receive riluzole.
- Shorter riluzole treatment periods were associated with longer survival times when compared to longer treatment periods, demonstrating a time-dependent effect.

Criticisms and Limitations:

- The financial and administrative claims used in this analysis lacked certain clinical metadata, which has the potential to introduce selection bias.

- These data reflect the care that was coded, not necessarily the care that was consumed or delivered. For example, prescription claims for riluzole reflect that a medication was dispensed, not that it was necessarily consumed by the person according to the directions.
- The hospital discharge and prescription databases used are not population-based registries. Therefore, certain subsets of the ALS population may not be reflected in the data. For example, people with mild symptoms managed on an outpatient basis may not be captured. On the other hand, patients who had advanced disease may also be missed, introducing selection bias. This may have particular relevance in the palliative care setting when caring for people early or late in the disease process.

Other Relevant Studies and Information:

- As of 2021 there were 5 drugs approved by the US Food and Drug Administration to treat ALS. Three of these involve some formulation of riluzole, edavarone (Radicava™), and a combination of dextromethorphan HBr and quinidine sulfate (Nuedexta®).
- A populated-based outcome study concluded that riluzole reduced the mortality rate by 23% and 15% at 6 and 12 months, respectively. The study also reported that riluzole prolonged median survival by 4.2 months.[2]
- Several retrospective studies have published results similar to Cetin et al., with Kaplain-Meier curves crossing at time points ranging from 11 to 26 months.[3–5]
- A Cochrane review of riluzole for ALS published in 2012 reported: "Riluzole 100 mg daily probably prolongs median survival by two to three months in patients with probable and definite amyotrophic lateral sclerosis with symptoms less than five years, forced vital capacity greater than 60% and aged less than 75 years."[6]

Summary and Implications: This observational study suggests that riluzole has a time-dependent effect on ALS, with shorter treatment periods being associated with longer survival times. Riluzole's impact on survival appears to decline over time, with most of the benefit being derived within the first 6 months of treatment. After 18 months of riluzole treatment, the survival curves of riluzole-treated and untreated patients cross, indicating potential harm from continued treatment beyond this point.

CLINICAL CASE: DETERMINING HOW TO GET THE MOST OUT OF RILUZOLE

TR is a 54-year-old man diagnosed with ALS 2.5 years ago. At the time of diagnosis he was started on riluzole 50 mg orally every 12 hours. Now, upon hospice admission you are performing a medication reconciliation with TR and his caregiver. Before you can ask him what medications he is taking, the caregiver says: "You better not think about stopping his riluzole just so you can save money. That's the drug that has kept him alive for the past few years!"

Is this patient likely to continue to benefit from treatment with riluzole?

Suggested Answer

Based on the study by Cetin et al.,[1] the patient likely derived any survival benefit from riluzole within the first 6 months of treatment. The patient in this case scenario has ALS meeting hospice criteria and has been receiving riluzole for approximately 30 months. This is past the time point where the Kaplan-Meir curves crossed in similar studies, suggesting that continuing riluzole at this point may be associated with decreased survival.[2–5]

Given the perceived importance of riluzole to the family and the limited treatment options available for ALS, the hospice clinician performing the medication reconciliation will need to establish trust and should assess the family's willingness to receive additional information about the value of riluzole at this point in TR's journey. It may be helpful to highlight that TR has likely gotten all the benefit he can from this medication—in other words, riluzole may no longer be providing him protection, and continued use may be causing more harm than benefit. The patient, family, and clinical care team will need to consider these data in the context that we don't fully understand some of the reasons why this unique situation occurs but that data continue to emerge questioning the optimal time and duration of treatment.[6]

Overall, while riluzole cannot stop or reverse the progressive nature of ALS, evidence has shown that it can prolong survival in people with ALS by 2–3 months and that the timing of treatment and diagnosis of ALS plays a key role in obtaining positive outcomes.[7] Each decision will need to be individualized based on patient-specific factors (e.g., stage of disease, comorbidities).

References

1. Cetin H, Rath J, Füzi J, Reichardt B, et al. Epidemiology of amyotrophic lateral sclerosis and effect of riluzole on disease course. *Neuroepidemiology.* 2015;44(1):6–15. doi:10.1159/000369813. Epub 2015 Jan 7. PMID: 25571962.
2. Traynor BJ, Alexander M, Corr B, Frost E, Hardiman O. An outcome study of riluzole in amyotrophic lateral sclerosis—a population-based study in Ireland, 1996–2000. *J Neurol.* 2003 Apr;250(4):473–479. doi:10.1007/s00415-003-1026-z. PMID: 12700914.
3. Zoccolella S, Beghi E, Palagano G, et al. Riluzole and amyotrophic lateral sclerosis survival: a population-based study in southern Italy. *Eur J Neurol.* 2007;14:262–268.
4. Lee CT, Chiu YW, Wang KC, et al. Riluzole and prognostic factors in amyotrophic lateral sclerosis longterm and short-term survival: a population based study of 1149 cases in Taiwan. *J Epidemiol.* 2013;23:35–40.
5. Bensimon G, Lacomblez L, Delumeau JC, Bejuit R, Truffinet P, Meininger V. A study of riluzole in the treatment of advanced stage or elderly patients with amyotrophic lateral sclerosis. *J Neurol.* 2002;249:609–615.
6. Thakore NJ, Lapin BR, Mitsumoto H, Pooled Resource Open-Access ALS Clinical Trials Consortium. Early initiation of riluzole may improve absolute survival in amyotrophic lateral sclerosis. *Muscle Nerve.* 2022 Sep 18. doi:10.1002/mus.27724. Epub ahead of print. PMID: 36117390.
7. Miller RG, Mitchell JD, Moore DH. Riluzole for amyotrophic lateral sclerosis (ALS)/ motor neuron disease (MND). *Cochrane Database Syst Rev.* 2012;(3):CD001447. Published 2012 Mar 14. doi:10.1002/14651858.CD001447.pub3.

28

Topical Lorazepam, Diphenhydramine, and Haloperidol for Nausea in Cancer Patients

MARY LYNN MCPHERSON

> Although ABH [Ativan, Benadryl, Haldol] gel is relatively inexpensive, widely used, and easy to apply in patients who cannot take oral medications, it has no scientific basis for continued use for treatment of nausea in cancer patients based on these pharmacologic and clinical studies.
>
> —FLETCHER ET AL.[1]

Research Question: Using a noninferiority clinical trial approach, to determine any difference in the effectiveness of Ativan, Benadryl, Haldol (ABH) versus a placebo gel in the treatment of nausea in patients with cancer.

Funding: This work was supported by the American Cancer Society (Grant No. PEP 10-174-01) (T. J. Smith).

Year Study Began: Not indicated

Year Study Published: 2014

Study Location: Virginia Commonwealth University

Who Was Studied: Patients 18 years or older with a current diagnosis of cancer, and a self-reported nausea score of at least 4 of 10, able to complete a medical screening questionnaire, and with no allergies to ingredient medications. Patients also could not have had changes to their antiemetic regimen within the past 12 hours nor received any chemotherapy in the past 5 days (unless it was a stable oral chemotherapy drug).

Who Was Excluded: Patients not meeting the inclusion criteria.

How Many Patients: 40

Study Overview: This was a randomized, double-blind, placebo-controlled, noninferiority trial. Participants were randomized to 1 of 2 sequences of treatments: ABH gel first, then placebo, versus placebo gel first, then ABG gel. Randomization was done by the investigational drug pharmacy. Patients self-rated their nausea on a 0–10 scale before intervention and 1 hour after each intervention (Figure 28.1).

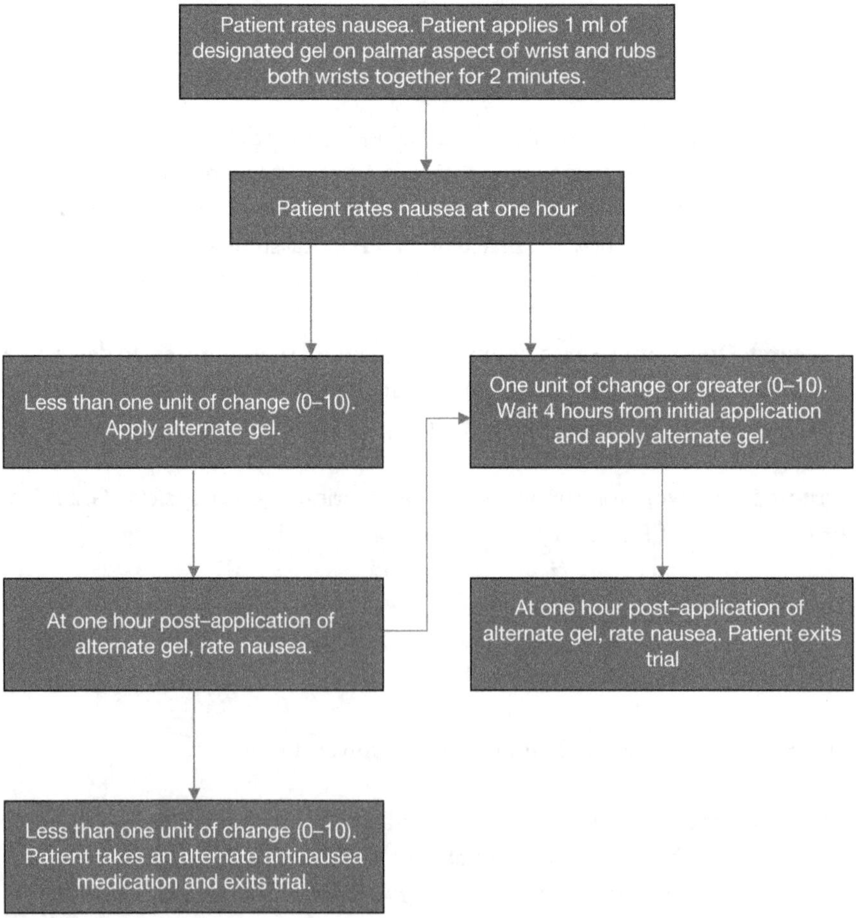

Figure 28.1. Noninferiority trial methods.

Study Intervention: Study gel (ABH) consisted of lorazepam (20 mg), diphenhydramine (250 mg), haloperidol (20 mg), lecithin organogel (2 mL), ethoxydiglycol (0.83 mL), water (0.2 mL) and pluronic gel (20%). Placebo gel was pluronic lecithin organogel alone. Usual medical care was given throughout this study. Twenty patients completed both arms of the study.

Follow-up: 2–5 hours

Endpoints: The primary endpoint was the difference in the patient's self-rated nausea score from baseline to 1 hour after treatment application. Secondary outcomes included completion of the Memorial Symptom Assessment Scale-Condensed (MSAS-C), number of vomiting episodes, and side effects from treatment application.

RESULTS

Primary Outcome:

The placebo gel was shown to be noninferior to the ABH gel.

Measure	ABH Gel	Placebo Gel	Significance
Mean change in nausea score from baseline to 60 minutes	1.7 ± 2.05	0.9 ± 2.45	*P* = .42

- Difference in the change between the 2 treatment groups was 0.8 ± 3.25; 95% CI: –0.72 to 2.32.
- Noninferiority test assessed by paired *t*-test, *P* = .0115.

Secondary Outcomes:

- ABH gel did not decrease vomiting events better than placebo (*P* = .34).
- No side effects were reported by 20/21 patients in the active treatment arm (1 patient reported drowsiness).
- Only 1 patient stated a change in MASA-C score attributable to study gels.
- 14/21 (66.67%) of patients said "no" when asked if the treatment was effective; 7/21 reported "yes" (similar to the placebo response).
- Only 9/16 patients could correctly identify the active treatment; 7/16 could not.

Criticisms and Limitations:

- This trial wasn't adequately powered to meaningfully assess the risks and benefits of ABG gel.
- The study did not specify the etiology the nausea, making it hard to interpret the findings in real-world practice.

Other Relevant Studies and Information:

- Not all medications are suitable for systemic absorption when applied topically or transdermally.[2,3] Factors that affect drug delivery include the drug's partition coefficient, molecular size, solubility/melting point, ionization, diffusion coefficient, and physiochemical properties of the drug delivery system.[2]
- The results of this noninferiority study in patients with cancer are unsurprising because a previous study evaluated the absorption and systemic serum levels obtained by application of the same ABH active treatment in 10 healthy volunteers. No lorazepam or haloperidol was detected in any blood sample from any of the 10 volunteers (samples drawn at 0, 30, 60, 90, 120, 180, and 240 minutes postapplication). Five of the 10 volunteers had a detectable diphenhydramine level in 1 or more samples, but it was a subtherapeutic concentration and highly erratic.[4]
- Hospice and palliative care practitioners would really like this topical formulation to be effective in treating nausea, where oral medication administration is not practical and parenteral administration is more invasive. Despite evidence to the contrary, providers have a strong history of recommending topical ABH (and sometimes ABHR, where R stands for Reglan [metoclopramide]) for nausea in serious or advanced illness. One study reported in excess of 11 000 prescriptions for 8 600 hospice patients over a 1-year period.[5]
- Nausea can be a very complicated complaint, involving a variety of potential neurotransmitters and receptors (e.g., acetylcholine, histamine, serotonin, dopamine). It would be more prudent to do a careful symptom assessment and select an antinausea medication that most likely targets the cause instead of combining a cocktail of antinausea medications in hopes that 1 or more of the medications will provide relief.
- There is no advantage to guideline management of nausea and vomiting in advanced cancer patients compared with single-agent

haloperidol based on a recently published randomized trial.[1] There are no randomized trials of single versus multiple antiemetics, so sequential trials of single antiemetics should be the standard approach to managing nausea in advanced cancer.[6]

- The Multinational Association of Supportive Care in Cancer guidelines updated in 2021 recommend oral or parenteral metoclopramide or haloperidol as first-line therapy and methotrimeprazine and olanzapine as second-line antiemetics for nausea and/or vomiting in advanced cancer.[7]

Summary and Implications: ABH gel is poorly absorbed via topical administration in healthy volunteers. When administered to cancer patients with nausea, ABH gel was no better than placebo gel in relieving symptoms. If the medications are not absorbed, it seems reasonable that there is a low likelihood of therapeutic success. Continuing to encourage use of a medical intervention without supporting evidence is inappropriate, and use should be discouraged.

CLINICAL CASE: NAUSEA IS THE WORST FEELING IN THE WORLD!

NV is a 52-year-old man with non–small cell lung cancer who has been experiencing nausea and vomiting for several weeks. He has not received any chemotherapy or radiation for the past several weeks and is not constipated, although he is taking scheduled low-dose opioids. He denies nausea with position changes or any relationship to meals. He has no notable chemical or metabolic imbalances. On examination his vital signs are normal, bowel sounds are present, and there is no evidence of dehydration. "Can't you do something about this nausea?" he asks. "This is a miserable way to live. Anything that goes in my stomach threatens to come right back up!" Would you recommend ABH topical gel for NV?

Suggested Answer

Based on the evidence reviewed in this chapter, it is unlikely that topical lorazepam, diphenhydramine, or haloperidol would be sufficiently absorbed systemically to provide NV any relief. NV's symptoms do not give us a particular clue as to the neurotransmitters involved in the nausea he is experiencing. Barring that, antidopaminergic agents have been shown to be useful in treating nausea that is likely due to stimulation of the chemoreceptor trigger zone.[8]

Given NV's nausea, however, it would be preferable to avoid the oral route of administration. One option is prochlorperazine by rectum, which may not be met with great enthusiasm from the patient. Another alternative is administration of oral haloperidol by high concentrate solution (2 mg/mL) in the buccal cavity. It would be reasonable to start with 0.5 or 1 mg of haloperidol, which would be a very small volume and hopefully would not worsen the nausea. A third option is use of the 5-mg oral disintegrating tablet of olanzapine. The use of olanzapine to treat nausea in cancer patients has also been reviewed in this publication.[9]

The bottom line is that a careful symptom assessment should be done and antinausea medications selected that best target the cause of the nausea and vomiting. While topical administration is not feasible, we have several other options short of parenteral administration.

References

1. Fletcher DS, Coyne PJ, Dodson PW, Parker GG, Wan W, Smith TJ. A randomized trial of the effectiveness of topical "ABH Gel" (Ativan(®), Benadryl(®), Haldol(®)) vs. placebo in cancer patients with nausea. *J Pain Symptom Manage.* 2014;48(5):797–803. doi:10.1016/j.jpainsymman.2014.02.010.
2. Marwah H, Garg T, Goyal AK, Rath G. Permeation enhancer strategies in transdermal drug delivery. *Drug Deliv.* 2016;23(2):564–578. doi:10.3109/10717544.2014.935532.
3. Paudel KS, Milewski M, Swadley CL, Brogden NK, Ghosh P, Stinchcomb AL. Challenges and opportunities in dermal/transdermal delivery. *Ther Deliv.* 2010;1(1):109–131. doi:10.4155/tde.10.16.
4. Smith TJ, Ritter JK, Poklis JL, et al. ABH gel is not absorbed from the skin of normal volunteers. *J Pain Symptom Manage.* 2012;43(5):961–966. doi:10.1016/j.jpainsymman.2011.05.017.
5. Weschules DJ. Tolerability of the compound ABHR in hospice patients. *J Palliat Med.* 2005;8(6):1135–1143. doi:10.1089/jpm.2005.8.1135.
6. Hardy J, Skerman H, Glare P, et al. A randomized open-label study of guideline-driven antiemetic therapy versus single agent antiemetic therapy in patients with advanced cancer and nausea not related to anticancer treatment. *BMC Cancer.* 2018;18(1):510.
7. Davis M, Hui D, Davies A, et al. MASCC antiemetics in advanced cancer updated guideline. *Support Care Cancer.* 2021;29(12):8097–8107.
8. Henson LA, Maddocks M, Evans C, Davidson M, Hicks S, Higginson IJ. Palliative care and the management of common distressing symptoms in advanced cancer: pain, breathlessness, nausea and vomiting, and fatigue. *J Clin Oncol.* 2020;38(9):905–914. doi:10.1200/JCO.19.00470.
9. Navari RM, Pywell CM, Le-Rademacher JG, et al. Olanzapine for the treatment of advanced cancer-related chronic nausea and/or vomiting: a randomized pilot trial. *JAMA Oncol.* 2020;6(6):895–899. doi:10.1001/jamaoncol.2020.1052.

29

Gabapentin for Uremic Itching

LYDIA MIS AND ARIF KAMAL

> Studies in this review showed the efficacy of gabapentin in the treatment of uremic pruritus.
>
> —EUSEBIO-ALPAPARA ET AL.[1]

Research Question: Is gabapentin an effective pharmacologic intervention for uremic pruritus?

Funding: None

Year Study Began: 2003–2016

Year Study Published: 2020

Study Location: Articles indexed worldwide

Who Was Studied: Randomized trials of adult patients with chronic kidney disease on hemodialysis who were treated with gabapentin for uremic pruritus.

Who Was Excluded: Pilot studies, reviews, protocols, editorials, and non–randomized controlled trial clinical studies.

How Many Patients: 315 participants across 7 studies

Study Overview: See Figure 29.1. The authors conducted a systematic review and meta-analysis that included:

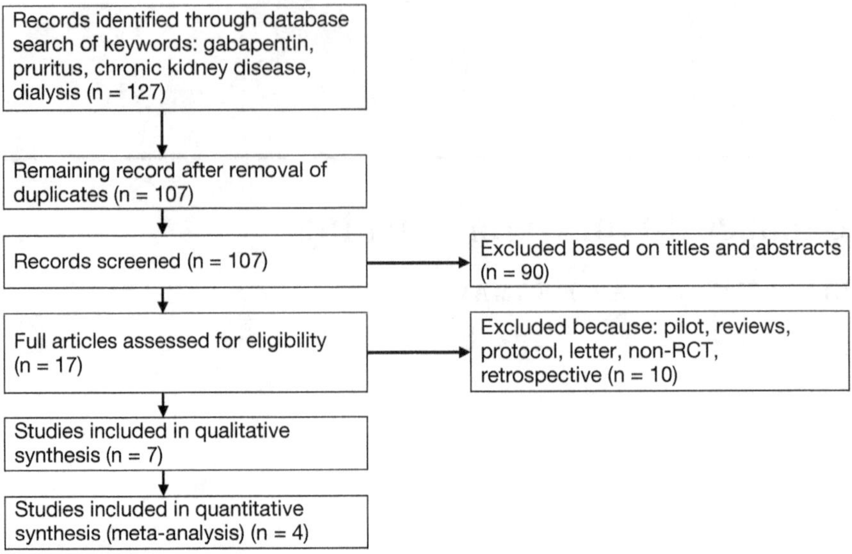

Figure 29.1. Study selection process.

- Five randomized, double-blind controlled trials
- One randomized, single-blind clinical trial
- One open-label, prospective, randomized clinical trial

Study Intervention: Gabapentin 100 mg daily or gabapentin 100–400 mg given 2–4 times weekly after dialysis (compared to placebo or an active comparator).

Follow-Up: 2–4 weeks

Endpoints:

- The primary endpoint was pruritus reduction by ≥ 50% as measured using a pruritus visual analog scale in patients on dialysis receiving gabapentin as compared to placebo or comparator agent.
- Secondary outcomes were the incidence of adverse drug effects due to study medication.

RESULTS

- Gabapentin at a dose of at least 300 mg was either as effective as or superior to other comparators (pregabalin, hydroxyzine, dexchlorpheniramine) or placebo with respect to reducing pruritus scores as shown in Table 29.1.
- One study of gabapentin 100 mg daily versus ketotifen 1 mg twice daily demonstrated no overall difference in pruritus scores as shown in Table 29.1.

Table 29.1 STUDIES INCLUDED IN QUALITATIVE SYNTHESIS

Study	**Sample Size**	**Gabapentin Dosage**	**Comparator**	**Notable Outcome**
Gobo-Oliveira et al.[2]	60	300 mg 3 times weekly after HD	Dexchlorpheniramine 6 mg twice daily	Significant reduction in pruritus scores in both groups from baseline with no significant difference between comparators
Amirkhalou et al.[3]	52	100 mg daily	Ketotifen 1 mg twice daily	Significant decrease in pruritus scores, but overall no difference between the groups; gabapentin significantly better in males aged 30–60 years old ($P = .008$)
Nofal et al.[4]	54	100–300 mg 3 times weekly after HD	Placebo	The mean pruritus VAS scores decreased from 7.6 to 1.8 in the gabapentin group and from 6.9 to 6.8 in the placebo group ($P = .001$)
Solak et al.[5]	50	300 mg 3 times weekly after HD	Pregabalin 75 mg daily	Significant decrease in pruritus scores from baseline in both groups but no significant difference between comparators
Noshad and Nazari[6]	40	100–200 mg 4 times weekly after HD	Hydroxyzine 10 mg/day 4 times per week	At end of 4 weeks, only 10% of gabapentin patients had pruritus vs. 80% in the hydroxyzine group
Naini et al.[7]	34	400 mg 2 times weekly after HD	Placebo	From baseline mean pruritus score of 7.2 (range: 3–10), mean pruritus scores decreased by 6.7 in the gabapentin group and 1.5 in the placebo group ($P < .001$)
Gunal et al.[8]	25	300 mg 3 times weekly after HD	Placebo	Gabapentin superior: 96% had pruritus reduced with 16% by ≥ 50%

Abbreviations: HD, hemodialysis; VAS, visual analog scale.

Criticisms and Limitations:

- Of the 7 studies included in the meta-analysis, 4 (57%) had moderate and 2 (29%) had high risk of bias.
- There was significant variability in the dosing and frequency of gabapentin, and the optimal dosing of gabapentin for treating pruritus is uncertain.

Other Relevant Studies and Information:

- Rayner et al. studied the effect of gabapentin or pregabalin in a consecutive cohort study in 71 patients with refractory pruritus.[9] Patients were initiated on gabapentin and offered pregabalin if intolerant of gabapentin. Gabapentin relieved itching in 47 patients (66%). Pregabalin was offered to 16 of the 21 patients intolerant of gabapentin, with 81% of patients experiencing relief of pruritus. Overall, gabapentin or pregabalin relieved itching in 85% of patients.
- Ravindran et al. studied the effect of gabapentin 100 mg or pregabalin 25 mg in a randomized single-blind prospective-interventional study.[10] Both gabapentin and pregabalin significantly decreased itching intensity ($P < .001$). While there was no statistically significant difference in efficacy, gabapentin was associated with statistically significantly more adverse effects, with 11 of 21 patients (52.3%) experiencing fatigue, dizziness, or somnolence ($P \leq .001$).

Summary and Implications: Pruritus is a distressful symptom experienced by many patients receiving regular hemodialysis. In this meta-analysis and systematic review of randomized controlled trials comparing gabapentin to other agents for the treatment of this condition, the results favored gabapentin, with a lower pooled incidence of uremic pruritus, and a similar adverse effect profile compared to the comparators. The authors of this analysis suggest treating patients with dialysis-related pruritus with gabapentin, initially at a dose of 100 mg 3 times weekly after dialysis (which was effective in some of the included studies) and gradually titrating up to find the optimal dose for each patient with respect to efficacy and tolerability.

CLINICAL CASE: REDUCING IRRITABLE ITCHING

Case History

A 70-year-old man receives 3 times weekly, facility-based hemodialysis for stage V chronic kidney disease. He reports 8/10 pruritus, particularly in his arms and legs, throughout much of the day. His comorbidities include insulin-dependent diabetes, which has been complicated by vision changes and numbness and tingling in his fingers and toes. He is interested in a pharmacologic option for management of the pruritus.

Suggested Answer

The systematic review by Eusebio-Alpapara et al. presents several positive individual studies and pooled analysis highlighting the efficacy and safety of gabapentin for management of uremic pruritus. Studies were dose adjusted for low renal function and ranged from 100 to 300 mg after each dialysis session. For patients not tolerant to gabapentin, 2 studies demonstrate a role for pregabalin. Overall, the number needed to treat from studies suggest high efficacy, with high likelihood of benefit at the individual patient level.

References

1. Eusebio-Alpapara KMV, Castillo RL, Dofitas BL. Gabapentin for uremic pruritus: a systematic review of randomized controlled trials. *Int J Derm.* 2020;59:412–422. doi:10.1111/ijd.14708.
2. Gobo-Oliveria M, Pigari VG, Ogata MS, et al. Gabapentin versus dexchlorpheniramine as treatment for uremic pruritus: a randomized controlled trial. *Eur J Dermatol.* 2018;28:488–495.
3. Amirkhalou S, Rashedi A, Taherian J, et al. Comparison of gabapentin and ketotifen in treatment of uremic pruritus in hemodialysis patients. *Pak J Med Sci.* 2016;32:22–26.
4. Nofal E, Farag F, Nofal A, et al. Gabapentin: a promising therapy for uremic pruritus in hemodialysis patient: a randomized-controlled trial and review of literature. *J Dermatolog Treat.* 2016;27:515.
5. Solak Y, Biyik Z, Atalay H, et al. Pregabalin versus gabapentin in the treatment of neuropathic pruritus in maintenance haemodialysis patients: a prospective, crossover study. *Nephrology.* 2012;17:710–717. doi:10.1111/j.1440-1797.2012.01655.x.

6. Noshad H, Nazari KS. Comparison of gabapentin and an antihistamine in the treatment of uremic pruritus and its psychological problems. *J Urmia Univ Med Sci.* 2010;21:286–292.
7. Naini A, Harandi A, Khanbabapour S, et al. A promising drug for treatment of uremic pruritus. Saudi Center of transplantation. *J Kidney Dis Transplant.* 2007;18:378–381.
8. Gunal AI, Ozalp G, Yoldas TK, et al. Gabapentin therapy for pruritus in hemodialysis patients: a randomized, placebo-controlled, double-blind trial. *Nephrol Dial Transplant.* 2004;19:3137–3139.
9. Rayner H, Haharani J, Smith S, Suresh V, Dasgupta I. Uraemia pruritus: relief of itching by gabapentin and pregabalin. *Nephron Clin Pract.* 2012;122:75–79. doi:10.1159/000349943.
10. Ravindran A, Kunnath RP, Sunny A, Vimal B. Comparison of safety and efficacy of pregabalin versus gabapentin for the treatment of uremic pruritus in patients with chronic kidney disease on maintenance haemodialysis. *Indian J Palliat Care.* 2020;26(3):281–286. doi10.4103/IJPC.IJPC_212_19.

30

Treatment of Malodorous Tumors With Topical Metronidazole

LYDIA MIS AND ARIF KAMAL

> In summary, this clinical study showed that MTZ 0.75% gel is safe and highly effective in reducing the intensity of malodors from fungating wounds in breast cancer patients. After 14 days of application, the drug increased levels of satisfaction among the patients, their families, and medical personnel.
>
> —WATANABE ET AL.[1]

Research Question: Can application of metronidazole (MTZ) 0.75% gel to malodorous tumors successfully decrease purulent exudate, odor, pain, and microbial growth and improve patient quality of life (QOL) with acceptable side effects?

Funding: Funded by Galderma. All study drugs were provided by Galderma Company, Tokyo, Japan.

Year Study Began: April 2012

Year Study Published: 2015

Study Location: Japan (multiple centers)

Who Was Studied: Patients aged ≥ 20 years with fungating wounds ± infection; malodor ≥ 2 (scale 0–4); skin ulceration requiring daily dose ≤ 30 g MTZ 0.75%

gel; Eastern Cooperative Oncology Group (ECOG) performance status ≤ 3; anticipated survival ≥ 3 months.

Who Was Excluded: Patients who received systemic antibiotics within 2 weeks prior to study; other topical treatments to wound; anticipated change in concurrent cancer therapy; wounds not in contact with tumor; wounds invading bone; allergy to MTZ; concurrent alcohol or interacting medications.

How Many Patients: 21

Study Overview: This was an uncontrolled pre-/postevaluation (Figure 30.1).

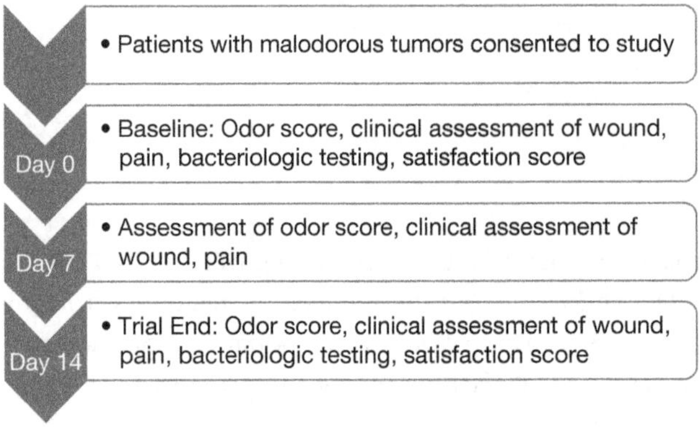

Figure 30.1. Summary of trial's design.

Study Intervention: MTZ 0.75% gel was applied 1–2 times daily up to a maximum of 30 g daily for 14 days. The fungating wounds were cleaned and covered with appropriate dressing material. Odor was scored by patients and investigators (or nurses or study coordinators), and wounds were clinically examined for the amount and type of exudate and scored based on the frequency of needed dressing changes. Pain was assessed using a 100-mm visual analog scale (VAS). Bacteriologic testing was performed at baseline and at the end of the study for identification and quantification of causal bacteria. Patients were given a survey at baseline and the conclusion of the study to categorize the change in satisfaction (markedly improved to worsened).

Follow-Up: Patients were followed for the duration of the study period (including a patient who discontinued treatment at 7 days).

Endpoints: The primary outcome was improvement of odor score. Secondary outcomes included clinical findings of fungating wounds, pain, bacteriologic findings, patient satisfaction, and pharmacokinetics (to determine extent of systemic absorption).

RESULTS

- Odor control to a score of 0 to 1 (0 = no smell, 1 = smell not offensive, slight smell about 20 cm from ulcer) was achieved in 95.2% of patients (20 of 21), as shown in Table 30.1. Scores between investigators and nurses were similar and higher than patient self-scores.
- Clinical examination of wounds demonstrated an overall decrease in purulent fluid drainage and an increase in serous fluid drainage.
- There was no significant change in pain as measured by VAS from baseline to day 7 or 14 of the trial period, as shown in Table 30.1.

Table 30.1 SUMMARY OF TRIAL'S INVESTIGATOR RESULTS

	Baseline *n* = 21	**Day 7** *n* = 21	**Day 14**[a] *n* = 20
Odor Score	Number (percentage, %)		
0	0	11 (52.4)	13 (61.9)
1	0	5 (52.4)	7 (33.3)
2	13 (61.9	2 (9.5)	0
3	3 14.3)	3 (14.3)	1 (4.8)
4	5 (23.8)	0	0
Clinical Characterization of Wound Drainage			
Purulent	6	ND	ND
Serous with blood	5	ND	ND
Serous	4	12	10
Patient Satisfaction	**Number (percentage, %)**		
Markedly improved			9 (42.9)
Moderately improved			6 (28.6)
Slightly improved			5 (23.8)
No change			1 (4.8)
Worsened			0
Pain			
VAS (± SD)	28.3 (± 29.1)	25.9 (± 27.1)[b]	22.2 (± 25.3)[b]

Abbreviations: VAS, visual analog scale; SD, standard deviation; ND, not described
[a] On day 14 or at the time of premature study discontinuation.
[b] No difference from day 7 to 14.

- There was a decrease in the numbers of anaerobic (odor-causing) bacteria from baseline to the end of the study period (42.9% to 4.8%, respectively), with no significant changes in the profiles of the aerobic bacteria.
- Patient satisfaction was improved by day 14, with 15 patients (71.4%) indicating satisfaction with topical MTZ 0.75% gel to control fungating tumor odor, as indicated in Table 30.1 by markedly or moderately improved.
- Pharmacokinetics demonstrated that there was wide variability in the amount of systemically absorbed MTZ, which did not exceed the systemic exposure of 250 mg MTZ orally as a single dose.
- Topical MTZ 0.75% gel was well tolerated except for 2 cases of bleeding due to removal of dried, adherent gel with the wound dressing changes.

Criticisms and Limitations: This was an open-label, noncontrolled, industry-sponsored trial in a very small number of patients. Thus, it is not clear from this study whether the MTZ gel caused the improvements in odor and patient satisfaction.

Additionally, while MTZ 0.75% gel was effective in decreasing odor by day 14, there was no follow-up at the conclusion of the trial to determine how long patients maintained this benefit, nor the frequency at which redosing (if needed) would be applied.

Other Relevant Studies and Information:

- Bower and colleagues evaluated a 0.8% MTZ gel for the treatment of open, malodorous fungating tumors using a VAS from 1 to 10.[2] There was a statistically significant improvement (investigator and patient report) in odor control without adverse effects.
- Peng and Dai found a significant decrease in wound malodor in patients using a combination of MTZ powder with an autolytic debridement gel as compared to silver sulfadiazine.[3]
- Case reports by Hu and colleagues reported an immediate decrease in odor in patients who crushed a 500-mg tablet and sprinkled the powder on the wounds.[4]
- Treatment of fungating malodorous wounds is often standardized per institution. Topical administration of MTZ as either crushed tablets or as topical 0.75%–1% gel is frequently utilized in patient-centered approaches.[1–5] Tolerability, application ease, and cost may dictate the formulation applied.

Summary and Implications: Topical use of MTZ 0.75% gel on fungating wounds decreased purulent drainage and increased serous fluid drainage through the decrease in the number of anaerobic bacteria from baseline to the end of the study.[1] Acceptable odor control was achieved in 95.2% of patients, and patient satisfaction improved.[1–5] Topical administration of MTZ is preferred over oral administration of MTZ due to the potential for nausea, vomiting, and alcohol intolerance, leading to poor patient satisfaction and QOL.

CLINICAL CASE: MALODOROUS SKIN TUMOR—METRONIDAZOLE GEL VERSUS POWDER

Case History

A patient presents with squamous cell cancer of the rectum complicated by progressive disease, recurrent Fournier gangrene, and recurrent polymicrobial skin infections due to resistant gram-negative and gram-positive aerobic and anaerobic organisms. The wound management team examined the wound and found scattered open-cratered lesions noted from the scrotum to the mons pubis. There was a moderate amount of yellow, foul drainage. Recommendations included nonstick dressings, protectant barriers, and MTZ application to scrotal lesions for odor control daily and dressing changes as needed. The patient is saturating his dressings multiple times daily, requiring frequent daily dressing changes. Odor is present only when doing dressing changes. Both MTX gel and tablets are on formulary. Which product would you recommend?

Suggested Answer

Both MTZ powder and gel significantly decrease odor associated with fungating tumors. The choice of either MTZ gel or tablets is based on availability, ease of application, and amount of drainage. MTZ gel application would be difficult as it would not adhere adequately to the wound as the drainage required frequent daily dressing changes. MTZ powder (crushed tablets or powder) is easy to sprinkle onto the wounds and absorbent dressings. Since the wounds were anterior, MTZ powder would be easy and affordable for the patient to use as an outpatient. Had the wounds been posterior, it would have been appropriate to apply gel directly to the dressing with application directly onto the wound.

References

1. Watanabe K, Shimo A, Tsugawa K, et al. Safe and effective deodorization of malodorous fungating tumors using topical metronidazole 0.75% gel (GK567): a multicenter, open-label, phase III study (RDT.07.SRE.27013). *Support Care Cancer.* 2016;24:2583–2590. doi:10.1007/s00520-015-3067-0.
2. Bower M, Stein R, Evans TRJ, et al. A double-blind study of the efficacy of metronidazole gel in the treatment of malodorous fungating tumours. *Eur J Cancer.* 1992;28A(4/5):888–889.
3. Peng L, Dai Y. Effect of metronidazole combined with autolytic debridement for the management of malignant wound malodor. *J Int Med Res.* 2019;48(4):1–7. doi:10.1177/0300060519889746.
4. Hu J, Ligtenberg K, Leventhal J, Bunick C. Successful management of malodor from fungating tumors using crushed metronidazole tablets. *JAAD Case Reports.* 2020;6:26–29. doi.org/10.1016/j.jdcr.2019.10.025.
5. Rupert K, Fehl A. A patient-centered approach for the treatment of fungating breast wounds. *J Adv Pract Oncol.* 2020;11(56):503–510.

31

The Effect of Cannabis on Appetite and Quality of Life in Patients With Cancer-Related Anorexia-Cachexia Syndrome

BALAKRISHNAN NATARAJAN AND BAVNA BHAGAVAT

> We found no differences between the three groups over 6 weeks of treatment for the primary end points of appetite and [quality of life], for cannabinoid-related toxicity, or for secondary end points such as mood or nausea.
>
> —Strasser et al.[1]

Research Question: In patients with cancer-related anorexia-cachexia syndrome (CACS), what are the effects of cannabis extract (CE), delta-9-tetrahydrocannabinol (THC), and placebo on appetite and quality of life and how do they compare with each other?

Funding: Institute for Clinical Research (Berlin, Germany)

Year Study Began: 1999

Year Study Published: 2006

Study Location: Division of Oncology/Hematology, Department of Internal Medicine, Cantonal Hospital, St. Gallen, Switzerland; Departments of Medical Oncology and Anesthesiology/Pain Management, University Hospital Charité, Central Campus; Institute for Clinical Research, Berlin; Department of Anesthesiology and Intensive Care, Friedrich-Schiller-University, Jena; and Medizinische Poliklinik, University, Hospital, Bonn, Germany

Who Was Studied: 243 adults with CACS with 5% involuntary weight loss within the past 6 months, estimated life expectancy of 3 months, Eastern Cooperative Oncology Group (ECOG) performance status (PS) of 2, unchanged antineoplastic therapy for 4 weeks, and unchanged supportive treatment for 1 week before baseline assessments.

Who Was Excluded: Patients unable to consent to research; unable to feed themselves; use of enteral/parenteral nutrition, anabolic agents, gestagens, cannabinoids, or corticosteroids (except for 20 mg prednisolone for 5 days) within the past month; or secondary anorexia or psychiatric disorder.

How Many Patients: 243

Study Overview: This is a multicenter, phase 3, double-blind, 3-arm, parallel-design, randomized controlled trial in which patients were randomized to receive either placebo, CE, or THC for a period of 6 weeks (Figure 31.1). Treatment allocation was done in a 1:2:2 ratio and stratified by center.

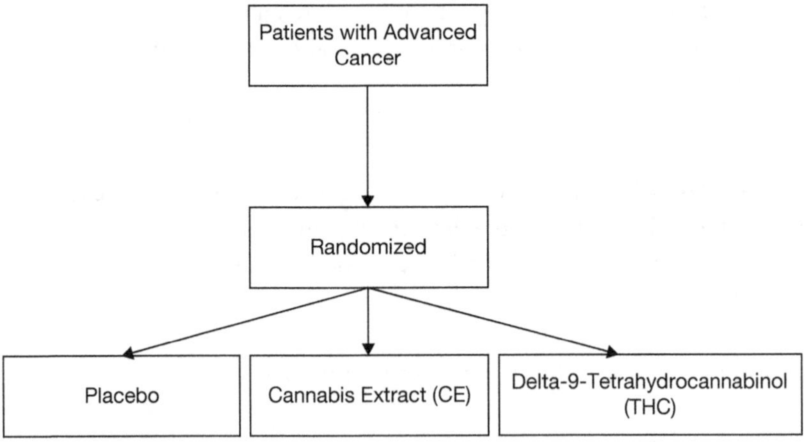

Figure 31.1. Summary of study design.

Study Intervention:

- Patients were randomized to twice-daily oral doses of either placebo, CE, or THC. Patients in the placebo arm received standardization medium capsules indistinguishable from the capsules used in the other treatment arms.

- Patients were assessed at initial screening, when treatment commenced (week 0), and at weeks 2, 4, and 6. Vital signs, ECOG PS, and urinary cannabinoids test were measured at each session.

Follow-Up: 6 weeks

Endpoints:

Primary outcomes: Appetite change from week 0 to 6 (mean of daily appetite visual analog scale [VAS] scores), change in QOL from baseline to week 6 (European Organization for Research and Treatment of Cancer Quality of Life Questionnaire C30 [EORTC QLQ-C30]).

Secondary outcomes: Weight, estimation of food intake during prior 24 hours, current nausea, mood.

Adverse events: Adverse effect hazard rate, anorexia-cachexia, and cannabinoid toxicity (CannTox).

RESULTS

- There were no significant differences in body weight between the treatment and placebo groups at baseline or week 6 (mean of 61 kg) or in weight loss (mean of 600 g in 6 weeks).
- All treatment arms indicated a 5% improvement in the overall score on the Anorexia-Cachexia EORTC QLQ-C30 module until week 2, and an additional 5% improvement until week 6 in the placebo group, steady state with THC, and worsening by 2.5% with CE. This was illustrated in the following parts of this assessment: physical, role, emotional, cognitive, social functioning, dyspnea, diarrhea, and financial problems.

Primary outcome:

- The mean overall QOL after 6 weeks was not significantly different between the CE, THC, and placebo groups (Table 31.1).
- The mean increase in appetite was comparable between the CE and placebo groups, and lower in the THC group. However, this was not clinically significant (Table 31.1).

Secondary outcome:

- Average weight loss among all patients recruited was 11.9%.
- No clinically significant improvement in nausea, mood, baseline body weight, week 6 body weight, or weight loss between groups was elicited (Table 31.1).

Table 31.1 SUMMARY OF KEY FINDINGS

Outcome	PL (n = 48)	CE (n = 95)	P Value	THC (n = 100)	P Value
Mean increase in appetite (mm ± SD)	5.8 ± 23.8	5.4 ± 24.7	.46	0.6 ± 18.5	.95
Quality of life (mean score change ± SD)	3.0 ± 19.5	1.1 ± 19.2	.80	5.1± 21.2	.43
Nausea improvement (% with VAS score < 30 mm)	40	61	.367	50	.367
Mood (%)	64	60	.461	46	.461

Abbreviations: CE, cannabis extract; PL, placebo; SD, standard deviation; THC, delta-9-tetrahydrocannabinol; VAS, visual analog scale.

Adverse effects:

- There were 526 adverse events in total, with CE having the largest number overall (n = 238), followed by THC (n = 197) and placebo (n = 91). Temporary or permanent dose reductions were necessary in 78 patients.
- Adverse effects that occurred more than 10 times in absolute frequency over all groups were nausea, fatigue, pain, anemia, vertigo, dyspnea, diarrhea, and obstipation.
- Of the adverse effects, 241 were mild, 227 were moderate, 57 were severe, and 1 was undetermined.
- Severe adverse events were dizziness, nausea/vomiting, and dyspnea.

Criticisms and Limitations:

- This study ended at 6 weeks, potentially masking the benefit of THC or CE over a longer period.
- Other limitations included a 20% dropout rate, small sample size, and early trial closure due to insufficient differences between study arms.

Other Relevant Studies and Information:

- With respect to appetite increase, the Jatoi trial[2] illustrated that megestrol acetate alone was significantly superior to dronabinol and the combination therapy (megestrol acetate and dronabinol). No statistical difference in severity of nausea or vomiting was present between the megestrol acetate and dronabinol treatment arms.

- Regarding QOL, (anorexia-specific Functional Assessment of Anorexia/Cachexia Therapy [FAACT-AN]) scores were significantly greater in the megestrol acetate–treated group versus the dronabinol-treated group.
- In the THC treatment arm of the Brisbois trial,[3] patients reported clinically significant improvements in appetite, taste, and protein consumption.
- Patients were allowed to modify their own THC doses and take a higher THC dose in the Brisbois trial,[3] unlike this Strasser trial,[1] which may have influenced an increased appetite and caloric intake, more than a standardized low dose in the Strasser trial.[1]
- The 2020 American Society of Clinical Oncology (ASCO) guideline[4] on the management of cancer cachexia recommended that there is insufficient evidence to strongly support cannabinoids.

Summary and Implications: This was the first phase 3 trial in patients with CACS, comparing the effects of CE with placebo and THC.[1] Over 6 weeks of treatment, there were no statistically significant differences between the 3 groups in appetite, QOL, mood, nausea, or cannabinoid-related toxicity. Unlike in HIV patients, there is currently no significant evidence to suggest a benefit of CE or THC in improving appetite and QOL in patients with advanced cancer experiencing cachexia. With the increasing availability of THC and cannabidiol products, more extensive studies with a larger sample size are needed.

CLINICAL CASE: IS THERE AN INDICATION FOR CANNABINOIDS IN PALLIATION OF APPETITE AND QOL IN PATIENTS WITH CANCER-RELATED ANOREXIA-CACHEXIA SYNDROME?

Case History

A 52-year-old female diagnosed with cervical cancer has received 2 out of three 21-day cycles of topotecan and cisplatin chemotherapy.[5] She has a body mass index of 24 kg/m^2 and a 6% weight loss over the past year. She reports decreased appetite. Physical exam is notable for loss of bulk and atrophy of the bilateral temporalis, deltoid, and quadriceps muscles. She has an ECOG PS of 2.

Should this patient receive cannabinoids to stimulate her appetite?

Suggested Answer

The Strasser trial investigated the effect of CE (cannabidiol + THC), THC, and placebo on appetite and QOL in patients with CACS.

The Strasser trial did not demonstrate significant evidence to support the recommendation of cannabinoids for palliation of appetite and QOL. Some evidence is present that suggests a benefit of THC in improving chemosensory alterations according to the Brisbois trial, which can encourage increased food intake; however, this trial is limited based on sample size. Significant improvements in appetite[6] and caloric intake[7] are present in HIV patients, although evidence is low quality.[8]

Based on the above studies, ASCO guidelines[4] do not recommend cannabinoids or any other pharmacologic agent in directly treating cancer-related cachexia. Thus, this patient should not receive cannabinoids.

References

1. Strasser F, Luftner D, Possinger K, et al. Comparison of orally administered cannabis extract and delta-9-tetrahydrocannabinol in treating patients with cancer-related anorexia-cachexia syndrome: a multicenter, phase III, randomized, double-blind, placebo-controlled clinical trial from the Cannabis-In-Cachexia-Study-Group. *J Clin Oncol.* 2006;24(21):3394–3400.
2. Jatoi A, Windschitl HE, Loprinzi CL, et al. Dronabinol versus megestrol acetate versus combination therapy for cancer-associated anorexia: a North Central Cancer Treatment Group study. *J Clin Oncol.* 2002;20(2):567–573.
3. Brisbois TD, de Kock IH, Watanabe SM, et al. Delta-9-tetrahydrocannabinol may palliate altered chemosensory perception in cancer patients: results of a randomized, double-blind, placebo-controlled pilot trial. *Ann Oncol.* 2011;22(9):2086–2093.
4. Roeland EJ, Bohlke K, Baracos VE, et al. Management of cancer cachexia: ASCO guideline. *J Clin Oncol.* 2020;38(21):2438–2453.
5. Dillon EL, Basra G, Horstman AM, et al. Cancer cachexia and anabolic interventions: a case report. *J Cachexia Sarcopenia Muscle.* 2012;3(4):253–263.
6. Beal JE, Olson R, Laubenstein L, et al. Dronabinol as a treatment for anorexia associated with weight loss in patients with AIDS. *J Pain Symptom Manage.* 1995;10(2):89–97.
7. Haney M, Gunderson EW, Rabkin J, et al. Dronabinol and marijuana in HIV-positive marijuana smokers. Caloric intake, mood, and sleep. *J Acquir Immune Defic Syndr.* 2007;45(5):545–554.
8. Mucke M, Weier M, Carter C, et al. Systematic review and meta-analysis of cannabinoids in palliative medicine. *J Cachexia Sarcopenia Muscle.* 2018;9(2):220–234.

32

Olanzapine for the Treatment of Advanced Cancer-Related Chronic Nausea and/or Vomiting

CINDY NGUYEN

> Olanzapine significantly reduced nausea and vomiting after 1 day and 7 days of treatment initiation and is relatively well tolerated.
>
> —Navari et al.[1]

Research Question: Does olanzapine decrease nausea/vomiting, unrelated to chemotherapy, in patients with advanced cancer?

Funding: National Cancer Institute of the National Institutes of Health under award no. UG1CA189823 to the Alliance for Clinical Trials in Oncology NCI Community Oncology Research Program Research Base

Year Study Began: 2017

Year Study Published: 2020

Study Location: Mayo Clinic Rochester, Minnesota; University of Indiana, Indianapolis, Indiana; University of Alabama, Birmingham, Alabama; Washington University, St. Louis, Missouri

Who Was Studied: Adult patients with malignant disease in an advanced, incurable stage with at least 1 week of chronic nausea (worst daily score of > 3 on a 0–10 numeric rating scale).

Who Was Excluded: Patients who received chemotherapy or radiotherapy during the previous 14 days, antipsychotic medications within the last 30 days, or any of the previously mentioned planned during the study's duration.

How Many Patients: 30

Study Overview: This study is a double-blind, randomized, placebo-controlled clinical trial of participants receiving an assigned study treatment in addition to rescue antiemetics for persistent nausea and/or vomiting. Baseline evaluation assessed the intensity of appetite, nausea, fatigue, sedation, pain, and well-being on a 0–10 numeric rating scale (0 indicated the best possible, 10 the worst possible). Subsequently, each day for 7 days, the intensity of symptoms was recorded, including the number of emesis episodes in the previous 24 hours, medication administration, and any rescue medications utilized (Figure 32.1).

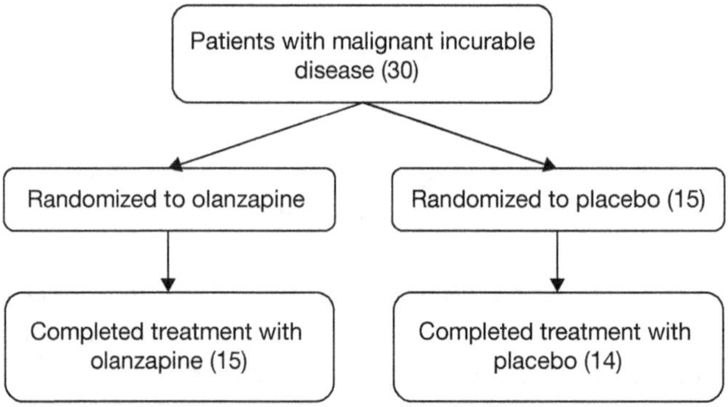

Figure 32.1. Summary of study design.

Study Intervention: Olanzapine (5 mg) or placebo, orally, daily for 7 days

Follow-up: 7 days

Endpoints: Patient-reported outcomes were collected at baseline and daily for 7 additional days. The study trial's primary objective was the estimated effect of olanzapine and placebo on chronic nausea and vomiting. The primary endpoints were the change in nausea score, based on a numerical scale, from baseline to day 7 of treatment. The emesis episodes were recorded from baseline and daily for

7 days after each study participant's treatment initiation. Additional endpoints collected were the numerical rating scores of nausea, appetite, fatigue, sedation, pain, and well-being.

RESULTS

- After day 1 and day 7 of placebo or olanzapine, the median nausea scores in the placebo arm were 9 out of 10 (range, 8–10) on both days and in the olanzapine arm were 2 out of 10 (range, 2–3) on day 1 and 1 out of 10 (range, 0–3) on day 7 (Table 32.1).
- The intervention group receiving olanzapine 5 mg daily had statistically significantly reduced nausea scores than the control group by 8 points ($P < .001$).
- The intervention group reported less emesis, less use of rescue medications, better appetite, less sedation, less fatigue, and better well-being (Table 32.1).

Table 32.1 SUMMARY OF STUDY'S KEY FINDINGS

	Median (Range) Olanzapine Arm (n = 15)	Placebo Arm (n = 15)	Difference Between Arms Effect Estimate (95% CI)	P Value
Nausea scores (NRS): 0 indicated the best possible, 10 the worst possible				
Baseline	9 (9–10)	9 (8–10)		.87
Day 1	2 (2–3)	9 (8–10)		
Day 7	1 (0–3)	9 (8–10)		
Δ of day 0 to day 7	−8 (−10 to −6)	−1 (−2 to 1)	−8 (−8 to −7)	< .001
Vomiting episodes/day: Higher values indicate worse quality of life				
Baseline	2 (1–5)	3 (2–4)		
Day 1	0 (0–0)	2 (1–3)		
Day 7	0 (0–0)	2 (1–3)		
Δ of day 0 to day 7	−2 (−5 to −1)	−1 (−3 to 1)	−2 (−2 to −1)	.001
Rescue antiemetic doses/day: Higher values indicate worse quality of life				
Baseline	2 (0–2)	2 (1 to > 2)		N/A[b]
Day 1	0 (0–0)	2 (1–2)		
Day 7	0 (0–1)	1.5 (1 to > 2)		
Δ of day 0 to day 7	−2 (−2 to 0)	1[a]	N/A[b]	N/A[b]

[a] Range not calculated due to 1 patient reporting > 2.0 doses at baseline and day 7.
[b] CIs and P values not available due to patient being given the option of choosing "> 2 antiemetic doses per day," which they chose.

- Following the 7 days of the study trial, the protocol code was broken and patients were permitted to receive olanzapine prescriptions from their clinicians and continue treatment. The study investigators followed up with the patient's clinicians and found that every patient in the treatment group continued olanzapine with efficacy and none reported any adverse drug events at weeks 3–12. Additionally, 93% of the placebo group patients started on olanzapine therapy after the study protocol concluded.

Criticisms and Limitations:

- This study's small sample size warrants the need for a larger study to determine the broader utility and significance of olanzapine for chronic nausea and vomiting in advanced cancer.
- Baseline differences in cancer types, disease, and treatments were not studied to determine the efficacy of olanzapine for specific cancer types.
- The implication of long-term use of olanzapine is unknown. This study followed patients for 7 days, and it is unclear if there are concerns for adverse effects, including sedation, with long-term use > 7 days.

Other Relevant Studies and Information:

- Prior to this study, Navari et al. studied the efficacy and safety of olanzapine 10 mg compared to placebo, which demonstrated favorable results for nausea prevention for patients receiving highly emetogenic chemotherapy. However, some patients in the treatment group experienced increased sedation.[2] Following evidence of this, future studies explored the utility of low-dose olanzapine 5 mg to prevent chemotherapy-associated nausea and vomiting while minimizing associated adverse effects.
- To compare the efficacy and safety of 2 doses of olanzapine (5 mg and 10 mg), a multi-institutional, double-blind trial randomized patients receiving highly emetogenic chemotherapy to either 10 mg or 5 mg and combined antiemetic therapy. Both study groups experienced a significant improvement in the delayed phase of emesis; however, the olanzapine 5-mg arm reported lower somnolence rates than olanzapine 10 mg (45.5% vs. 53.3%).[3]
- Several case reports have revealed the efficacy of olanzapine in refractory nausea and vomiting in patients with advanced cancer. Due to its antagonism at multiple key receptor sites, olanzapine has a role as a single agent over a multiple-agent antiemetic regimen.[4]

Summary and Implications: This small, double-blind, randomized, placebo-controlled trial found that low-dose olanzapine 5 mg was effective in reducing symptoms of nausea and vomiting unrelated to chemotherapy among patients with advanced cancer. Low-dose olanzapine was well tolerated, and no excess adverse events or sedation was observed in the treatment group.

CLINICAL CASE: ANOTHER STRING TO ONE'S BOW OF ANTIEMETICS

Case History

A 45-year-old female with a past medical history significant for advanced cancer presents with refractory nausea and vomiting. She is no longer pursuing operative or curative treatments, and her goals of care are focused on symptom control and comfort. She continues to experience significant nausea and frequent emesis episodes on ondansetron 8 mg orally disintegrating tablet every 8 hours and lorazepam 1 mg intravenously every 6 hours as needed and has required 4 doses in the last 24 hours. She has previously trialed and not tolerated metoclopramide and prochlorperazine.

What medication would you recommend next?

Suggested Answer

The patient in this case could start low-dose olanzapine 5 mg by mouth once daily at bedtime for her refractory nausea and vomiting. Although there are concerns for gastrointestinal absorption of medications with significant emesis, olanzapine has multiple dosage forms including oral tablets, intramuscular solution, and orally disintegrating tablets. She may trial olanzapine 5 mg administered under the tongue at bedtime daily for about 4–5 days to allow the drug levels to approach steady state (approximate half-life: ~30 hours). Medication safety considerations include prolonged QT interval, anticholinergic effects, and extrapyramidal symptoms, especially with patients concurrently on other high-dose antipsychotics and those with Parkinson disease.

In the 2017 Update of Antiemetic Guidelines, the National Comprehensive Cancer Network included a 4-drug antiemetic regimen containing olanzapine as a category 1 recommendation (intervention is appropriate based on high-level evidence) for patients on highly emetogenic chemotherapy.[5] Both Navari et al. trials have evaluated the efficacy and demonstrated a clear benefit of olanzapine for nausea prevention, independently and dependently of chemotherapy, in patients with advanced cancer.

References

1. Navari RM, Pywell CM, Le-Rademacher JG, et al. Olanzapine for the treatment of advanced cancer-related chronic nausea and/or vomiting: a randomized pilot trial. *JAMA Oncol.* 2020;6(6):895–899. doi:10.1001/jamaoncol.2020.1052.
2. Navari RM, Qin R, Ruddy KJ, et al. Olanzapine for the prevention of chemotherapy-induced nausea and vomiting. *N Engl J Med.* 2016;375(2):134–142. doi:10.1056/NEJMoa1515725.
3. Yanai T, Iwasa S, Hashimoto H, et al. A double-blind randomized phase II dose-finding study of olanzapine 10 mg or 5 mg for the prophylaxis of emesis induced by highly emetogenic cisplatin-based chemotherapy. *Int J Clin Oncol.* 2018;23(2):382–388. doi:10.1007/s10147-017-1200-4.
4. Srivastava M, Brito-Dellan N, Davis MP, Leach M, Lagman R. Olanzapine as an antiemetic in refractory nausea and vomiting in advanced cancer. *J Pain Symptom Manage.* 2003;25(6):578–582. doi:10.1016/s0885-3924(03)00143-x.
5. Berger MJ, Ettinger DS, Aston J, et al. NCCN guidelines insights: antiemesis, version 2.2017. *J Natl Compr Cancer Netw.* 2017;15(7):883–893. doi:10.6004/jnccn.2017.0117.

33

Safety and Benefit of Discontinuing Statin Therapy in Advanced Life-Limiting Illness

JESSICA NYMEYER

> This study provides evidence that suggests that survival is not affected when statins prescribed for primary or secondary prevention of cardiovascular disease are discontinued in this population.
>
> —Kutner et al.[1]

Research Question: Does discontinuation of statin therapy impact life expectancy, incidence of cardiac events, or quality of life in individuals with a life expectancy of 1 year or less without active cardiovascular disease?

Funding: Funding provided by the National Institute of Nursing Research with support and facilities provided by the Veterans Affairs Health Care System

Year Study Began: 2011

Year Study Published: 2015

Study Location: Multicenter study took place at 15 Palliative Care Research Cooperative Group sites in the United States.

Who Was Studied: English-speaking adults with a life expectancy estimated between 1 month and 1 year and Australia-Modified Karnofsky Performance Scale (AKPS) score < 80% who were on statin therapy for primary or secondary cardiac prevention for at least 3 months prior to enrollment without evidence of active cardiovascular disease.

Who Was Excluded: Individuals whose physician felt they had active cardiovascular disease requiring ongoing statin therapy, contraindications to continuing statin therapy including myositis or liver function tests or creatine kinase levels more than 2.5 times normal range, or lack of willingness to consent to enrollment by patient, proxy, or treating physician.

How Many Patients: 381

Study Overview: This is a multicenter, parallel-group, unblinded, randomized, pragmatic clinical trial with 381 individuals with a life expectancy of 1 month to 1 year currently receiving statin therapy randomized to either continue therapy or discontinue in a 1:1 ratio stratified by study site and cardiovascular disease history (Figure 33.1).

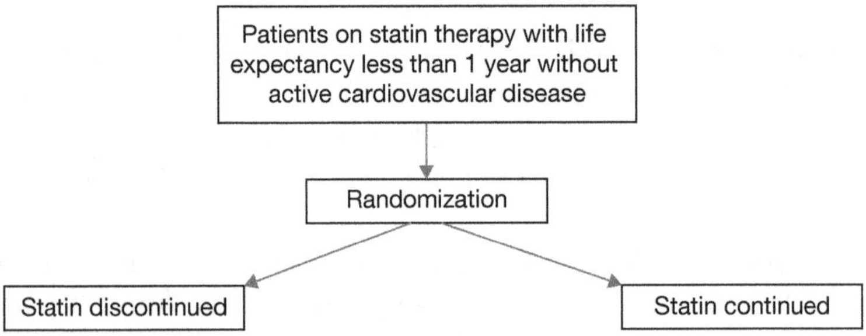

Figure 33.1. Summary of study design.

Study Intervention: Participants in the study group had their statin discontinued, and those in the control group continued statin therapy as ordered by their physician. All participants completed baseline assessments. Data on survival, performance status, and health resource utilization (number of medications taken and adverse events including hospitalizations and cardiovascular events) were collected weekly during the first month and monthly until death or 1 year. Patient-reported outcomes including quality of life, symptoms, and satisfaction were obtained at weeks 2, 4, 8, 12, 16, 20, and 24.

Quality of life was measured with the McGill Quality of Life Questionnaire with subscales for physical symptoms, psychological symptoms, existential well-being, and support. Symptoms of pain, fatigue, nausea, depression, anxiousness, drowsiness, appetite, well-being, and breathing were assessed using the Edmonton Symptom Assessment Scale, with symptoms of muscle-related pain, weakness, headache, and fever added to assess for side effects of statin use.

Follow-Up: Median of 18 weeks

Endpoints: The primary endpoint was proportion of deaths within 60 days of trial enrollment. Secondary endpoints included survival and time to first cardiovascular-related event, performance status, quality of life, symptom burden, number of nonstatin medications, statin-related adverse events, and satisfaction with health care.

RESULTS

- Study groups were equally divided between cancer and noncancer diagnoses. Most participants were older, White, and insured with Medicare; 69% took statins for over 5 years, and 58% had cardiovascular disease.
- The proportion of patients who died within 60 days was not significantly different between the groups. Median survival was 7 months.
- There was no significant difference in the time to first cardiovascular-related event, with only 24 participants in the study experiencing an event (discontinuation group: 13; continuation group: 11).
- Overall well-being based on the McGill Quality of Life Questionnaire was significantly higher for individuals who discontinued statin therapy, although a single question measuring quality of life was not significantly different between the groups.
- The total number of nonstatin medications was significantly lower in the group discontinuing statin therapy by 0.7 medications.
- There were no statistically significant differences in symptom burden between the groups.
- Most patients had high satisfaction with their health care with no significant difference between the study and control groups (Table 33.1).

Table 33.1 SUMMARY OF KEY FINDINGS

Outcome	Discontinued Statin *n* = 189	Continued Statin *n* = 192	*P* Value
Death within 60 days	45 (23.8%)	39 (20.3%)	.36
Cardiovascular events	13 (6.8%)	11 (5.7%)	.64
Median time to death	229 days	190 days	.6
Patient-reported outcomes[a]			
Quality of life (baseline 6.94)[b]	7.07	6.74	.03
Symptoms (baseline 34.6)[c]	32.4	34.9	.23
Nonstatin medications (baseline 10.9)[d]	10.1	10.8	.03

[a] Baseline compared to week 20 mean.
[b] McGill Quality of Life Questionnaire total score.
[c] Edmonton Symptom Assessment Scale rating of 13 symptoms.
[d] Includes daily and as-needed medications.

Criticisms and Limitations:

- The primary endpoint and sample size were changed midway through the study when it was recognized that median survival was about 3 times longer than initially anticipated for study design. This resulted in decreased power to assess secondary endpoints and highlights the difficulty in prognosticating for patients with advanced illness.
- There may have been some imbalances between study arms. Individuals in the withdrawal arm had greater cognitive impairment ($P = .02$, 27% vs. 17%), suggesting greater disease severity.

Other Relevant Studies and Information:

- A separate publication details participant perception of statin deprescribing. A 9-question survey was administered prior to randomization at time of baseline data collection. Results reveal that < 10% of participants were concerned that discontinuing statin therapy represented their doctor "giving up" or thinking they were "about to die."[2]
- Secondary data analysis of participants aged 65–75 in the randomized control Antihypertensive and Lipid-Lowering Treatment to Prevent Heart Attack Trial–Lipid-Lowering Trial (ALLHAT-LLT) found no benefit when older adults received statin therapy for primary cardiovascular prevention.[3]

- The American Heart Association 2018 Guideline on the Management of Blood Cholesterol notes the "feasibility and utility of deprescribing" statin therapy in patients receiving palliative care and recommends shared decision-making between patients and their prescribers regarding the appropriateness of continued statin therapy.[4]

Summary and Implications: This randomized clinical trial provides important evidence for clinicians discussing discontinuation of statin therapy with patients living with advanced illness. The analysis suggests that discontinuing statin therapy at the end of life for patients without active cardiovascular disease may not adversely impact life expectancy or the incidence of cardiovascular events. The trial also suggests that discontinuing statin therapy may result in improved quality of life, use of fewer nonstatin medications, and an associated reduction in medication cost.

CLINICAL CASE: ARE THESE MEDICATIONS HELPING ME?

Case History

Ms. Hernandez is a 72-year-old woman with a history of chronic obstructive pulmonary disease, hypertension, hyperlipidemia, and advanced metastatic lung cancer. She has received multiple lines of disease-modifying treatment, but unfortunately her cancer has progressed and she has had a significant decline in her functional status in the past month, now requiring occasional assistance with daily tasks (AKPS score 60%). She has good insight into the severity of her condition and is accepting that her life expectancy may only be months. She knows she will no longer be taking chemotherapy and asks if she needs to continue all of her other medications, including her statin, which she has been taking for 8 years.

Suggested Answer

Medication deprescribing should be approached on a case-by-case basis with consideration of the patient's goals and their medical history. The Kutner trial demonstrates that patients with life expectancy < 1 year who are receiving statin therapy for primary or secondary prevention of cardiovascular disease can safely discontinue therapy without an increased risk of cardiovascular events or impact on survival. Discontinuing Ms. Hernandez's statin will reduce the number of medications she is taking each day and may contribute to improved quality of life and monetary savings.

References

1. Kutner JS, Blatchford PJ, Taylor DH, et al. Safety and benefit of discontinuing statin therapy in the setting of advanced, life-limiting illness: a randomized clinical trial. *JAMA Intern Med.* 2015;175(5):691–700. doi:10.1001/jamainternmed.2015.0289.
2. Tjia J, Kutner JS, Ritchie CS, et al. Perceptions of statin discontinuation among patients with life-limiting illness. *J Palliat Med.* 2017;20(10):1098–1103. doi:10.1089/jpm.2016.0489.
3. Han BH, Sutin D, Williamson JD, et al. Effect of statin treatment vs usual care on primary cardiovascular prevention among older adults: the ALLHAT-LLT randomized clinical trial. *JAMA Intern Med.* 2017;177(7):955. doi:10.1001/jamainternmed.2017.1442.
4. Grundy Scott M., Stone Neil J., Bailey Alison L., et al. 2018 AHA/ACC/AACVPR/AAPA/ABC/ACPM/ADA/AGS/APhA/ASPC/NLA/PCNA guideline on the management of blood cholesterol: a report of the American College of Cardiology/American Heart Association Task Force on Clinical Practice Guidelines. *Circulation.* 2019;139(25):e1082–e1143. doi:10.1161/CIR.0000000000000625.

34

Corticosteroids for Cancer-Related Pain, Fatigue, and Anorexia

JUDITH A. PAICE

> This study found no evidence of any additional analgesic effect of methylprednisolone 32 mg daily for 7 days in patients with advanced cancer treated with opioids.
>
> —PAULSON ET AL.[1]

Research Question: Is oral methylprednisolone safe and effective for managing cancer-related pain, fatigue, appetite loss, and satisfaction with treatment?

Funding: Financial support provided by the lead author

Year Study Began: 2008

Year Study Published: 2014

Study Location: 5 palliative care units and outpatient oncology services in Norway: Telemark Hospital, Haraldsplass Deaconess Hospital, Sørlandet Hospital, St. Olav's University Hospital, and Oslo University Hospital

Who Was Studied: Patients with cancer, aged ≥ 18 years of age, with an average pain intensity ≥ 4 (on a 0–10 numeric rating scale) in the previous 24 hours, with > 4 weeks expected survival and receiving an opioid for moderate to severe cancer pain.

Who Was Excluded: Patients with average pain intensity ≥ 8 for the last 24 hours, use of corticosteroids in the last 4 weeks, diabetes, peptic ulcer disease, use of nonsteroidal anti-inflammatory drugs, radiotherapy or systemic cancer treatment started < 4 weeks prior, spinal cord compression, need for bone surgery, or severe cognitive impairment.

How Many Patients: 49

Study Overview: This is a randomized, placebo-controlled, parallel-group, multicenter phase 3 trial (Figure 34.1).

Study Intervention: Patients received identical-appearing capsules of either methylprednisolone 16 mg or placebo twice daily for 7 days. No changes were allowed in the scheduled opioid intake for 48 hours prior to inclusion and throughout the study, although breakthrough opioids were allowed.

Follow-Up: 7 days

Endpoints: Primary outcome: Difference in average pain intensity of 1.5 points (on 0–10 scale) between the intervention and placebo groups. Secondary aims included the effects of therapy on fatigue, appetite loss, satisfaction with treatment, and adverse effects associated with treatment.

RESULTS

- There were no differences between groups in average pain intensity at day 7 (methylprednisolone group = 3.6; placebo group = 3.7).
- There were no differences between groups in opioid consumption.
- Methylprednisolone treatment was associated with statistically significant improvements in symptoms of fatigue, appetite, and satisfaction with treatment as compared to placebo (Table 34.1).
- There were no statistically significant differences between the number of adverse events between groups.

Criticisms and Limitations: A key concern of the trial is the heterogeneity of the pain syndromes included; limiting to those with bone pain might have yielded different results. Despite randomization, the steroid group included more patients with neuropathy and higher baseline opioid doses.

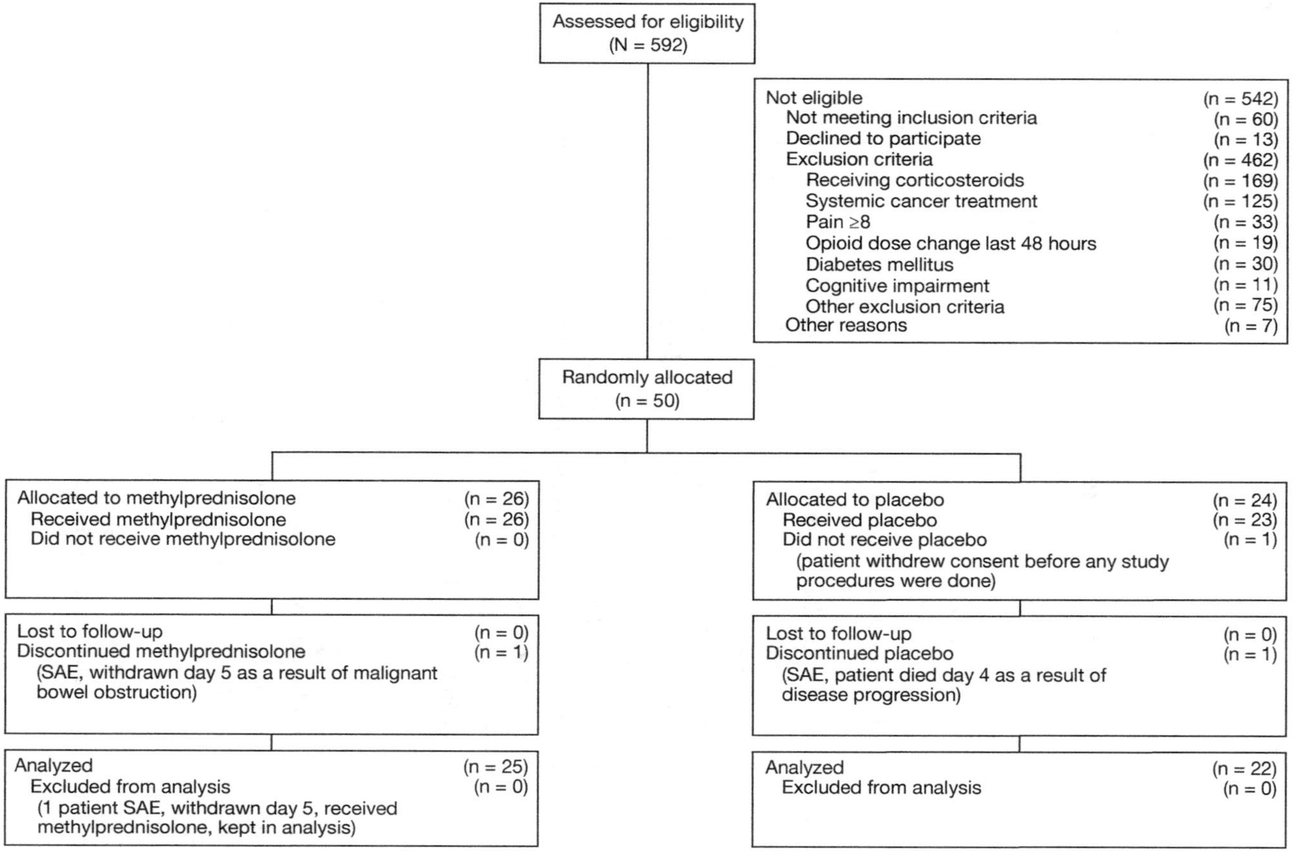

Figure 34.1. Study overview.

From Paulsen O, Klepstad P, Rosland JH, et al. Efficacy of methylprednisolone on pain, fatigue, and appetite loss in patients with advanced cancer using opioids: a randomized, placebo-controlled, double-blind trial. *J Clin Oncol.* 2014;32(29):3221–3228. Reprinted with permission from Wolters Kluwer Health Inc.

Table 34.1 SUMMARY OF METHYLPREDNISOLONE RANDOMIZED CONTROLLED TRIAL

Outcome	Methylprednisolone	Placebo	*P* Value
Average pain intensity (0–10): day 7	3.6	3.68	.88
Morphine consumption (OME): day 7	318.6	188.2	.08
Mean difference	44.8	22.4	.51
Relative difference	1.19	1.20	.95
Fatigue (0–100): day 7	60.4	70.5	.16
Mean difference	−16.7	3.3	.003
Appetite loss (0–100): day 7	49.3	65.2	.10
Mean difference	−24.0	1.5	.003
Patient satisfaction with treatment	5.4	2.0	.001

Abbreviation: OME, oral morphine equivalent.

Other Relevant Studies and Information:

- Few studies exist regarding the analgesic effects of corticosteroids in cancer pain. A systematic review found scarce studies, and most of the evidence was of low quality.[2]
- A Cochrane review of corticosteroids for cancer pain found a paucity of studies, high risk of bias, small sample sizes, and other limitations. The authors concluded that the evidence is weak and further trials are needed to determine optimal dose, duration, and route.[3]
- Despite limited evidence, corticosteroids are commonly employed by palliative care providers, with 66% of respondents to an online survey ordering these agents for people with painful bone metastases.[4]
- Most clinical practice guidelines recommend corticosteroids for cancer-related pain.[5–7]

Summary and Implications: In this small randomized trial involving patients with active cancer, methylprednisolone was not associated with significant improvements in pain, but it was associated with improvements in secondary outcomes of fatigue and appetite. Patient satisfaction with treatment was also higher in the methylprednisolone group, and there were no differences in adverse effects between groups. Though evidence is limited, this and other studies support the use of palliative methylprednisolone for patients with a variety of cancer-related symptoms.

CLINICAL CASE: CANCER PAIN

Case History

A 35-year-old man was diagnosed with synovial sarcoma in the right proximal femur, which initially responded to chemotherapy, radiation, and resection. He is now presenting 2 years later with severe pain in the right hip and upper thigh, exacerbated by weight bearing. Imaging reveals local recurrence and new lung lesions. He also reports severe fatigue that he attributes to the opioids that have been prescribed to relieve pain while treatment planning takes place. He has had significant adverse effects to opioids in the past, including nausea and constipation, and is reluctant to take these medications.

Suggested Answer

Current evidence supporting the efficacy of corticosteroids for cancer pain control is weak. The results of this study would argue against using methylprednisolone for cancer pain. However, many oncologists and palliative care providers would consider a short course of 7–10 days of dexamethasone for this patient. Additionally, this patient is fatigued and has had gastrointestinal adverse effects to careful rotation of opioids. Corticosteroids may provide adjuvant therapy to allow reduced doses of opioids while potentially reducing fatigue and nausea, serving as a bridge until definitive cancer treatment can be planned.

References

1. Paulsen O, Klepstad P, Rosland JH, et al. Efficacy of methylprednisolone on pain, fatigue, and appetite loss in patients with advanced cancer using opioids: a randomized, placebo-controlled, double-blind trial. *J Clin Oncol.* 2014;32(29):3221–3228.
2. Paulsen O, Aass N, Kaasa S, Dale O. Do corticosteroids provide analgesic effects in cancer patients? A systematic literature review. *J Pain Symptom Manage.* 2013;46(1):96–105.
3. Haywood A, Good P, Khan S, et al. Corticosteroids for the management of cancer-related pain in adults. *Cochrane Database Syst Rev.* 2015;(4):CD010756.
4. White P, Arnold R, Bull J, Cicero B. The use of corticosteroids as adjuvant therapy for painful bone metastases: a large cross-sectional survey of palliative care providers. *Am J Hosp Palliat Care.* 2018;35(1):151–158.
5. Swarm RA, Paice JA, Anghelescu DL, et al. Adult cancer pain, version 3.2019, NCCN clinical practice guidelines in oncology. *J Natl Compr Canc Netw.* 2019;17(8):977–1007.

6. World Health Organization. *WHO Guidelines for the Pharmacological and Radiotherapeutic Management of Cancer Pain in Adults and Adolescents.* World Health Organization; 2018.
7. Fallon M, Giusti R, Aielli F, et al. Management of cancer pain in adult patients: ESMO Clinical Practice Guidelines. *Ann Oncol.* 2018;29(Suppl 4):iv166–iv191.

35

Role of Paracetamol (Acetaminophen) for Cancer Pain Requiring High-Dose Opioids

SHILA PANDEY

> Our study is the first to restrict the patient population to those requiring high-dose "strong opioids" and finds no evidence to support the use of adjuvant paracetamol.
>
> —ISRAEL ET AL.[1]

Research Question: Does the addition of paracetamol (acetaminophen) to a high-dose opioid regimen improve analgesia or reduce opioid-related adverse effects in patients with cancer receiving palliative care?

Funding: Brisbane South Palliative Care Collaborative

Year Study Began: 2007

Year Study Published: 2010

Study Location: Australia

Who Was Studied: Adults with cancer receiving palliative care in the hospital or community requiring high-dose opioids (oral morphine equivalent of 200 mg/day) with a baseline pain score ≥ 2 and a Mini-Mental State Examination score of at least 22 out of 30.

Who Was Excluded: Patients unable to consent in English, with primary neuropathic pain, who are regularly febrile, or with a prognosis of < 2 weeks.

How Many Patients: 22

Study Overview: This is a prospective, double-blind, randomized, crossover trial in which cancer patients receiving palliative care received 5 days of paracetamol 500 mg by mouth 4 times a day and 5 days of placebo. The order in which the paracetamol or placebo was delivered was determined by a computer-generated randomization schedule (Figure 35.1). This design allowed for participants to contrast their perceived pain control.

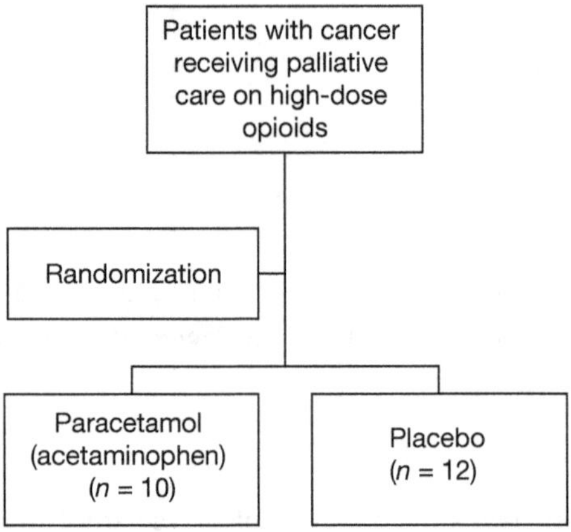

Figure 35.1. Summary of study design.

Study Intervention: Patients were randomly assigned to receive 5 days of paracetamol (two 500-mg tablets by mouth 4 times daily) and 5 days of placebo or vice versa based on a randomization schedule. All medications containing paracetamol were discontinued after study enrollment. Patients continued all other usual medications. Any patient who developed a fever was withdrawn from the study.

All patients were asked to keep a daily diary for 10 days that included subjective measures on pain, nausea and vomiting, cognitive impairment, and feeling of overall well-being using an 11-point numeric rating scale (NRS). A detailed log of all breakthrough medications was recorded. A research nurse visited community patients at last 2 times and called every other day, whereas hospitalized patients had daily visits.

Follow-Up: 10 days

Endpoints:

Primary outcomes: Daily overall level of pain using an 11-point NRS, ranging from 0 (none) to 10 (unbearable), and number of daily breakthrough analgesics required.

Secondary outcomes: subjective nausea, vomiting, cognitive impairment, constipation, and overall well-being using the same NRS, as well as whether pain was better controlled during the first or second part of the study.

RESULTS

- Overall, there were no statistically significant differences between the placebo and paracetamol groups on rated pain, use of breakthrough analgesics, well-being, nausea, drowsiness, unclear thinking, or constipation (Table 35.1).

Table 35.1 SUMMARY OF STUDY'S KEY FINDINGS

Treatment	**Placebo Mean (SD)**	**Paracetamol Mean (SD)**	**Mean Difference (SD)**	**95% CI**	d^a	P^b
Rated pain	3.59 (1.58)	3.43 (1.44)	0.16 (1.42)	−0.47 to 0.79	0.11	.60
Breakthroughs	1.41 (1.45)	0.99 (1.26)	0.42 (1.02)	−0.03 to 0.97	0.41	.07
Well-being	5.26 (1.40)	5.26 (1.63)	−0.21 (1.42)	−0.83 to 0.42	0.15	.50
Nausea	0.86 (1.46)	0.83 (1.22)	0.03 (1.48)	−0.62 to 0.69	0.02	.92
Drowsiness	2.31 (2.19)	1.88 (1.93)	0.43 (1.30)	−0.15 to 1.01	0.33	.14
Unclear thinking	1.06 (1.38)	0.94 (1.09)	0.12 (0.85)	−0.26 to 0.50	0.14	.52
Constipation	1.05 (1.68)	0.81 (1.23)	0.24 (1.29)	−0.34 to 0.81	0.17	.40

[a] Absolute value of standard mean difference.
[b] Value from paired *t*-test.

- None of the mean differences in pain or other secondary outcomes reached clinical significance.
- There was a small trend toward higher pain rating and use of more more breakthrough analgesics in the placebo group; however, this was not statistically significant.
- At the end of the trial, most patients were unable to decide during which part of the study, with or without paracetamol, pain was better controlled.

Criticisms and Limitations:

- This study did not include patients with changing analgesic requirements (± 30% daily requirements); therefore, the results have limited generalizability to these patients.
- There were 9 patients who withdrew from the trial, 8 of whom were in the placebo-first arm. Three of the withdrawals in the placebo-first arm were due to fever among people who had previously been regularly taking acetaminophen. Prior regular use of acetaminophen may have been masking fevers related to infection or other etiology. Other reasons for withdrawal included protocol violation, clinical deterioration, and unstable pain.
- Although mean symptom ratings were analyzed during the last 4 days of treatment, there is a potential for carryover effects—defined as when an initial treatment "carries over" to influence a person's response to a subsequent therapy—since there was no washout period.[2] Generally, a drug is considered to be eliminated after about 4–5 half-lives. In adults, the reported half-life of acetaminophen is ~2–3 hours. Therefore, it is possible the benefits of acetaminophen may have persisted for 10–15 hours after the last dose.

Other Relevant Studies and Information:

- Two other studies, one double-blind randomized controlled study and a prospective study, assessing the added benefits of paracetamol in addition to opioid therapy have come to similar conclusions.[3,4]
- Alternatively, Stockler et al.[5] found paracetamol significantly improved pain and well-being when compared to placebo; however, the mean difference was 0.4 on an NRS, and these benefits are of uncertain clinical benefit.
- A 2017 Cochrane review[6] determined there was insufficient high-quality evidence to support or oppose the use of paracetamol alone or in combination with opioids for the first 2 steps of the 3-step World Health Organization cancer pain ladder.
- Given the mixed results on the role of paracetamol for cancer patients on high-dose opioids, paracetamol is still included in the National Comprehensive Cancer Network adult cancer pain guidelines[7] for opioid-naïve and opioid-tolerant patients. The European Society for Medical Oncology[8] recommends the use of paracetamol for the management of mild pain.

Summary and Implications: Among patients with advanced cancer, this randomized controlled trial failed to demonstrate an added benefit of paracetamol when added to a high-dose opioid regimen (> 200 mg morphine per day) with respect to pain control, adverse effects, or overall well-being. However, there were significant methodological limitations to the study—including the withdrawal of a disproportionate number of patients in the paracetamol study arm—that may have undermined the results. Despite these findings, there may still be a role for paracetamol in cancer pain management, warranting palliative care providers to consider a time limited to determine its benefit in an individual patient.

CLINICAL CASE: SHOULD PARACETAMOL BE CONTINUED?

Case History

A 67-year-old man with metastatic lung cancer on immunotherapy has chronic back pain from osseous metastasis to the thoracic spine and ribs. He is currently on a transdermal fentanyl patch 125 mcg/hour every 72 hours, morphine immediate release 15 mg orally every 4 hours as needed, pregabalin 75 mg orally nightly, and paracetamol 1000 mg by mouth every 8 hours around the clock. He uses about 3 breakthrough doses of morphine immediate release 15 mg per day and reports his pain is well controlled. He has been taking the paracetamol for several months now and questions its continuation.

Should the paracetamol be continued?

Suggested Answer

The results of this study by Israel et al. do not support the continued use of paracetamol in this patient who is receiving > 200 mg morphine per day. A discussion with the patient about pill burden and overall satisfaction with the analgesic regimen is warranted. If the patient agrees, a trial period discontinuing the paracetamol and continuing to assess pain can be an effective method to assess its analgesic role. If pain and other associated symptoms remain the same, there is no need to continue the paracetamol. If the pain worsens, the paracetamol may be restarted.

Additional considerations with ongoing paracetamol use include potential for masking a fever, which may delay treatment of an infection, and monitoring of other medications that may contain paracetamol (e.g., over-the-counter cough and cold products), which could cause liver damage.

References

1. Israel FJ, Parker G, Charles M, Reymond L. Lack of benefit from paracetamol (acetaminophen) for palliative cancer patients requiring high-dose strong opioids: a randomized, double-blind, placebo-controlled, crossover trial. *J Pain Symptom Manage.* 2010;39(3):548–554. doi:10.1016/j.jpainsymman.2009.07.008.
2. Cleophas TJ. Carryover bias in clinical investigations. *J Clin Pharmacol.* 1993 Sep;33(9):799–804. doi:10.1002/j.1552-4604.1993.tb01954.x. PMID: 8227475.
3. Axelsson B, Christensen SB. Is there an additive analgesic effect of paracetamol at step 3? A double-blind randomized controlled study. *J Palliat Med.* 2003;18:724e725.
4. Axelsson B, Stellborn P, Ström G. Analgesic effect of paracetamol on cancer related pain in concurrent strong opioid therapy. A prospective clinical study. *Acta Oncol.* 2008;47(5):891–895. doi:10.1080/02841860701687259.
5. Stockler M, Vardy J, Pillai A, Warr D. Acetaminophen (paracetamol) improves pain and well-being in people with advanced cancer already receiving a strong opioid regimen: a randomized, double-blind, placebo-controlled cross-over trial. *J Clin Oncol.* 2004;22(16):3389–3394. doi:10.1200/JCO.2004.09.122.
6. Wiffen PJ, Derry S, Moore RA, et al. Oral paracetamol (acetaminophen) for cancer pain. *Cochrane Database Syst Rev.* 2017;(7):CD012637.
7. National Comprehensive Cancer Network. NCCN guidelines version 2.2021 adult cancer pain. 2021. https://www.nccn.org/professionals/physician_gls/pdf/pain.pdf. Accessed December 21, 2021.
8. Fallon M, Giusti R, Aielli F, et al. Management of cancer pain in adult patients: ESMO clinical practice guidelines. *Ann Oncol.* 2018;29(Suppl 4):iv166–iv191. doi:10.1093/annonc/mdy152.

36

Treatment of Painful Wounds With Topical Morphine

BRIDGET MCCRATE PROTUS AND JONI BRINKER

The use of topical opioids for skin ulcer analgesia bears great potential.

—TWILLMAN ET AL.[1]

Research Question: Does topical application of a morphine-hydrogel preparation provide clinically significant improvement in patient reports of wound pain?

Funding: No funding source identified

Year Study Began: Not identified in article

Year Study Published: 1999

Study Location: Cancer Pain Management Service, University of Kansas Cancer Center, Kansas City, Kansas, United States

Who Was Studied: Adult patients with painful skin ulcers due to a variety of underlying medical conditions admitted to the University of Kansas Cancer Center.

Who Was Excluded: No inclusion or exclusion criteria provided.

How Many Patients: 9

Study Overview: This is an open-label treatment case series of 9 patients seen by the Cancer Pain Management Service (CPMS) at the study location to determine the effectiveness of a topical morphine-infused IntraSite® gel (MIG) preparation for treating painful wounds. Findings of a painful skin ulcer were incidental to the intent of the initial patient referral. Only 1 patient (case 5) was referred specifically for a painful skin lesion following determination of a beneficial effect of the study treatment from the first patient case report (Figure 36.1).

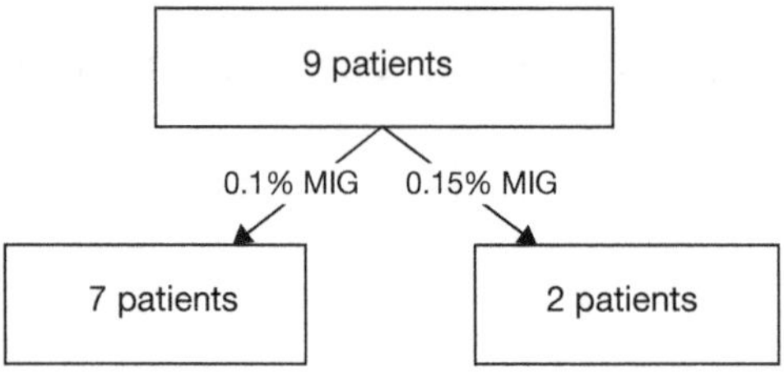

Figure 36.1. Summary of study design.

Study Intervention: Patients referred to the CPMS were provided a thorough pain assessment. When a painful skin lesion was discovered during assessment, MIG at either 0.1% or 0.15% was ordered for twice-daily application with dressing changes. MIG was prepared in the hospital pharmacy by adding 1 mg morphine per 1 mL IntraSite® gel to reach a 0.1% weight-to-weight (w/w) product, or 1.5 mg morphine per 1 mL IntraSite® for a 0.15% w/w product. IntraSite® is an amorphous hydrogel wound dressing on the wound care formulary at the study hospital. Approximately 1 mL of MIG was applied directly to each painful wound site after cleansing and a 4"×4" gauze pad was used as a secondary dressing. Alternately, the MIG was applied to the 4"×4" gauze pad and the pad was applied to directly contact and cover the wound bed. A series of 9 consecutive patients received the open-label treatment and were followed for the course of their hospital stay. Patient use of systemic analgesics and adjuvant medications both scheduled and "as needed" were continued as ordered and the additional intervention of MIG was provided when systemic analgesia was insufficient to provide pain relief at the site of the wound.

Follow-Up: Patient follow-up was not standardized as part of the case series and ranged from about 48 hours to 1 year postdischarge from hospital.

Endpoints: Primary outcome: Improved control of wound pain as determined by subjective report of the patient.

RESULTS

- All but 1 patient reported improvement in pain after treatment with MIG (Table 36.1).
- No patients reported any adverse events such as sedation or skin irritation with use of MIG, and there appeared to be no difference in wound healing.
- In general, patients who had difficulty adhering to wound care regimens due to pain were reported to have some improved wound healing when pain was better controlled for them with MIG use.

Criticisms and Limitations:

- Very small, open-label case series with no placebo control or blinding[1]

Other Relevant Studies and Information:

- Topical morphine does not work on superficial burns or neuropathic pain. Despite a small case series suggesting systemic pain relief from topical application of morphine in pluronic lecithin organogel (PLO), systemic absorption or clinical benefit for pain relief when morphine is applied topically to intact skin is unlikely.[2–4]
- Hydrogels are designed to maintain moisture balance and soften necrotic tissue to aid in wound healing.[5] Release of medications, such as morphine, from a hydrogel into the wound environment may be impacted by many factors—presence of wound exudate, slough, and eschar—that have not been adequately studied. Additionally, even nonmedicated hydrogels have demonstrated pain relief in wounds through a soothing or cooling effect.[5]
- If mixed under sterile conditions, morphine in IntraSite® gel is stable for up to 28 days at room temperature or refrigerated. As expected, other opioids may have different stability. For example, under similar conditions, diacetylmorphine (diamorphine, heroin) in IntraSite® gel acts as a pro-drug and degrades to morphine.[6,7]
- Morphine in hydrogel may have some systemic absorption from large wounds. In a case series report, 1 patient with a skin ulceration of 60 cm^2 demonstrated systemic bioavailability of morphine at nearly 20% after topical application.[7] No additional systemic absorption/bioavailability studies for topical application of morphine in hydrogel to open wounds have been published.

Table 36.1 SUMMARY OF KEY FINDINGS

Patient Case	Painful Wound Description	MIG Use	Outcome
1-A; 36 yo female	Chronic ulcers from pyoderma gangrenosum hospitalized for painful, nonhealing skin graft site on right arm	0.1% BID at dressing changes	Pt reported pain improvement with first application and continued BID treatment for 13-day hospital stay and 2 weeks after discharge
2-B; 45 yo male	Esophageal cancer with painful sacral pressure injury	0.1% BID at dressing changes	Pt able to distinguish pain severity at different sites; after MIG initiated no further pain at site of pressure injury reported for remainder of hospitalization (15 days)
3-C; 67 yo male	Metastatic renal cell carcinoma with painful sacral pressure injury	0.1% BID at dressing changes	Prior to MIG application, pain rated at 6.5 on 0–10 scale; after single application, pain reported at 0 until personal hygiene caused discomfort, but pain returned to 0 after next MIG application until hospital discharge
4-D; 78 yo female	Stage IV ductal carcinoma of right breast with painful ulcerated lesion at tumor site	0.1% single application	Prior to application, pain reported at 6 on 0–10 scale; after application, pain reported at 0 for remainder of 8-day hospital stay
5-E; 49 yo female	Painful diabetic foot ulcer with peripheral vascular disease	0.1% with titration to 0.15%; frequency not specified	Pt reported "good pain relief" with use of MIG for 6 months, then reported MIG less effective; when dose increased to 0.15%, pain control returned for more than 1 year
6-F; 31 yo female	Hidradenitis suppurativa outbreak with painful lesions	0.15% BID at dressing changes; application of 1 mL/site	Pt noted pain relief at 15 minutes after application; pain reported at 0 on 0–10 scale until lesions healed
7-G; 48 yo female	Painful melanoma lesions on foot and lower leg	0.1% applied as needed	Pt reported each MIG application provided a couple of hours of pain relief; pt continued as-needed use for more than 1 year
8-H; 51 yo male	Multiple sclerosis with stage 1 bilateral scapula pressure injuries	0.15% BID at dressing changes	Pt reported scapula site pain as 7 on 0–10 scale, reduced to 2/10 after MIG application, and continued treatment for 6 weeks
9-I; 81 yo male	Colorectal cancer with pain related to swelling, redness, bruising of scrotum; no open wound	0.1% application; frequency not specified	Pt reported no change in pain level

Abbreviations: BID, twice a day; MIG, morphine-infused IntraSite® gel; Pt, patient; yo, year old.

- Although generally well tolerated, case studies subsequent to Twillman et al. have reported some adverse effects from topical morphine in hydrogel, primarily pruritus and/or a burning sensation localized to the site of application, which in some cases also occurred with a placebo (plain hydrogel) application.[8–13]
- Peripherally acting mu-opioid receptor antagonists (PAMORAs) such as methylnaltrexone, naloxegol, and naldemedine may reduce the effectiveness of topical opioids due to the PAMORAs' ability to inhibit opioid response in the peripheral nervous system.[14] Clinicians should be aware that patients taking PAMORAs for opioid-induced constipation or off-label uses of systemic opioid-induced, cholestatic, or uremic pruritus may not experience relief of wound pain with topical morphine application.
- In vitro studies of lung, breast, and liver cancer cell lines demonstrate expression of opioid receptors. In vitro studies suggest a possible tumor cell growth-promoting effect of morphine at these opioid receptors; however, the clinical significance of this receptor effect has not been explored.[15–18]
- Tayeb et al. performed a scoping review of the literature on topical analgesics used in hospice, palliative, and cancer care, finding 9 articles on topical morphine and 6 on topical methadone. Study formats included randomized controlled trials, prospective cohort studies, and case series or case reports. Their review concluded that while evidence is very limited, it may be reasonable to trial topical analgesics when pain is refractory to Food and Drug Administration–approved medications and routes.[19]
- After the 1999 case series, Zeppetella et al. completed a 5-patient pilot study with a double-blind, placebo-controlled, crossover trial in a hospice inpatient unit. Patients had painful sacral pressure injuries and were concurrently taking systemic opioid analgesics. Results were positive and morphine appeared to improve pain rating on a visual analog scale more than placebo. No systemic adverse effects were reported, and no difference was noted in local side effects (pruritus, burning) between the morphine or placebo gels.[8] The researchers' attempts at a larger-scale clinical trial were unsuccessful; however, a small sample of positive results was published as a letter to the editor.[9]
- Cialkowska-Rysz and Dzierzanowski compared pain intensity and pain relief in cancer patients using nonhydrogel formulations of topical morphine—a 0.2% morphine-triethanolamine in carbomer polymer gel (for mucosal lesions) or 0.2% morphine glycerol–Eucerin

(petrolatum)-based ointment (for skin lesions) in a 2-phase placebo-controlled crossover trial followed by an open-label trial. Thirty-five patients were included in the study, 22 with skin lesions. Mean pain intensity (MPI) prior to the study was 5.9 on a numerical rating scale (0–10). On day 7, the morphine treatment group's MPI score was 2.5 versus the placebo group's score of 4.9. By day 14, the morphine treatment group maintained an MPI score of 2.5 versus the placebo group at 5.2 ($P < .0001$). Two patients experienced moderate pruritus.[12]

- Palliative wound care practices, focusing on pain and symptom management, and often in nonhealing wounds, are commonly based on anecdotal report and smaller case studies. While the trend for benefit of topical MIG is positive and the reported side effects, when present, are very mild, a definitive recommendation for MIG is difficult. Systematic reviews trend toward benefit based on low-quality evidence.[10,11]
- In 2021, Jyothi et al. published a comparison of 10 mg morphine or 10 mg loperamide compounded in 15 g of a hydrogel-colloidal silver formulation (Megaheal®). While 13 patients were randomized, only 9 patients—4 in the loperamide arm and 5 in the morphine arm—completed the study, and there was no placebo arm. Patient scores on the numerical rating scale showed statistically significant reduction in pain for both treatment arms at 12 and 24 hours; however, due to limitations in study design, results may not be useful in most clinical settings.[13]
- A retrospective study evaluated a 0.125% concentration of morphine in VersaBase® hydrogel for 23 hospitalized patients with painful chronic pressure injuries or malignant wounds. A total of 371 topical morphine doses were administered to the patients over their hospital stay and the morphine equivalent daily dose (MEDD) as well as a pain intensity score was documented. While study results demonstrated no change in pain intensity score, there was a downward trend in total MEDD at 24 hours, 48 hours, and 1 week after topical morphine was initiated. The authors concluded a potential systemic opioid-sparing effect from the topical application of morphine to painful wounds.[20]

Summary and Implications: This small case series provides some evidence to support use of topical morphine in hydrogel (MIG) for painful wounds. Since the study was published in 1999, a small number of other papers have reported similar beneficial results. However, due to the data limitations, the role of MIG for painful wounds remains uncertain.

CLINICAL CASE: WHO SHOULD RECEIVE MIG?

Case History

A 75-year-old female is newly admitted to hospice with a diagnosis of chronic respiratory failure. She has a stage 3 pressure injury of the sacrum and incontinence-associated dermatitis (IAD) to the perianal area. The stage 3 pressure injury presents with red, nongranulating tissue and < 25% yellow slough. Moderate serous exudate is present. There is no evidence of bacterial infection, and pressure is adequately offloaded. Treatment includes cleansing with a commercial wound cleanser followed by the application of a nonadherent dressing. The IAD presents as intact but reddened skin secondary to persistent loose stools. Treatment includes cleansing with a perineal cleanser followed by the application of a zinc oxide–based barrier cream. Pain is present with dressing changes and incontinence care. Should this patient receive MIG?

Suggested Answer

The Twillman open-label treatment case series introduced the use of MIG to ameliorate pain in open, inflamed wounds. The patient in this case series presents with 2 painful skin concerns—a stage 3 pressure injury and IAD; however, the IAD presents as intact skin. Although both skin concerns are associated with pain, the Twillman open-label treatment case series suggests that MIG is only appropriate to manage the pain of the stage 3 pressure injury. The clinician may want to trial alternative treatments to manage the pain associated with IAD and incontinence care, such as gentle cleansing, prompt incontinence care, frequent application of a zinc oxide–based barrier cream, as-needed use of topical anesthetics, and pharmacological management of the loose stools.

References

1. Twillman RK, Long TD, Cathers TA, Mueller DW. Treatment of painful skin ulcers with topical opioids. *J Pain Symptom Manage.* 1999;17(4):288–292.
2. Welling A. A randomised controlled trial to test the analgesic efficacy of topical morphine on minor superficial and partial thickness burns in accident and emergency departments. *Emerg Med J.* 2007;24(6):408–412.
3. Wilken M, Ineck JR, Rule AM. Chronic arthritis pain management with topical morphine: case series. *J Pain Palliat Care Pharmacother.* 2005;19(4):39–44.
4. Paice JA, Von Roenn JH, Hudgins JC, et al. Morphine bioavailability from a topical gel formulation in volunteers. *J Pain Symptom Manage.* 2008;35(3):314–320.

5. Jones A, Vaughan D. Hydrogel dressings in the management of a variety of wound types: a review. *J Orthop Nurs.* 2005;9(Suppl 1):S1–S11.
6. Zeppetella G, Joel SP, Ribeiro MD. Stability of morphine sulphate and diamorphine hydrochloride in IntraSite gel. *Palliat Med.* 2005;19(2):131–136.
7. Ribeiro MD, Joel SP, Zeppetella G. The bioavailability of morphine applied topically to cutaneous ulcers. *J Pain Symptom Manage.* 2004;27(5):434–439.
8. Zeppetella G, Paul J, Ribiero M. Analgesic efficacy of morphine applied topically to painful ulcers. *J Pain Symptom Manage.* 2003;25(6):555–558.
9. Zeppetella G, Ribiero M. Morphine in IntraSite gel applied topically to painful ulcers. *J Pain Symptom Manage.* 2005;29(2):118–119.
10. LeBon B, Zeppetella G, Higginson I. Effectiveness of topical administration of opioids in palliative care: a systematic review. *J Pain Symptom Manage.* 2009;37(5):913–917.
11. Farley P. Should topical opioid analgesics be regarded as effective and safe when applied to chronic cutaneous lesions? *J Pharm Pharmacol.* 2011;63(6):747–756.
12. Cialkowska-Rysz A, Dzierzanowski T. Topical morphine for treatment of cancer-related painful mucosal and cutaneous lesions: a double-blind, placebo-controlled cross-over clinical trial. *Arch Med Sci.* 2019;15(1):146–151.
13. Jyothi B, Mitragotri MV, Kurugodiyavar MD, Shaikh SI, Korikanthimath VV. Morphine versus loperamide with IntraSite gel in the treatment of painful dermal ulcers: a randomized, crossover study. *Pain Physician.* 2021;24(1):e37–e44.
14. Barnett V, Twycross R, Mihalyo M, Wilcock A. Opioid antagonists. *J Pain Symptom Manage.* 2014;47(2):341–352.
15. Chen DT, Pan JH, Chen YH, et al. The mu-opioid receptor is a molecular marker for poor prognosis in hepatocellular carcinoma and represents a potential therapeutic target. *Br J Anaesth.* 2019;122(6):e157–e167.
16. Fujioka N, Nguyen J, Chen C, et al. Morphine-induced epidermal growth factor pathway activation in non-small cell lung cancer. *Anesth Analg.* 2011;113(6):1353–1364.
17. Ecimovic P, Murray D, Doran P, McDonald J, Lambert DG, Buggy DJ. Direct effect of morphine on breast cancer cell function in vitro: role of the NET1 gene. *Br J Anaesth.* 2011;107(6):916–923.
18. Gach K, Piestrzeniewicz M, Fichna J, Stefanska B, Szemraj J, Janecka A. Opioid-induced regulation of mu-opioid receptor gene expression in the MCF-7 breast cancer cell line. *Biochem Cell Biol.* 2008;86(3):217–226.
19. Tayeb BO, Winegarden JA, Alashari RA, et al. Scoping review of off-label topical analgesia in palliative, hospice and cancer care: towards flexibility in evidence-based medicine. *J Pain Res.* 2021;14:3003–3009.
20. Klosko RC, Saphire ML. Topical morphine gel as a systemic opioid sparing technique. *J Pain Palliat Care Pharmacother.* 2022;36(3):159–165.

37

Dexamethasone in the Prophylaxis of Radiation-Induced Pain Flare After Palliative Radiotherapy for Bone Metastases

MEREDITH MAXWELL AND TAMMIE E. QUEST

> Dexamethasone reduces radiation-induced pain flare in the treatment of painful bone metastases.
>
> —CHOW ET AL.[1]

Research Question: In patients with bone metastases from a nonhematological malignancy, does treatment with oral dexamethasone prior to and shortly after radiation therapy decrease the risk of having a pain flare?

Funding: Canadian Cancer Society

Year Study Began: 2011

Year Study Published: 2015

Study Location: 23 Canadian Cancer Centers located in Ontario, Quebec, Manitoba, and Alberta

Who Was Studied: Adults with pain related to radiologically confirmed bone metastases from a nonhematological cancer who received a single 8-Gy fraction of palliative radiotherapy to 1 or 2 target volumes.

Who Was Excluded: Patients who used any corticosteroid medication other than topical or inhaled preparations concurrently or within the 7 days prior to the anticipated radiation treatment; had medical contraindications to corticosteroids; had a Karnofsky Performance Status of < 40; had plans for cytotoxic chemotherapy within 10 days of radiotherapy; had evidence of spinal cord compression, pathological fracture, or impending fracture requiring surgical fixation; required nonsteroidal anti-inflammatory drugs (NSAIDs) other than low-dose daily aspirin; or had received radiotherapy previously to the study site(s).

How Many Patients: 298

Study Overview: This study was a double-blinded, placebo-controlled phase 3 randomized control trial (RCT) in which patients were randomized to receive either 8 mg dexamethasone or placebo by mouth just prior to a single-fraction radiation treatment and for 4 days thereafter (Figure 37.1).

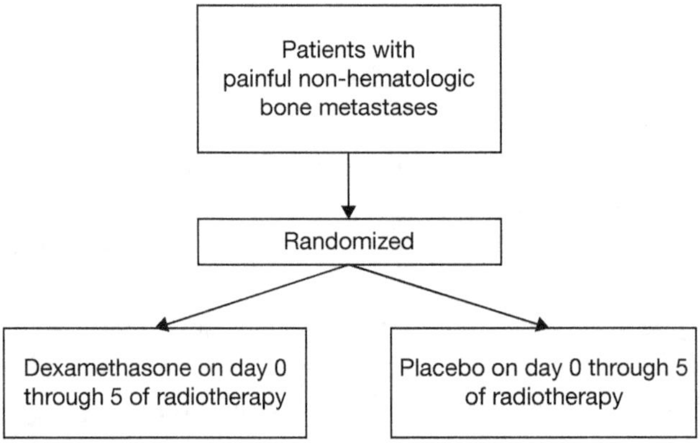

Figure 37.1. Study intervention.

Study Intervention: Patients were randomly assigned to receive either two 4-mg tabs of dexamethasone or 2 tablets of placebo at least 1 hour prior to a single fraction of radiation and on days 1–4 after radiotherapy. Patients recorded the worst pain scores daily from day 0 to 10 after treatment, how pain compared to pain prior to radiotherapy, and their opiate intake. At baseline and at day 10 and day 42 after treatment, patients also completed the European Organization for Research and Treatment of Cancer (EORTC) Quality of Life QLQ-C15-PAL questionnaire, the bone metastases module (EORTC QLQ-BM22), and the Dexamethasone Symptom Questionnaire (DSQ).

Follow-up: 42 days after radiotherapy treatment

Endpoints:

Primary outcome: Per-patient incidence of pain flare days from day 0 to 10 of radiotherapy.

Secondary outcomes: Proportion of patients achieving partial or full response to radiotherapy at day 42, toxicity of dexamethasone, quality of life (as measured by day 0, day 10, and day 42 scores on the EORTC QLQ-C15-PAL, EORTC QLQ-BM22, and DSQ), and evaluation of the relationship between pain flares and overall response to radiotherapy.

RESULTS

- Fewer patients in the dexamethasone treatment group experienced pain flares on days 1–5 than in the placebo group. There was no difference in the incidence of pain flares on days 6–10.
- Similarly, dexamethasone significantly reduced mean pain scores for days 1–5, but not days 6–10.
- There was no difference in median cumulative oral morphine equivalents.
- There was no difference in overall response to radiotherapy.
- Several patients in the treatment group experienced hyperglycemia; however, no patients required hospitalization for these events.
- At day 10, patients treated with dexamethasone had significantly less nausea, less interference in functional status, and better appetite.
- There was no significant difference in DSQ scores at baseline or day 10.
- Significantly more patients treated with dexamethasone reported depression at day 42.

Criticisms and Limitations:

- As noted by Ishiwata and colleagues,[2] patients taking NSAIDs were excluded, which limits generalizability as these medications are standard of care for treatment of pain related to bone metastases.
- Failure to assess all secondary related endpoints in a detailed time study as demonstrated in Figure 37.2—this study does not address radiological features or comorbidities that could increase risk of pain flares.

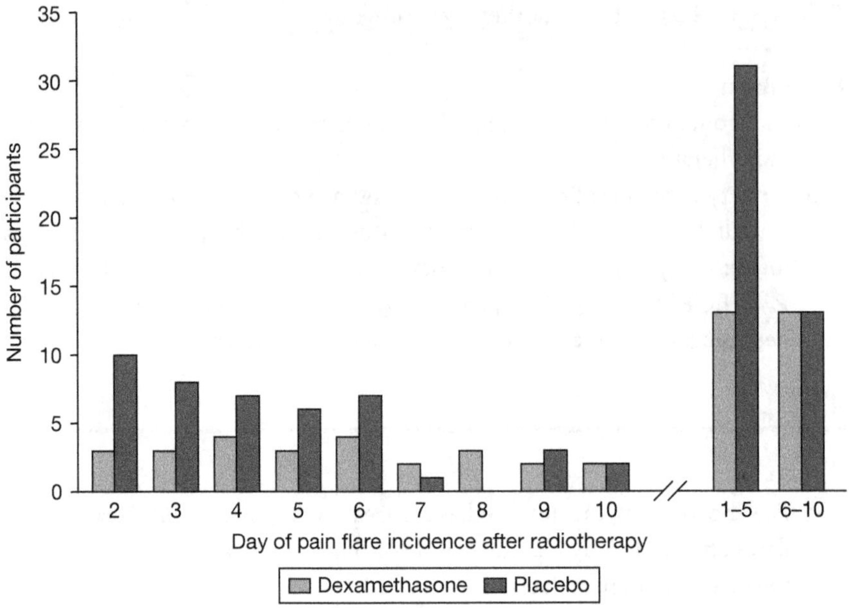

Figure 37.2. Daily pain flare incidence.

Other Relevant Studies and Information:

- In a secondary analysis of the original data, Chow et al.[3] explored differences between genders in terms of baseline characteristics, pain levels, and response to radiotherapy. The majority of patient-reported outcomes and response to radiation were not significantly different according to gender. Differences included the psychosocial domain on the QLQ-BM22 and nausea, vomiting, and a change in degree of dyspnea on the QLQ-C15-PAL.
- Further secondary analysis by Chow et al.[4] examined differences in study participants according to age (< 75 years old vs. 75+ years old). At baseline, younger patients had better performance status, worse nausea, insomnia, and functional interference and consumed more opiates. Older patients had a higher frequency of prostate cancer. Between the 2 age groups there were no significant differences in patient-reported outcomes or response to radiation.

- A systematic review by Fabregat et al.[5] of 5 studies including Chow et al.[1] supported glucocorticoids as effective prophylaxis for pain flares resulting from radiotherapy with a moderate level of evidence.
- In 2020, van der Linden et al.[6] completed a multicenter, double-blind, placebo-controlled 3-arm trial that randomized 295 patients into 1 of 3 groups: 8 mg dexamethasone before radiotherapy followed by 3 daily doses thereafter, 8 mg of dexamethasone before radiotherapy followed by 3 doses of placebo, and 4 doses of placebo. Unlike Chow et al.,[1] the difference in the incidence of pain flares between the groups did not quite achieve statistical significance ($P = .07$), nor did the difference in mean duration of pain flares ($P = .0567$). The authors did find, however, that dexamethasone postponed the occurrence of pain flares and resulted in lower mean pain scores on days 2–5.

Summary and Implications: This double-blinded, placebo-controlled RCT demonstrated that oral dexamethasone given just prior to a single-fraction radiation treatment and for 4 days thereafter reduced the number of patients reporting pain flares and mean pain scores on days 1–5 following radiation treatment. Other studies have largely supported these findings. The potential benefit of avoiding a pain flare should be weighed against patient-specific potential for risks that arise with use of steroids.

CLINICAL CASE: WHO SHOULD RECEIVE DEXAMETHASONE FOR PREVENTION OF PAIN FLARES RELATED TO RADIOTHERAPY?

Case History

A 68-year-old woman with a history of well-controlled insulin-dependent diabetes mellitus as well as metastatic breast cancer presents with a history of pain related to a bony metastasis in her pelvis. The pain has been poorly responsive to her current medication regimen for pain, which includes long- and short-acting oxycodone in addition to scheduled ibuprofen several times per day. She has never received radiation treatment to this area previously and is considering palliative single-fraction radiation treatment. Should this patient be prescribed 8 mg of oral dexamethasone on days 0–5 of her radiation treatment?

Suggested Answer

The incidence of pain flares after radiation treatment of painful bone metastases is approximately 30%–40%. In this study, dexamethasone treatment lowered the number of pain flares and mean pain scores on days 1–5 after radiation treatment, with a number needed to treat of 11 in their intention-to-treat analysis. Although these results support a plan for treatment with dexamethasone, mutual decision-making with this patient should include discussion of potential risks of steroid treatment. This would include risk of hyperglycemia as well as potential for gastrointestinal bleeding if NSAIDs were to be continued.

References

1. Chow E, Meyer RM, Ding K, et al. Dexamethasone in the prophylaxis of radiation-induced pain flare after palliative radiotherapy for bone metastases: a double-blind, randomized placebo-controlled, phase 3 trial. *Lancet Oncol.* 2015;16:1463–1472.
2. Ishiwata T, Iwasawa S, Kurimoto R, Ebata T, Takiguchi Y. Prophylactic dexamethasone for radiation-induced bone-pain flare [letter to author]. *Lancet Oncol.* 2016;17:e39–e40.
3. Chow S, Ding K, Wan BA, et al. Gender differences in pain and patient reported outcomes: a secondary analysis of the NCIC CTG SC. 23 randomized trial. *Ann Palliat Med.* 2017;6(Suppl 2):S185–S194.
4. Chow S, Ding K, Wan BA, et al. Patient reported outcomes after radiation therapy for bone metastases as a function of age: a secondary analysis of the NCIC CTG SC-twenty three randomized trial. *Am J Hosp Palliat Care.* 2018;35(4):718–723.
5. Fabregat C, Almendros S, Navarro-Martin A, Gonzalez J. Pain flare-effect prophylaxis with corticosteroids on bone radiotherapy treatment: a systematic review. *Pain Pract.* 2020;20(1):101–109.
6. Van der Linden YM, Westhoff PG, Stellato RK, et al. Dexamethasone for the prevention of a pain flare after palliative radiation therapy for painful bone metastases: the multicenter double-blind placebo-controlled 3-armed randomized Dutch DEXA study. *Int J Radiation Oncol Biol Phys.* 2020;108(3):546–553.

38

Psilocybin for Depression and Anxiety in Cancer Patients

TAMMIE E. QUEST AND ALI JOHN ZARRABI

> When administered under psychologically supportive, double-blind conditions, a single dose of psilocybin produced substantial and enduring decreases in depressed mood and anxiety along with increases in quality of life and decreases in death anxiety in patients with a life-threatening cancer diagnosis.
>
> —GRIFFITHS ET AL.[1]

Research Question: Does high-dose psilocybin administered under supportive conditions improve depression, anxiety, and other quality-of-life outcomes in patients with a life-threatening cancer diagnosis?

Funding: Grants from the Heffter Research Institute, the Riverstyx Foundation, William Linton, the Betsy Gordon Foundation, the McCormick Family, the Fetzer Institute, George Goldsmith, and Ekaterina Malievskaia. Effort for Dr. Griffiths in writing the paper was partially funded by the National Institutes of Health.

Year Study Began: 2007

Year Study Published: 2016

Study Location: Johns Hopkins University, Baltimore, Maryland

Who Was Studied: Cancer patients with a *Diagnostic and Statistical Manual of Mental Disorders*, fourth edition (DSM-IV) diagnosis that included anxiety and/or depression symptoms. Sixty-five percent of participants had recurrent or metastatic cancer. All had a DSM-IV diagnosis (from most common to least): chronic adjustment disorder with anxiety, chronic adjustment disorder with mixed anxiety and depressed mood, dysthymic disorder, generalized anxiety disorder (GAD), major depressive disorder (MDD), or a dual diagnosis of GAD and MDD, or GAD and dysthymic disorder.

Who Was Excluded: Patients with central nervous system (CNS) involvement of their cancer, significant hepatic dysfunction, renal insufficiency, uncontrolled hypertension, epilepsy, pregnant women, regular use of psychoactive prescription medications (including benzodiazepines), severe depression or anxiety symptoms warranting immediate treatment, and personal or family history of certain psychiatric conditions like schizophrenia, psychotic disorder, and bipolar disorder.

How Many Patients: 56 randomized (51 finished first psilocybin dosing session)

Study Overview: This is a randomized, double-blind, crossover trial in which 56 cancer patients with a concomitant DSM-IV diagnosis including anxiety or depression symptoms were randomized to receive either high-dose psilocybin or low-dose psilocybin (control). Both groups received supportive psychotherapy (Figure 38.1).

Study Intervention: Participants were randomly assigned to 1 of 2 groups: the low-dose-first group received the low dose of psilocybin during the first session and the high dose on the second session. The high-dose-first group received the high dose first and the low dose second. The first dosing session occurred approximately 1 month after study enrollment, and the second session occurred approximately 5 weeks later. Participants met with session monitors (the staff who would be present with them during psilocybin dosing) on 2 or more occasions prior to the first dosing session, the day after the first session, between the first and second dosing sessions, and between the dosing session and 6-month follow-up (mean total of 14.9 hours of therapy). Monitors were nondirective and supportive during the drug sessions. Preparatory sessions prior to the first drug dosing included discussion of meaning in the participant's life and functioned to establish rapport and prepare the participant for the psilocybin session. Dosing sessions occurred in a living-room-like environment where participants ingested

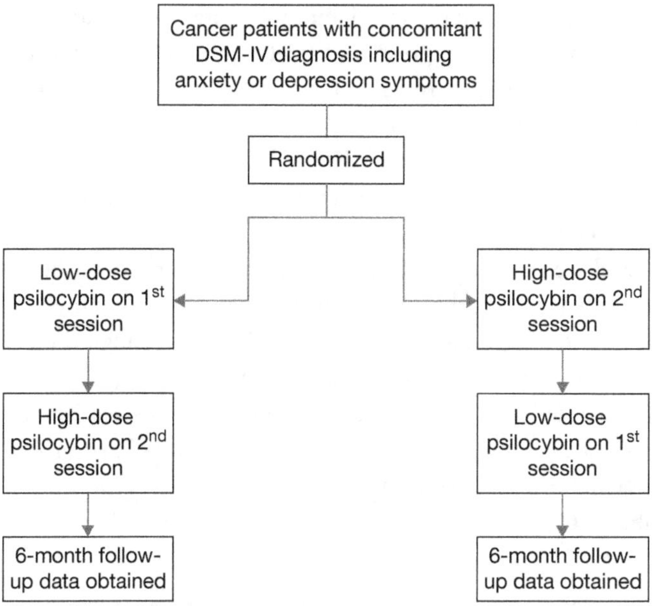

Figure 38.1. Flow diagram of trial design.

a psilocybin capsule and were encouraged to lie down on the couch, wear an eye mask to block visual distractions, and use headphones playing a preselected soundtrack. Participants were encouraged to "trust, let go, and be open" and focus their attention on inner experiences throughout the session.

Follow-Up: Approximately 9 months (mean 275 days)

Endpoints: Two primary therapeutic outcomes: Clinician-rated measure of depression (Hamilton Depression Rating Scale, GRID-HAM-D-17) and anxiety (Hamilton Anxiety Rating Scale, HAM-A). Subjective drug effect measures were assessed, including the Mystical Experience Questionnaire (MEQ30). Fifteen secondary measures focused on psychiatric symptoms, moods, and attitudes including the McGill Quality of Life Questionnaire (MQOL) and the Death Transcendence Scale. Cardiovascular outcomes such as blood pressure and heart rate were also measured.

RESULTS

- No serious adverse effects (cardiovascular or psychiatric) attributed to psilocybin administration occurred.

- Psilocybin produced large and significant decreases in clinician-rated and self-rated measures of depression, anxiety, or mood disturbance.
- Psilocybin produced increases in measures of quality of life, life meaning, death acceptance, and optimism.
- The mystical-type experience (MEQ30) during session 1 was significantly associated with the enduring change in therapeutic outcome measures 5 weeks later.
- At 5 weeks, 62% of high-dose psilocybin participants described the experience as among the top 5 *meaningful* experiences of their lives compared to 24% in the low-dose group. Among the high-dose group, the result was durable at 67.4% at 6-month follow-up.
- At 5 weeks, 66% of high-dose psilocybin participants described the experience as among the top 5 *spiritually significant* of their lives compared to 24% in the low-dose group. Among the high-dose group, the result was durable in 69.6% at 6-month follow-up. (See Table 38.1).

Table 38.1 SUMMARY OF STUDY'S KEY FINDINGS: PERCENTAGE OF PARTICIPANTS WITH CLINICALLY SIGNIFICANT RESPONSE RATE AND SYMPTOM REMISSION RATE AS ASSESSED BY CLINICIAN-RATED MEASURES

		Assessment Timepoint					
Measure	**Group**	**After Session 1**		**After Session 2**		**6 Months**[c]	
		CR[a]	**SR**[b]	**CR**	**SR**	**CR**	**SR**
GRID-HAMD-17 (Depression)	Low Dose First (High Dose Second)	32%	16%	75%	58%	77%	59%
	High Dose First (Low Dose Second)	92%[d]	60%[e]	84%	68%	79%	71%
HAM-A (Anxiety)	Low Dose First (High Dose Second)	24%	12%	83%	42%	82%	50%
	High Dose First (Low Dose Second)	76%[d]	52%[e]	80%	60%	83%	63%

Abbreviations: CR, clinical response; SR, symptom remission.

[a] For the clinician-rated measures (GRID-HAM-D-17 and HAM-A), a clinically significant response was defined as a ≥ 50% decrease in measure relative to baseline.

[b] Symptom remission is defined as a ≥ 50% decrease in measure relative to baseline and a score of ≤ 7 on the GRID-HAM-D or HAM-A.

[c] Effects of psilocybin on response and remission were sustained at 6 months (as indicated by a lack of significant difference, or $P > .05$).

[d] $P < .001$.

[e] $P < .01$.

Criticisms and Limitations:

- Participants were crossed over to the alternate-dose condition (i.e., low-dose to high-dose psilocybin) after 5 weeks, which precluded double-blind assessment of efficacy of the high-dose psilocybin after 5 weeks (as both groups received the high dose at that point)
- Participants were mostly highly educated and predominantly White (94%), limiting the generalizability of the study.

Other Relevant Studies and Information:

- Prior to the publication of this study, there were over 1000 publications studying psychedelic therapies that were conducted in the mid-20th century. These studies included use of psilocybin and lysergic acid diethylamide (LSD) for pain, death anxiety, anxiety, and depression in cancer populations. These studies came to a halt with the Controlled Substances Act (CSA) and limitations on funding for these types of trials.[2]
- A similar double-blind, placebo-controlled, crossover trial at New York University (NYU) was also published in 2016 in which 29 patients with cancer-related anxiety and depression were randomized to treatment with single-dose psilocybin or niacin (placebo) with concomitant psychotherapy.[3] Crossover was at 7 weeks. The results were similar to the Hopkins study: the pre-crossover psilocybin group reported immediate, substantial, and sustained (at 6.5 months) improvements in anxiety and depression as well as demoralization, hopelessness, spiritual well-being, and quality of life. As in the Hopkins trial, mystical experience mediated the therapeutic effect of psilocybin on anxiety and depression.
- Since the publication of the Johns Hopkins and NYU studies, other palliative care-oriented psychedelic studies have been published, including a 2020 pilot study using an adapted supportive expressive group therapy combined with psilocybin for demoralized older AIDS survivors.[4]
- To date, psilocybin and other classic psychedelics remain Schedule I drugs per the CSA and thus are defined as drugs with no currently accepted medical use and a high potential for abuse. No major American clinical societies recommend psilocybin for treatment of the symptoms and stress of a serious illness. However, significant private investment has led to the formation of several institutes dedicated to studying psychedelics, including at Johns Hopkins and NYU.

Summary and Implications: This seminal paper reintroduced psilocybin as a potential therapeutic for cancer-related anxiety and distress after decades of dormancy due to lack of funding and laws restricting study of classic psychedelic medicines. This small, randomized, double-blind, crossover trial demonstrated significant and sustained reductions in anxiety and depression and improvements in quality of life in a cancer population with predominantly recurrent or metastatic disease. This study, combined with the similar NYU trial, has led to multiple ongoing studies investigating the role of psychedelic drugs to potentially treat the symptoms and stress of a serious illness.

CLINICAL CASE: WHO SHOULD BE CONSIDRED FOR A PSYCHEDELIC-ASSISTED THERAPY CLINICAL TRIAL?

Case History

A 58-year-old woman with newly diagnosed metastatic breast cancer on cancer-directed therapy reports symptoms of anxiety, depression, and spiritual distress since her cancer diagnosis. You refer her to a mental health specialist, who diagnoses her with adjustment disorder with anxiety. As her palliative care clinician, you believe she is also demoralized with existential distress. During a clinic visit, she reports that she has heard about psychedelic therapy as a potential intervention for cancer patients with anxiety and depression. Should this patient undergo psychedelic-assisted psychotherapy?

Suggested Answer

Given that classic psychedelics (e.g., psilocybin, LSD, dimethyltryptamine [DMT]) are Schedule I drugs per the CSA and thus illegal for medical or recreational use outside of a clinical trial, you can help her identify clinical trials for which she meets inclusion/exclusion criteria. It would be unwise to recommend her to undergo psychedelic treatment outside the supportive context of a clinical trial. In general, cancer patients with CNS involvement, uncontrolled hypertension, psychiatric symptoms necessitating immediate treatment, or personal or family history of psychosis, bipolar disorder, or schizophrenia are generally excluded from these studies. The patient can be directed to clinicaltrials.gov to identify studies enrolling patients like her. As her clinician, you can also assist her in identifying studies. In the interim, you can facilitate access to a multidisciplinary team of professionals to help her manage the symptoms and stress related to her serious illness, regardless of whether she can or does ultimately enroll in a psychedelic-assisted psychotherapy clinical trial.

References

1. Griffiths RR, Johnson MW, Carducci MA, et al. Psilocybin produces substantial and sustained decreases in depression and anxiety in patients with life-threatening cancer: a randomized double-blind trial. *J Psychopharmacol.* 2016;30(12):1181–1197.
2. Carhart-Harris RL, Roseman L, Haijen E, et al. Psychedelics and the essential importance of context. *J Psychopharmacol.* 2018;32(7):725–731.
3. Ross S, Bossis A, Guss J, et al. Rapid and sustained symptom reduction following psilocybin treatment for anxiety and depression in patients with life-threatening cancer: a randomized controlled trial. *J Psychopharmacol.* 2016;30(12):1165–1180.
4. Anderson BT, Danforth A, Daroff PR, et al. Psilocybin-assisted group therapy for demoralized older long-term AIDS survivor men: an open-label safety and feasibility pilot study. *EClinicalMedicine.* 2020;27:100538. Published 2020 Sep 24.

39

The Use of Opioids for Breakthrough Pain in Acute Palliative Care Unit by Using Doses Proportional to Opioid Basal Regimen

JIMI S. MALIK AND TAMMIE E. QUEST

> The findings of this study suggest that in patients receiving opioids for chronic cancer pain, the risks of administering doses of opioids proportional to the basal opioid regimen, even though relatively high, are minimal, either with opioids at fast or slow onset of action.
>
> —MERCADANTE ET AL.[1]

Research Question: Are doses of opioids for breakthrough pain proportional to the basal opioid regimen safe and effective in clinical practice?

Funding: Information not provided in the manuscript

Year Study Began: 2008

Year Study Published: 2010

Study Location: La Maddalena Cancer Center, Palermo, Italy

Who Was Studied: All cancer patients consecutively admitted to La Maddalena Cancer Center Pain Relief and Palliative Care Unit over a period of 6 months (January 2008 to June 2008) were surveyed.

Who Was Excluded: Patients without cancer who were not admitted to the La Maddalena Cancer Center Pain Relief and Palliative Care Unit.

How Many Patients: 66

Study Overview: This is a prospective, observational study in which 66 consecutive patients admitted to a pain relief and palliative care unit over a 6-month period were surveyed. Of those surveyed, patients who were receiving opioids in doses of oral morphine equivalents of ≥ 60 mg daily and prescribed opioids for breakthrough pain of a different nature were included in the study.

Study Intervention: Patients were encouraged to call when their pain became severe, either during the titration phase or when basal pain was controlled (considered when the mean pain intensity was ≤ 4/10 on a 0–10 severity scale) and superimposed episodes of breakthrough pain occurred. Department policy suggested the breakthrough pain dose given be one-fifth of the oral morphine equivalent to daily doses, taking into account the route conversion ratios. Opioid conversion ratios used were based on the ratios conventionally used in that particular unit where the study was conducted (conversion ratios are included in Table 1 of the paper).

Numerical pain intensity scores, as well as differences in pain intensity after administration of different breakthrough opioids, are illustrated in Table 39.1. For each episode of breakthrough pain, trained nurses recorded pain intensity on a 0–10 severity scale at the time of the initial patient call (T0) and 15 minutes after administering the breakthrough pain dose of the opioid (T15). If a further breakthrough pain medication was required in the subsequent 2 hours, the administration of the initial opioid medication was considered unsuccessful.

Follow-up: 2 hours from delivery of the breakthrough pain medication

Endpoints:

- Primary outcome was the measurement of change in pain intensity among patients given opioids for breakthrough pain.
- Secondary outcome was the percentage of pain reduction.

Table 39.1 CHANGES IN PAIN INTENSITY IN PATIENTS TREATED WITH DIFFERENT OPIOIDS FOR BREAKTHROUGH PAIN

	Intravenous Morphine	Oral Transmucosal Fentanyl	Oral Morphine	Intravenous Methadone	Oral Methadone	Oral Oxycodone
Evaluable BTP episodes	248	124	31	15	4	5
T0 pain intensity (0–10 scale)	7.2	6.9	6.7	6.9	7.75	7.14
T15 pain intensity (0–10 scale)	2.72	2.53	2.39	2.86	3.5	3.4
Difference after 15 minutes	4.48	4.37	4.31	4.04	4.25	3.74
P value	.0005	.0005	.0005	.0005	.003	.001

Abbreviation: BTP, breakthrough pain.

RESULTS

- There were 624 episodes of breakthrough pain recorded during admission (5.3 d, SD ± 3.6), of which 503 were completely documented at both T0 and T15.
- Out of 503 episodes, 427 (84.9%) were successfully treated with the first opioid administration, without any further request, whereas 76 episodes (15.1%) required further opioid treatment within the subsequent 2 hours.
- Intravenous morphine and oral transmucosal fentanyl were the most frequently administered opioids.
- Pain intensity decreased at T15 in all the groups ($P \leq .001$) regardless of the drug modality used.
- The effects of opioid treatment were not modulated by gender or age ($P = .383$ and $P = .788$, for 33% and 50% of pain reduction, respectively, for gender, and $P = .288$ and $P = .218$, respectively, for age).

Criticisms and Limitations:

- First, and most importantly, this was a nonrandomized study without a control group; thus, it is not possible from this analysis to confirm that opioid treatment caused the observed improvements in pain symptoms.
- This is a single-center study in a cancer center, and it is unclear if the findings are generalizable to other settings.
- This study is at a high risk of having a placebo response since neither the patient nor the physician was blinded to the drug administration or the dose.[2,3]
- It is not possible to tell based on this analysis what the optimal opioid dosing is for maximizing pain control and minimizing side effects.
- This analysis provided minimal information on opioid safety and side effects.

Other Relevant Studies and Information:

- A 2007 study by Mercadante and colleagues[4] compared intravenous (IV) morphine and oral transmucosal fentanyl given for breakthrough pain. This study showed that IV morphine and oral transmucosal fentanyl, when given in a dose proportional to the basal opioid regimen, were comparable in treating breakthrough cancer pain, with IV morphine having a faster effect.
- A 2018 study of 592 patients by Azhar and colleagues[5] demonstrated that the majority of patients with advanced cancer with breakthrough pain reported good response to oral immediate-release opioids, supporting the use of these opioids in clinical practice. Among the minority with a suboptimal response, factors associated with a statistically significant association with poor response to immediate-release opioids for breakthrough pain were younger age and higher Edmonton Symptom Assessment System (ESAS) scores for pain, anxiety, and dyspnea.
- A double-blind, randomized, well-powered study tested 3 dose proportions between the breakthrough dose and the around-the-clock dose; 1/6, 1/8, and 1/12.[6] There was no difference in the 3 proportions and responses as determined by reduction in breakthrough pain intensity. There were no differences in harms. Therefore, the authors recommended using 1/12 of the morphine equivalent daily dose as the initial dose for breakthrough pain and adjusting the dose depending on response.
- According to a 2017 overview of Cochrane reviews,[7] the amount and quality of evidence around the use of opioids for treating cancer-related

pain is low. The evidence we do have, though, indicates that around 19 out of 20 people with moderate or severe pain who are given opioids and can tolerate them should have that pain reduced to mild or no pain within 14 days.

Summary and Implications: This 2010 Mercadante study demonstrates an improvement in patient perception of pain severity when breakthrough pain opioids are given at a dose one-fifth the basal opioid regimen, regardless of the specific opioid used.

CLINICAL CASE: WHICH OPIOID IS PREFERRED IN THE TREATMENT OF BREAKTHROUGH CANCER PAIN?

Case History

Palliative care is consulted to see a 55-year-old male with stage IV colon cancer for abdominal pain and symptom management. At home, he was initially taking as-needed short-acting morphine for pain for a couple months before a long-acting morphine was added to the regimen 3 weeks ago. With worsening cancer-related pain that was uncontrolled despite an increase in his morphine regimen as an outpatient, his long-acting opioid is rotated to a fentanyl patch. He does not have any trouble swallowing, there are no known drug allergies, and his kidney function is normal.

What is the superior opioid choice for reducing breakthrough cancer-related pain severity?

Suggested Answer

The 2010 study from Mercadante and colleagues demonstrated that the majority of patients with cancer who had a daily oral morphine equivalent need of > 60 mg/day could have a statistically significant improvement in perceived breakthrough pain severity with a number of breakthrough opioids, regardless of the opioid drug or modality of administration used. The dosages of opioids given for breakthrough pain were based on the protocol at the institution, which included a breakthrough pain dose that was one-fifth of the total daily oral morphine equivalent need.

Based on this study and for this particular patient case, then, it can be inferred that any opioid choice for breakthrough pain would be helpful in significantly reducing the patient's breakthrough pain severity.

References

1. Mercadante S, Villari P, Ferrera P, Mangione S, Casuccio A. The use of opioids for breakthrough pain in acute palliative care unit by using doses proportional to opioid basal regimen. *Clin J Pain*. 2010;26(4):306–309.
2. Hoenemeyer TW, Kaptchuk TJ, Mehta TS, Fontaine KR. Open-label placebo treatment for cancer-related fatigue: a randomized-controlled clinical trial. *Sci Rep*. 2018;8(1):2784.
3. Shaibani A, Frisaldi E, Benedetti F. Placebo response in pain, fatigue, and performance: possible implications for neuromuscular disorders. *Muscle Nerve*. 2017;56(3):358–367.
4. Mercadante S, Villari P, Ferrera P, et al. Transmucosal fentanyl versus intravenous morphine in doses proportional to basal opioid regimen for episodic-breakthrough pain. *Br J Cancer*. 2007;96:1828–1833.
5. Azhar A, Kim YJ, Haider A, et al. Response to oral immediate-release opioids for breakthrough pain in patients with advanced cancer with adequately controlled background pain. *Oncologist*. 2019;24(1):125–131.
6. Currow DC, Clark K, Louw S, Fazekas B, Greene A, Sanderson CR. A randomized, double-blind, crossover, dose ranging study to determine the optimal dose of oral opioid to treat breakthrough pain for patients with advanced cancer already established on regular opioids. *Eur J Pain*. 2020;24(5):983–991.
7. Wiffen PJ, Wee B, Derry S, Bell RF, Moore RA. Opioids for cancer pain—an overview of Cochrane reviews. *Cochrane Database Syst Rev*. 2017;(7):CD012592. Published 2017 Jul 6.

40

Perioperative Pregabalin for Prevention of Postmastectomy Pain Syndrome

RAVI PATHAK AND TAMMIE E. QUEST

> The present study showed a statistically and clinically significant reduction in the emergence of neuropathic postmastectomy pain syndrome by using a moderate dose of pregabalin for one week after breast cancer surgery.
>
> —REYAD ET AL.[1]

Research Question: Does perioperative use of pregabalin prevent postmastectomy pain syndrome (PMPS)?

Funding: No funding or grants, governmental coverage from the National Cancer Institute, Cairo University

Year Study Began: 2015

Year Study Published: 2018

Study Location: National Cancer Institute, Cairo University, Cairo, Egypt

Who Was Studied: Patients between the ages of 18 and 60 years and with American Society of Anesthesiologists physical status I, II, or III who are scheduled for elective breast surgery (either modified radical mastectomy or conservative breast surgery) combined with axillary dissection.

Who Was Excluded: Patients with allergies to gabapentinoids, nonsteroidal anti-inflammatory drugs (NSAIDs), or morphine; patients who are pregnant or lactating; patients with morbid obesity; patients with major medical disorders; and patients with history of gabapentinoid intake in the last 3 months.

How Many Patients: 200

Study Overview: This is a parallel-group, double-blind, randomized controlled trial in which 200 patients with breast cancer scheduled for elective breast cancer surgery were randomized to receive either perioperative pregabalin or placebo for 7 days (Figure 40.1).[1] The patients received standardized intraoperative

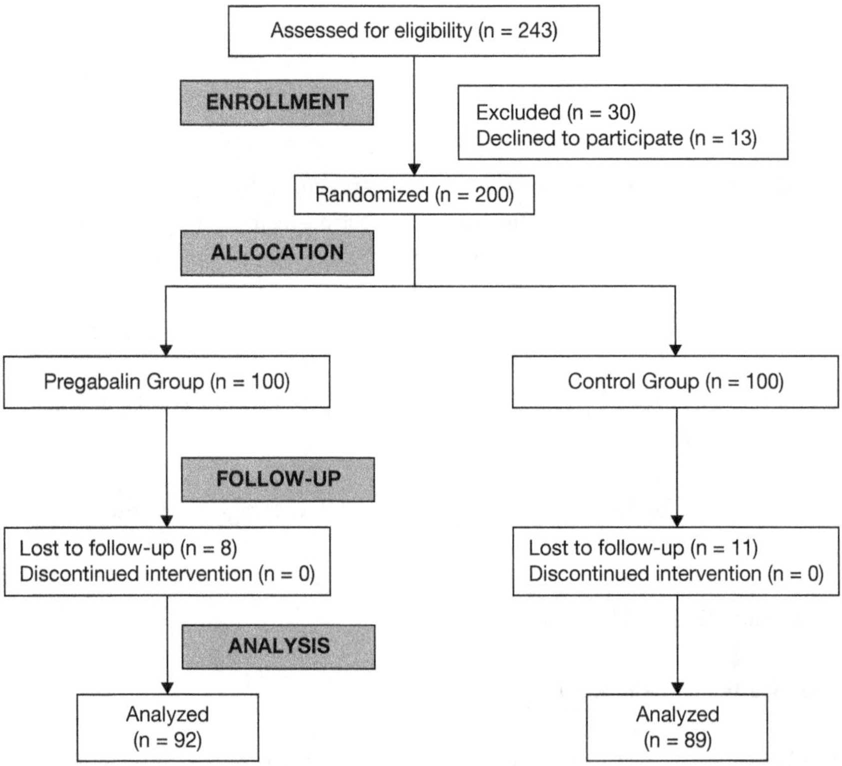

Figure 40.1. CONSORT flowchart.

Reprinted from Reyad RM, Omran AF, Abbas DN, et al. The possible preventive role of pregabalin in postmastectomy pain syndrome: a double-blinded randomized controlled trial [published correction appears in J Pain Symptom Manage. 2019 Jun;57(6):e11]. *J Pain Symptom Manage*. 2019;57(1):1–9. doi:10.1016/j.jpainsymman.2018.10.496. Copyright 2019, with permission from Elsevier.

anesthetic management, standardized in-hospital postoperative multimodal pain management (morphine, ketorolac), and standardized multimodal pain medications at discharge (acetaminophen, NSAIDs, tramadol). The primary outcome was development of neuropathic PMPS. Neuropathic pain was assessed using the Grading System for Neuropathic Pain (GSNP).

Study Intervention: The patients in the pregabalin group received a 75-mg dose 1 hour prior to induction of anesthesia and every 12 hours subsequently for 7 days. The control group received placebo at the same time points. The patients received standardized intraoperative anesthetic management, standardized in-hospital postoperative multimodal pain management (morphine, ketorolac), and standardized multimodal pain medications at discharge (acetaminophen, NSAIDs, tramadol) with a goal of < 40 mm on a visual analog scale (VAS). Patients were evaluated each hospital day and subsequently at postdischarge follow-up visits at 4, 12, and 24 weeks postoperatively. All data was collected by junior pain clinic physicians who were blinded to the study group.

Follow-Up: 24 weeks

Endpoints: Primary: Development of neuropathic PMPS, which was defined as intermittent or persistent numbness; tingling; burning, shooting, stinging, or stabbing pains; and hyperesthesia involving the anterior aspect of the chest, axilla, and/or upper arm at 12 weeks after surgery. These symptoms were graded according to the GSNP. Secondary: VAS scores, daily pain medication consumption, frequency of side effects or adverse events during 7-day period of pregabalin or placebo administration.

RESULTS

- Patients who received pregabalin had decreased incidence of PMPS at 12 weeks (Table 40.1).[1]
- Patients who received pregabalin had significantly less neuropathic pain at 4 weeks, 12 weeks, and 24 weeks (Table 40.1).[1]
- Patients in both the pregabalin group and placebo group had comparable VAS scores for the first 3 postoperative weeks. However, the pregabalin group had significantly lower VAS scores at 4 weeks, 12 weeks, and 24 weeks (Table 40.1).[1]
- There was no significant difference in adverse events or pain medication consumption between the pregabalin and control groups

Table 40.1 VISUAL ANALOG SCALE SCORE AND PROPORTION OF PATIENTS WITH NEUROPATHIC PAIN AND PMPS DURING FOLLOW-UP VISITS IN THE 2 STUDIED GROUPS

ITT Sample	Pregabalin Group $n = 100$	Control Group $n = 100$	*P* Value	RR (95% CI)
Visual analog scale score				
4 weeks	29 ± 14	35 ± 14	.001	
12 weeks	25 ± 12	34 ± 14	.007	
24 weeks	27 ± 18	35 ± 21	.002	
Probable neuropathic pain on GSNP≥Grade 3				
4 weeks	15 (15%)	32 (32%)	.005	0.38 (0.19–0.75)
12 weeks	14 (14%)	32 (32%)	.002	0.35 (0.17–0.70)
24 weeks	13 (13%)	35 (35%)	< .001	0.28 (0.14–0.57)
PMPS at 12 weeks	11 (11%)	29 (29%)	< .001	0.26 (0.12–0.56)

Abbreviations: GSNP, Grading System for Neuropathic Pain; PMPS, postmastectomy pain syndrome; RR, relative risk; ITT, Intention to Treat.

Criticisms and Limitations:

- This is a single-center study from a large center in Cairo, Egypt. It is unclear how generalizable the results are to other settings and populations.
- This study did not control for surgical technique (i.e., size of incision, extent of dissection, number of lymph nodes removed). Variation in surgical technique may contribute to the development of PMPS. A longer follow-up period may have provided data on how perioperative gabapentin affects the long-term incidence, duration, and evolution of PMPS.
- Persistent pain after surgery is associated with young age, alcohol or drug use disorder, pain prior to surgery (even if distant from the surgical site), and mood disorder which was not controlled for in the study.[2,3]

Other Relevant Studies and Information:

- A similar randomized controlled trial from an academic center in India comparing pregabalin versus placebo in women undergoing mastectomy found no difference in incidence or severity of chronic postmastectomy pain at 12 weeks ($P = .407$ and $P = .307$, respectively).[4] The significant difference in this study is that there was a lack of standardized pain management protocols in the perioperative period. In addition, the follow-up period was 12 weeks as compared to 24 weeks in the study by Reyad et al.

- A meta-analysis that reviewed preoperative pregabalin for acute and chronic postoperative pain after breast cancer surgery showed that preoperative pregabalin did not reduce chronic postoperative pain (odds ratio 0.23, 95% CI: 0.02–2.80, $P = .25$) at 3 months.[5] Only 2 studies met the criteria to be included in the meta-analysis to evaluate preoperative pregabalin for the prevention of chronic postoperative pain after breast cancer surgery.
- A Cochrane review on pharmacotherapy for the prevention of chronic pain after surgery published in 2013 identified 5 trials with long-term pain outcomes in which patients received pregabalin.[6] The study groups included cardiac surgery, total knee arthroplasty, spine surgery, and thyroidectomy, but notably no studies involving breast surgery were included. Based on the meta-analysis from the 5 studies included, the authors felt that data for pregabalin failed to demonstrate statistical significance when compared to placebo at 3 months postsurgery.

Summary and Implications: This randomized controlled trial demonstrates that in patients undergoing elective breast cancer surgery, perioperative pregabalin use decreased the incidence of PMPS at 12 weeks as well as decreased pain intensity (VAS) at several time points from 4 weeks to 24 weeks. However, other studies and meta-analyses with different pregabalin dosing strategies and different lengths of follow-up have not demonstrated similar results.[4–6] Therefore, this study prompts the need for larger multicenter trials with diverse populations, utilization of standardized intraoperative and postoperative pain management, and follow-up for at least 24 weeks to determine if there is a role for pregabalin in the prevention of PMPS.

CLINICAL CASE: PERIOPERATIVE PREGABALIN TO PREVENT POSTMASTECTOMY PAIN AFTER ELECTIVE BREAST CANCER SURGERY

Case History

A 50-year-old woman with breast cancer is scheduled for elective radical mastectomy with axillary lymph node dissection. She is classified as American Society of Anesthesiologists physical status II. She is not allergic to gabapentinoids and has not taken gabapentinoids for > 3 months. In addition, she is not pregnant, her body mass index is < 35, and she has no other major medical issues.

Should this patient be prescribed pregabalin 75 mg twice a day for 7 days starting with the morning of surgery?

Suggested Answer

Approximately 10% of all surgical patients develop chronic postsurgical pain. The incidence of chronic postsurgical pain is higher after surgical procedures where there is potential transection of nerves such as mastectomy, thoracotomy, and limb amputations. It is estimated that 20%–40% of patients who undergo mastectomy develop chronic postsurgical pain.[1] This study showed that a regimen of pregabalin 75 mg twice a day starting on the morning of surgery resulted in a risk reduction of 0.26 (95% CI: 0.12–0.56) of developing PMPS. In addition, patients who received pregabalin had a statistically significant reduction in neuropathic pain and pain intensity at 4, 12, and 24 weeks without an increase in adverse events or side effects associated with pregabalin. Therefore, this patient may benefit from a course of perioperative pregabalin.

References

1. Reyad RM, Omran AF, Abbas DN, et al. The possible preventive role of pregabalin in postmastectomy pain syndrome: a double-blinded randomized controlled trial [published correction appears in *J Pain Symptom Manage.* 2019 Jun;57(6):e11]. *J Pain Symptom Manage.* 2019;57(1):1–9. doi:10.1016/j.jpainsymman.2018.10.496.
2. Hah JM, Cramer E, Hilmoe H, et al. Factors associated with acute pain estimation, postoperative pain resolution, opioid cessation, and recovery: secondary analysis of a randomized clinical trial. *JAMA Netw Open.* 2019;2(3):e190168.
3. Gartner R, Jensen MB, Nielsen J, Ewertz M, Kroman N, Kehlet H. Prevalence of and factors associated with persistent pain following breast cancer surgery. *JAMA.* 2009;302(18):1985–1992.
4. Vig S, Kumar V, Deo S, Bhan S, Mishra S, Bhatnagar S. Effect of perioperative pregabalin on incidence of chronic postmastectomy pain syndrome: a prospective randomized placebo-controlled pilot study. *Indian J Palliat Care.* 2019;25(4):508–513. doi:10.4103/IJPC.IJPC_85_19.
5. Rai AS, Khan JS, Dhaliwal J, et al. Preoperative pregabalin or gabapentin for acute and chronic postoperative pain among patients undergoing breast cancer surgery: a systematic review and meta-analysis of randomized controlled trials. *J Plast Reconstr Aesthet Surg.* 2017;70(10):1317–1328. doi:10.1016/j.bjps.2017.05.054.
6. Chaparro LE, Smith SA, Moore RA, Wiffen PJ, Gilron I. Pharmacotherapy for the prevention of chronic pain after surgery in adults. *Cochrane Database Syst Rev.* 2013;(7):CD008307. Published 2013 Jul 24. doi:10.1002/14651858.CD008307.pub2.

41

Morphine for Chronic Breathlessness

ANNE ROHLFING AND ERIC WIDERA

> Present results do not support the use of morphine for chronic breathlessness in people with advanced disease but who are mostly ambulatory.
>
> —CURROW ET AL.[1]

Research Question: Does scheduled low-dose, sustained-release morphine improve breathlessness in patients with moderate to severe chronic breathlessness?

Funding: Palliative Care Program, Australia's Department of Health

Year Study Began: 2010

Year Study Published: 2020

Study Location: 14 inpatient and outpatient cardiorespiratory and palliative care services in Australia

Who Was Studied: English-speaking adults (≥ 18 years of age) with a prognosis of ≥ 2 months and a modified Medical Research Council (mMRC) breathlessness score ≥ 2 on a stable medication regimen.

Who Was Excluded: Patients with limited functional status (Australia-modified Karnofsky Performance Status [AKPS] < 40), ≥20 oral morphine equivalents per day, uncontrolled nausea, renal dysfunction, hepatic dysfunction, anemia requiring transfusions, history of opioid-related respiratory failure, or a recent cardiac/respiratory event.

How Many Patients: 287

Study Overview: In this multicenter, double-blind, randomized controlled trial, 287 patients with moderate to severe chronic breathlessness were randomized 1:1 to 20 mg once daily sustained-released (SR) morphine versus placebo (Figure 41.1).

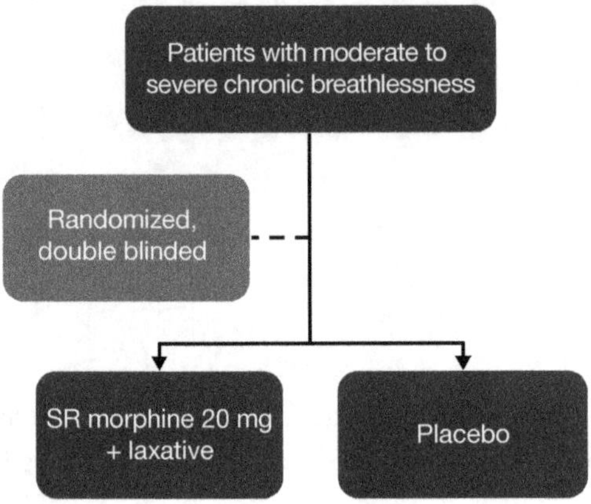

Figure 41.1. Summary of study design.

Study Intervention: Patients received either SR morphine 20 mg + laxative or placebo morphine + laxative daily for 1 week. Both groups were allowed to take ≤ 6 doses of as-needed immediate-release (IR) morphine during the treatment period. Patients completed diary entries twice daily to document breathlessness (*now* in morning entry; *now, worst, best, average* for evening entry) using a horizontal visual scale from *none* (0) to *worst possible* (100 mm). Study staff called patients to administer quality-of-life questionnaires, assess adverse events, and conduct in-person assessments of vitals, oxygen saturation, and end-tidal carbon dioxide at baseline, midway through the treatment period, and weekly for 4 weeks after the treatment period ended.

Follow-Up: 4 weeks

Endpoints:

Primary outcome: Change in intensity of breathlessness after 5–7 days.

Secondary outcomes: Intensity of *worst, best, now, average* breathlessness; health-related quality of life (European Organization for Research and Treatment of Cancer-Quality of Life Questionnaire Core 15 PAL [EORTC-QLQ-C15 PAL]); caregiver quality of life (Caregiver Quality of Life Index-Cancer [CQOLC]); use of as-needed IR morphine; change in functional status (AKPS).

RESULTS

- There was no difference between the treatment and placebo groups for the primary outcome of change in breathlessness *now*, and no difference was found for any of the secondary outcomes in *worst*, *best*, or *average* breathlessness scores (Table 41.1).

Table 41.1 SUMMARY OF STUDY'S KEY FINDINGS

	SR Morphine	Placebo	*P* Value
Change in breathlessness *now* (mm)	−5.00	−4.86	.95
Average IR morphine doses/day	5.8	8.7	.003
Constipation	15.8	2.3	.001
Nausea/vomiting (EORTC-QLQ-C15 PAL)	6.1	−1.4	.008
Fatigue (EORTC-QLQ-C15 PAL)	6.1	−4.8	< .001

Abbreviations: EORTC-QLQ, European Organization for Research and Treatment of Cancer-Quality of Life Questionnaire; IR, immediate release; SR, sustained release.

- Subgroup analysis of those patients with more severe chronic breathlessness (mMRC of 3 or 4) showed a trend toward reduction of *worst* breathlessness.
- Patients in the placebo group used 55% more doses of IR morphine per day compared to the treatment group on average, a statistically significant difference.
- Patients in the treatment group had more adverse events, specifically constipation, nausea/vomiting, and fatigue, based on reporting of events and quality-of-life scoring.
- There were no significant differences in oxygen saturation or end-tidal carbon dioxide, and no evidence for respiratory depression in the treatment group.

Criticisms and Limitations: While initially designed to focus on patients with severe chronic breathlessness (mMRC score 3–4), due to limited enrollment, the authors had to expand to include those with an mMRC score ≥ 2. Evolving evidence suggests that more severe breathlessness likely responds more to opioids than moderate breathlessness, which aligns with most clinical practice guidelines and makes this study harder to apply in practice. The applicability is also limited by the population itself: only 37% female with no data reported on race/ethnicity, average age 74.3 years, and majority chronic obstructive pulmonary disease (COPD) as etiology of breathlessness. Further limitations include its short timeframe (1 week), a dosing regimen not currently available in the United States (20 mg SR morphine), and exposure to morphine in both groups (via as-needed IR morphine).

Other Relevant Studies and Information:

- A randomized, double-blinded trial of SR morphine (10 mg twice daily) for patients with the same severity of chronic breathlessness (mMRC ≥ 2) but limited to COPD was published in 2020 by Verberkt et al., showing improvement in a COPD-specific health status score and a significant change in *worst* breathlessness but only for patients with severe dyspnea (mMRC ≥ 3).[2]
- Small, crossover trials have highlighted the safety of low-dose SR opioids in patients with chronic breathlessness, as well as some evidence of effect on chronic breathlessness.[3–5]
- While other guidelines have not yet been updated, the European Society of Medical Oncology released guidelines in 2020 for dyspnea management that cite this study and recommend SR morphine only for severe, debilitating breathlessness after failure of nonpharmacologic methods.[6]

Summary and Implications: In this randomized and double-blinded trial to assess efficacy of SR morphine on moderate to severe chronic breathlessness, no improvement in breathlessness scores was found. The treatment was overall well tolerated without any severe adverse events; patients did experience common opioid side effects of nausea, constipation, and fatigue. Given the evolving evidence that dyspnea is most responsive in those with severe dyspnea (mMRC grade 3 or 4), including the trend toward a positive effect in this trial, future studies should focus on the role of opioids for managing severe breathlessness.

CLINICAL CASE: HOW TO TREAT CHRONIC BREATHLESSNESS?

Case History

A 74-year-old woman with COPD on 2 L home oxygen presents to the clinic with severe breathlessness (mMRC of 4; too breathless to leave the house). She has been medically optimized per recent guidelines on an inhaler regimen, uses a pocket fan as well as guided imagery and meditation, and has already completed pulmonary rehabilitation. Her pulmonologist has referred her to your palliative care clinic given the severity of her disease and its effects on quality of life. Should you prescribe a SR opioid?

Suggested Answer

Based on the Currow study described in this chapter, as well as the subsequent trial by Verberkt, it is reasonable to consider adding a low dose of SR opioid to help manage severe chronic breathlessness after patients have been optimized for their disease treatment and using nonpharmacologic methods (i.e., pulmonary rehabilitation, fan, guided imagery, mindfulness meditation, acupuncture, etc.). While the opioids in these trials were a dose of SR morphine not currently available in the United States (20 mg daily or 10 mg twice daily), it would be reasonable to extrapolate to our lowest dose of 15 mg SR morphine once daily to start, with as-needed IR morphine of 5 mg, in addition to laxatives while on chronic opioids.

References

1. Currow D, Louw S, McCloud P, et al. Regular, sustained-release morphine for chronic breathlessness: a multicentre, double-blind, randomised, placebo-controlled trial. *Thorax*. 2020 Jan;75:50–56.
2. Verberkt C, van den Beuken-van Everdingen M, Schols J, et al. Effect of sustained-release morphine for refractory breathlessness in chronic obstructive pulmonary disease on health status: a randomized clinical trial. *JAMA Intern Med*. 2020;180(10):1306–1314.
3. Ekström M, Nilsson F, Abernethy A, Currow D. Effects of opioids on breathlessness and exercise capacity in chronic obstructive pulmonary disease: a systematic review. *Ann Am Thorac Soc*. 2015;12(7):1079–1092.
4. Abdallah S, Wilkinson-Maitland C, Saad N, et al. Effect of morphine on breathlessness and exercise endurance in advanced COPD: a randomised crossover trial. *Eur Respir J*. 2017;50(4):1701235.
5. Abernethy A, Currow D, Frith P, et al. Randomised, double blind, placebo controlled crossover trial of sustained release morphine for the management of refractory dyspnoea. *BMJ*. 2003 Sep;327(7414):523–528.
6. Hui D, Maddocks M, Johnson MJ, et al. Management of breathlessness in patients with cancer: ESMO Clinical Practice Guidelines. *ESMO Open*. 2020 Dec;5(6):e001038.

42

Hyoscine Butylbromide for the Management of Death Rattle

ELIZABETH SCHACK AND ELIZABETH CAPANO

> This study showed that hyoscine butylbromide, given prophylactically in the dying patient with a spontaneous decrease in level of consciousness or induced by palliative sedation, is an effective strategy in preventing death rattle. Hyoscine butylbromide given after the development of death rattle was frequently ineffective.
>
> —Mercadante et al.[1]

Research Question: Does the prophylactic use of hyoscine butylbromide (HB), an anticholinergic agent, improve outcomes in the management of death rattle in comparison to administration once death rattle starts?

Funding: This study did not receive any specific public, commercial, or not-for-profit grant or funding.

Year Study Began: Dates not included in article

Year Study Published: 2018

Study Location: 2 hospices located in Italy, 1 in Latina and the other in L'Aquila

Who Was Studied: Adults, 18 years and older, who were terminally ill and close to death with a decreased level of consciousness. In addition, the participants were required to have a score of ≤ 3 on the Richmond Agitation Sedation Scale—Palliative version (RASS-PAL).

Who Was Excluded: Patients who were actively being treated with another antimuscarinic medication, patients who already had death rattle, or those with an obvious secondary cause of death rattle, such as infection, aspiration, or cardiac failure.

How Many Patients: 132

Study Overview: This is a multicenter prospective and randomized trial in which patients with RASS-PAL scores of ≤ 3 were randomized to 1 of 2 treatment groups. In group 2, HB was the treatment given to actively dying patients prophylactically to determine if it is an effective treatment in preventing death rattle from starting or minimizing its effects. In group 1, patients were only treated with HB if they started to have death rattle (Figure 42.1).

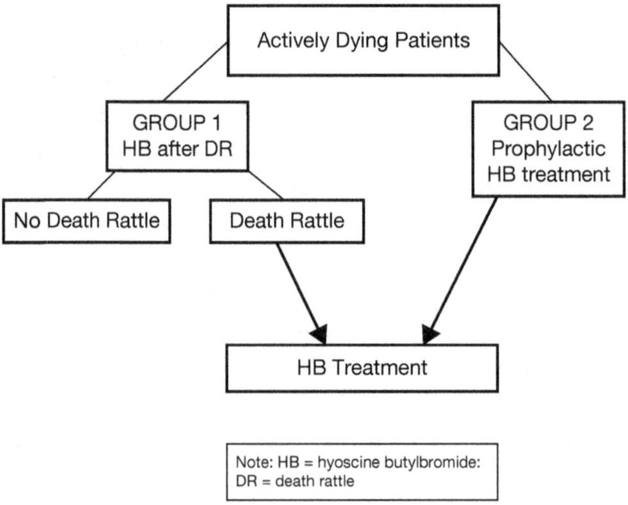

Figure 42.1. Study overview.

Study Intervention: In the first group, patients were administered HB only when death rattle developed. This study created a death rattle intensity scale from 0, which is not audible, to 3, indicating that the death rattle is audible at a distance of about 9.5 meters (31 feet) from the patient's door in a quiet room.

Group 2 received HB prophylactically in the absence of death rattle. Other symptomatic medications were continued including opioids, diuretics, sedatives, and neuroleptics when indicated, while patients receiving intravenous hydration were reduced to 10 mL/hour. Once the treatment (HB) was initiated (20-mg bolus followed by 60 mg/day), the patients were evaluated at predefined points: 30 minutes, 1 hour, and then every 6 hours until the patient died. The treatment was deemed effective if the patient didn't develop a death rattle in group 2 and if the intensity of the rattle was 0 or 1 on the death rattle scoring system in group 1.

Follow-Up: Until the participant's death

Endpoints:

Primary outcome: The presence of death rattle from the time of randomization and then at 30 minutes, 1 hour, and every 6 hours until death.

Secondary outcomes: Death rattle score (DRS) measuring intensity, death-rattle-free time (DRFT), and RASS-PAL also from randomization and then at 30 minutes, 1 hour, and every 6 hours until death.

RESULTS

- Overall, the study reveals that the prophylactic administration of HB in actively dying patients with reduced consciousness or induced palliative sedation is an effective preventative treatment for death rattle (see Table 42.1).

Table 42.1 SUMMARY OF KEY FINDINGS

Outcome	**Group 1**	**Group 2**	***P* Value**
Death rattle (from T0 to death)	*n* = 49 (60.5%)	*n* = 3 (5.9%)	.001
Death-rattle-free time	20.4 hours	27.3 hours	.0001
	SD (20.53)	SD (25.2)	
	Median 12 hours	Median 36 hours	
RASS-PAL and DRS	No difference	No difference	

Abbreviations: DRS, death rattle scale; RASS-PAL, Richmond Agitation-Sedation Scale—Palliative version; SD, standard deviation; T0, study start time.

- The treatment of HB once death rattle started was effective in a small percentage (approximately 20%) of patients. Effectiveness was measured by the patient having a DRS of 1 or less, meaning not audible at all or only audible near the patient.

- The secondary outcomes of DRS and RASS-PAL did not show statistical significance between the 2 groups.

Criticisms and Limitations:

- The study is not a traditional randomized controlled trial as HB was given in both arms of the study based on the administration inclusion criteria.
- Despite caregiver education and health care provider knowledge, the death rattle symptom can be distressing. While the lack of a placebo arm in this study could be considered a limitation, it is likely considered acceptable that the investigators chose the path of comparing traditional use versus prophylactic use based on the drug's mechanism of action.

Other Relevant Studies and Information:

- A study comparing HB and glycopyrrolate for patients experiencing death rattle in the dying process suggests that HB is the better agent for death rattle treatment. While the study only investigates the side-by-side comparison of 2 anticholinergic medications, it does suggest better efficacy of HB over glycopyrrolate.[2]
- A larger study done by Wildiers et al. comparing atropine, HB, and scopolamine for treatment of death rattle show that all 3 medications exhibit similar efficacy. The study's analysis suggests that earlier introduction of anticholinergics at a lower rattle intensity improves outcomes.[3]
- The SILENCE trial[4] demonstrates that subcutaneous scopolamine butylbromide, another anticholinergic agent, when compared to placebo was an effective prophylactic treatment in the reduction of the death rattle in patients at the end of life. This trial corroborates the study outcomes of Mercadante and colleagues.[1]

Summary and Implications: This trial comparing prophylactic use of HB for the prevention of death rattle versus use of HB to manage the condition once it has started found that HB can be effective treatment in minimizing death rattle. The implications of this study could lead to changes in the standards of care for end-of-life symptom management.

CLINICAL CASE: IS THERE BENEFIT TO STARTING ANTICHOLINERGICS BEFORE DEATH RATTLE IS PRESENT?

Case History

A 78-year-old woman with metastatic ovarian cancer who was participating in a clinical trial had a precipitous physical decline and developed overwhelming pain and other symptoms. She made a decision to focus on comfort after her symptom burden became too overwhelming for her to manage care at home. She decided with the support of her family to enter an inpatient hospice for aggressive symptom management. The inpatient hospice team is able to get her pain under control, and in the last 24 hours she becomes obtunded and is no longer able to interact with her health care providers or her family. She is only receiving opioids and occasional Ativan for agitation. Her significant other shares with the inpatient hospice team that he watched his own mother die and felt significant distress over hearing her "drown in her own secretions." He remembers the medical team explaining that it wasn't "distressing to her," but he is worried that the same thing will happen to his wife.

Should the inpatient hospice team initiate standing anticholinergics to reduce the possible occurrence of the death rattle symptom in this patient?

Suggested Answer

The Mercadante study suggests another paradigm of using anticholinergics prophylactically to either eliminate death rattle from occurring or minimize the risk of having the symptom at all. This patient would be eligible for the team to initiate the preemptive treatment of HB. The team would give the patient a bolus dose of 20 mg and then continue a daily amount of 60 mg/day to achieve the effectiveness simulated in the study. The inpatient hospice team would want to educate the patient's family that this may not completely prevent the sound from occurring but that it may reduce her risk of having it. The hospice team will continue to use the medication but will also use positioning to assist with minimizing the potential sound.

References

1. Mercadante S, Marinangeli F, Masedu F, et al. Hyoscine butylbromide for the management of death rattle: sooner rather than later. *J Pain Symptom Manage.* 2018;56(6):902–907.

2. Back IN, Jenkins K, Blower A, Beckhelling J. A study comparing hyoscine hydrobromide and glycopyrrolate in the treatment of death rattle. *Palliat Med.* 2001;15(4):329–336.
3. Wildiers H, Dhaenekint C, Demeulenaere P, et al. Atropine, hyoscine butylbromide, or scopolamine are equally effective for the treatment of death rattle in terminal care. *J Pain Symptom Manage.* 2009;38(1):124–133.
4. van Esch HJ, van Zuylen L, Geijteman ECT, et al. Effect of prophylactic subcutaneous scopolamine butylbromide on death rattle in patients at the end of life: the SILENCE randomized clinical trial. *JAMA.* 2021;326(13):1268–1276.

43

Randomized Controlled Trial of Oral Docusate in Patients on Hospice

ABBY STEVENS

> The study findings only suggest that there may be therapeutic equivalence between placebo and docusate, but do not prove this definitively.
>
> —TARUMI ET AL.[1]

Research Question: Does the addition of docusate to sennosides increase the stool frequency, volume, and consistency in patients on hospice with constipation?

Funding: College of Family Physicians of Canada, Caritas Research Trust Fund, Department of Family Medicine at the University of Alberta, Health Quality Council of Alberta, and Alberta Innovates-Health Solutions

Year Study Began: 2005

Year Study Published: 2012

Study Location: 3 inpatient hospice units in Edmonton, Alberta: St. Joseph's Auxiliary Hospital, Edmonton General Continuing Care Center, Capital Care Norwood

Who Was Studied: Adults newly admitted to inpatient hospice with malignancy, currently on or newly started on opioid analgesics, Palliative Performance Scale (PPS) score of at least 20% (able to tolerate sips or food, may or may not be bedbound, may or may not be confused), no difficulty swallowing, able to tolerate oral medications. In April 2006 (4 months after enrollment initiation), criteria were expanded to include patients without malignancy and no longer required patients to be currently receiving opioid therapy.

Who Was Excluded: Patients with gastrointestinal stoma, contraindication to docusate, prescribed docusate "as needed," if docusate was prescribed in liquid or crushed form, or if docusate was discontinued or withheld before the patient was screened.

How Many Patients: 74

Study Overview: This randomized, double-blind, placebo-controlled trial enrolled patients newly admitted to inpatient hospice and randomized to the docusate or placebo group. The study period lasted for 10 days (Figure 43.1).

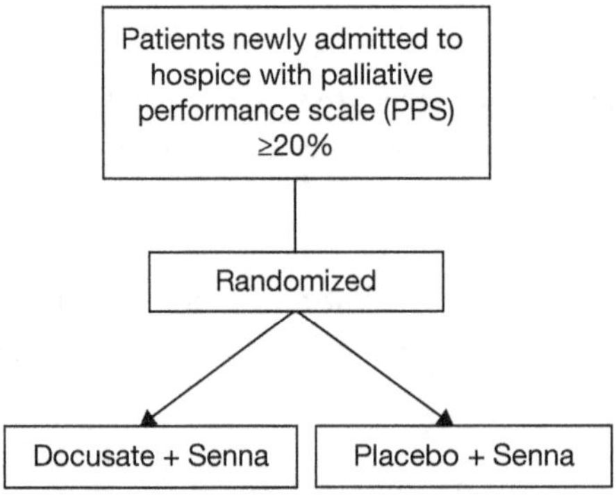

Figure 43.1. Summary of study design.

Study Intervention: Patients in the docusate group received two 100-mg docusate tablets twice daily plus 1–3 sennoside tablets (8.6 mg/tablet) 1–3 times daily. The placebo group received 2 cornstarch capsules twice daily, in addition to 1–3 sennoside tablets taken 1–3 times daily. After the 10-day study period, patients returned to their previous bowel regimen. During the study period, patients were allowed to take additional laxatives. Nursing staff at the inpatient hospice units received multiple educational sessions to standardize stool consistency and volume recordings.

Follow-Up: 10 days

Endpoints:

- Primary outcome measures
  - o Stool frequency
  - o Stool volume
    - Measured using standardized model of 3 sizes of stool: large = 1 full cup, medium = ½ cup, small = ¼ cup, or smear
  - o Stool consistency
    - Measured using Bristol Stool Form Scale[2]
- Secondary outcomes
  - o The need for additional bowel care interventions, such as bisacodyl suppository, sodium phosphate enema, oil retention enema followed by soapsuds cleansing edema, lactulose, polyethylene glycol, magnesium hydroxide, or mineral oil
  - o Patient's perception of difficulty and completeness of evacuation

RESULTS

- There were no significant differences found between the docusate and placebo groups in terms of stool frequency, volume, or consistency.
- At least 91.7% of patients in the docusate group received daily opioids compared with 100% of patients in the placebo group.
  - o Morphine equivalent daily dose (MEDD) of opioids was not significantly different between the groups: 92.9 mg MEDD in the docusate group and 154.3 mg MEDD in the placebo group.
- More patients in the docusate group had larger bowel movements.
- Patients in the docusate group had more type 3 (sausage, cracks in surface) and 6 (mushy stool, fluffy pieces with ragged edges) bowel movements according to the Bristol Stool Form Scale, and patients in the placebo group had more type 4 (smooth and soft, like a sausage or snake) and 5 (soft blobs with clear-cut edges) bowel movements (Figure 43.2).
- There was no significant difference between groups related to the perception of difficulty passing stools, sense of complete evacuation, or the administration of additional bowel care interventions (Figure 43.3).
- The Edmonton Symptom Assessment Score,[3] which assesses symptoms of constipation, were not statistically different between the study groups.

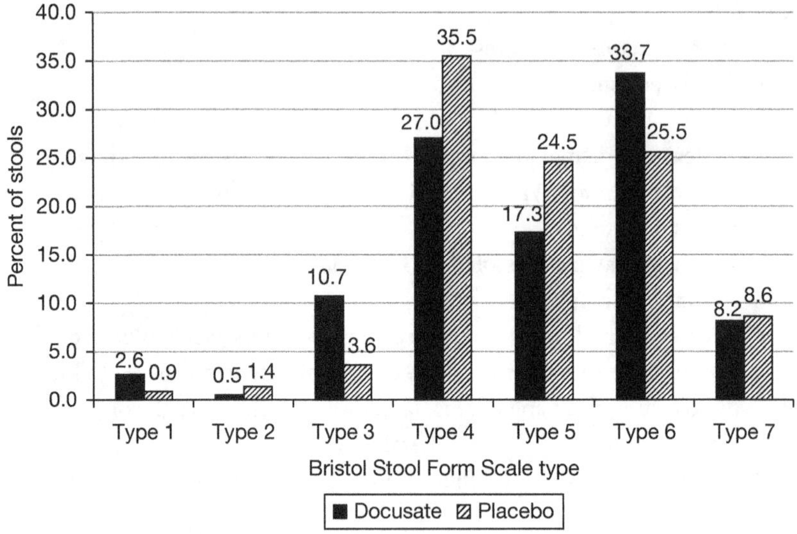

Figure 43.2. Stool consistency by study group.

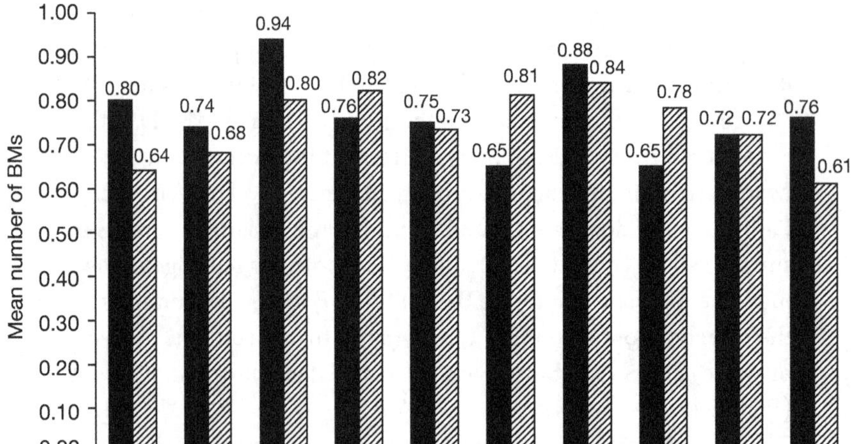

Figure 43.3. Mean number of bowel movements by day by study group.

Criticisms and Limitations:

- This study was conducted at inpatient hospice units, which generally admit patients with very serious illness who have a limited life expectancy. This may limit the generalizability of this study to the diverse population of people who receive palliative care.
- There were variations in achieving responses on sensation of completeness of evacuation after bowel movements due to timing of nurse administration of questions after bowel movement and whether patients required more assistance with bowel movements or not.
- This study took place over 5 years; the prescribers in the hospice units may have altered their prescribing habits due to the nature of the study taking place, contributing to the low number of patients eligible for study inclusion.
- Patients were able to receive rescue bowel care interventions, which could have contributed to the lack of difference observed in the groups.

Other Relevant Studies and Information:

- Hawley and Byeon[4] compared senna and docusate to senna alone in 60 hospitalized patients with cancer for 5–12 days. The senna-only cohort experienced more bowel movements, as defined by proportion of total days with at least 1 bowel movement or at least 40% or 50% of days with bowel movements, than the senna and docusate cohort, although not statistically significant. More patients in the senna and docusate group required additional bowel regimen interventions.
- As a result of these studies, the National Comprehensive Cancer Network 2019 Adult Cancer Pain guidelines[5] do not include stool softeners (i.e., docusate) in their recommendation for prophylaxis or treatment of opioid-induced constipation.

Summary and Implications: In this randomized controlled trial evaluating the benefit of docusate added to senna therapy for the treatment of constipation in patients admitted to an inpatient hospice unit, there was no added benefit of docusate with respect to stool frequency, volume, or consistency. Almost 92% and 100% of patients in the docusate and placebo groups, respectively, received concomitant opioids. These findings are similar to previous studies comparing bowel regimens for constipation management, and they are noticeably absent from recent clinical guidelines. The routine use of docusate as part of a bowel regimen for the treatment of constipation should continue to be questioned as it adds burden to patients and caregivers, may have limited clinical value, and increases the cost of care.

CLINICAL CASE: WHICH BOWEL REGIMEN IS BEST?

Case History

A patient with metastatic lung cancer was recently admitted to inpatient hospice for dyspnea management. He currently receives hydromorphone 1 mg intravenously every 3 hours as needed for shortness of breath (takes ~4 doses per day). He has been taking 1 docusate 100-mg capsule in the morning and at bedtime. He reports bowel movements every couple of days, which he describes as hard stools. He denies any other side effects of the docusate, such as abdominal pain or colic.

Is there anything that can be done to optimize the patient's bowel regimen?

Suggested Answer

Constipation is an expected side effect of opioids. For patients with serious illness, it is generally preferred to start a bowel regimen upon initiation of opioid therapy, irrespective of opioid dose. Docusate alone is not providing benefit to the patient, which is not surprising based on the results by Tarumi et al. It would be reasonable to stop docusate and start senna 2 tablets by mouth at night. Nighttime dosing has been recommended with the idea of allowing the senna to work overnight and produce bowel movement in the morning. Senna 8.6-mg tablets can be titrated up to 8 tablets per day in divided doses (i.e., 4 senna 8.6-mg tablets taken twice daily).

References

1. Tarumi Y, Wilson MP, Szafran O, Spooner GR. Randomized, double-blind, placebo-controlled trial of oral docusate in the management of constipation in hospice patients. *J Pain Symptom Manage*. 2013;45(1):2–13. doi:10.1016/j.jpainsymman.2012.02.008.
2. O'Donnell LJ, Virjee J, Heaton KW. Detection of pseudodiarrhoea by simple clinical assessment of intestinal transit rate. *BMJ*. 1990;300(6722):439–440.
3. Bruera E, Kuehn N, Miller MJ, Selmser P, Macmillan K. The Edmonton Symptom Assessment System (ESAS): a simple method for the assessment of palliative care patients. *J Palliat Care*. 1991;7(2):6–9.
4. Hawley PH, Byeon JJ. A comparison of sennosides-based bowel protocols with and without docusate in hospitalized patients with cancer. *J Palliat Med*. 2008;11(4):575–581. doi:10.1089/jpm.2007.0178.
5. Swarm RA, Youngwerth JM, Anghelescu DL. Adult Cancer Pain. National Comprehensive Cancer Network. https://www.nccn.org/professionals/physician_gls/pdf/pain.pdf. Published February 26, 2021. Accessed March 3, 2021.

Equianalgesic Conversion From Intravenous Hydromorphone to Oral Opioids

SCOTT A. STRASSELS AND JEFFREY FUDIN

> We determined that 1 mg of IV hydromorphone is equivalent to 2.5 mg of oral hydromorphone, approximately 11.5 mg of oral MEDD, 11 mg of oral morphine, and 8 mg of oral oxycodone. These new ratios may allow for more rapid opioid titration and optimization of pain in cancer inpatients and perhaps may even shorten the length of hospital stay.
>
> —REDDY ET AL.[1]

Research Question: What is the conversion ratio between intravenous (IV) and oral hydromorphone? What is the opioid rotation ratio between IV hydromorphone and morphine equivalent daily dose?

Funding: This study was supported in part by an MD Anderson Cancer Center (MDACC) support grant. As disclosed by the authors, "the funding organization had no role in the design and conduct of the study, in the collection, management, analysis, and interpretation of the data, or in the preparation, review, or approval of the manuscript."

Year Study Began: This chart review was conducted using 2010–2014 data.

Year Study Published: 2017

Study Location: University of Texas MDACC, Houston, Texas

Who Was Studied: Patients who received continuous infusions of IV hydromorphone for cancer-related pain were then converted to oral hydromorphone, morphine, or oxycodone and discharged home without readmission within 1 week for uncontrolled pain.

Who Was Excluded: People who underwent a subsequent opioid rotation (OR) after the initial rotation from IV hydromorphone to an oral opioid during the same inpatient stay; patients who underwent a following OR by the MDACC outpatient team within 1 week of discharge; individuals whose opioid was changed to methadone, hydrocodone, transdermal fentanyl, or to the transdermal rather than oral route.

How Many Patients: 394 (147 converted to oral hydromorphone, 163 converted to oral morphine, 84 converted to oral oxycodone)

Study Overview: The investigators examined the equianalgesic ratio of IV hydromorphone and oral hydromorphone, morphine, or oxycodone (used during hospitalization and prescribed for outpatient use) in people treated for cancer-related pain by an inpatient palliative care team at a National Cancer Institute–designated comprehensive cancer center. Patient charts were abstracted to summarize the individual's performance status, pain and symptom intensity during the previous 24 hours using the Edmonton Symptom Assessment Scale (ESAS), current delirium using the Memorial Delirium Assessment Scale (MDAS), and alcohol use using the Cut Down, Annoyed, Guilty, Eyeopener (CAGE) questionnaire, as well as pain descriptors, use of tobacco and illicit substances, and opioid dosing, including breakthrough medication use and calculated oral morphine equivalent daily dose using standard ratios and the total amount of IV hydromorphone and oral opioid used during the 24 hours prior to conversion.

Study Intervention: This was an observational study using data abstracted from medical charts. Aside from calculating the net IV hydromorphone use, the conversion ratio, and the opioid rotation ratio, there were no specific interventions.

Follow-up: None. Lack of readmission for pain within 1 week after discharge was used as a proxy for a successful conversion to oral opioids.

Endpoints: Estimated conversion ratio and opioid rotation ratios for IV hydromorphone to oral hydromorphone and oral morphine equivalent daily dose.

RESULTS

- Of the 394 individuals who received continuous infusions of hydromorphone, 147 were rotated to oral hydromorphone and the remaining 247 were converted to morphine or oxycodone.
- The median time from rotation to discharge was 2 days.
- The study participants were generally older (mean age 54 years), female, and White, and almost all had advanced-stage cancer.
- Nearly three-fourths of people had nociceptive pain, approximately 25% had mixed nociceptive and neuropathic pain, and 4% had only neuropathic pain.
- The median conversion ratio from IV to oral hydromorphone was 1:2.5 in people who were receiving < 30 mg of IV hydromorphone per day and 1:2.1 in individuals who received at least 40 mg of IV hydromorphone per day.
- The median opioid rotation ratio within the people who were rotated from IV hydromorphone to morphine or oxycodone was 11.46, expressed as morphine equivalent daily dose.
- The opioid rotation ratio from IV hydromorphone was lower for oral oxycodone than for oral morphine (8.06 vs. 11, $P = .0023$), as would be expected since oxycodone is more bioavailable than morphine.

Criticisms and Limitations:

- The people in this study were primarily younger and female and had advanced cancer. As a result, the generalizability of this work may be limited.
- Potentially important patient, disease, and treatment characteristics were not included, representing potential for confounding. These characteristics include genetic variability in terms of cytochrome P-450 (CYP) enzymes. Specifically, while neither hydromorphone nor morphine undergo CYP metabolism, oxycodone is metabolized to noroxycodone and oxymorphone by CYP3A4 and CYP2D6, respectively. As a result, it would have been useful to stratify the data to see if the conversion to morphine is more predictable than conversion to oxycodone.
- Additionally, it would have been useful to know the distribution of metastases and, specifically, the prevalence of painful bony metastases and use of corticosteroids or nonsteroidal anti-inflammatory drugs in the hospital or at home.

- The authors also do not specifically address the potential for challenges that clinicians at less specialized centers may face, including providing appropriate analgesia to people with respiratory (e.g., chronic obstructive pulmonary disease, sleep apnea) or cardiovascular comorbidities or people who are not hospitalized but require rotation to a different route of administration or a different opioid.
- Since this study was not designed to evaluate the conversion from oral hydromorphone/morphine/oxycodone to IV hydromorphone, we cannot draw conclusions about bidirectionality. This is particularly important, as a conservative conversion ratio in 1 direction could be a substantial overestimation in the other direction.

Other Relevant Studies and Information:

- This work by Reddy et al.[1] is needed because converting opioid therapy from 1 form of a drug to another or rotating from 1 opioid to another can be challenging and associated with significant risks, including death.[2]
- Furthermore, cancer pain is prevalent[3] and contributes to potentially avoidable medical resource use, including hospitalizations.[4]
- As prevention and treatment of cancer have improved, the incidence of these diseases has decreased, but prevalence has increased, resulting in more people living with chronic cancer yet still needing appropriate supportive and symptomatic care.
- Souter and Fitzgibbon[5] note that about 40% of people with cancer pain require rotation due to inadequate pain relief, genetic differences, and tolerance but that estimating the conversion ratio between drugs is notoriously imprecise.
- Souter and Fitzgibbon[5] also note that conversion ratios may differ based on the direction of the switch, an observation supported by Reddy et al.[6] and other authors, including McPherson[7] and Foxwell and Uritsky.[8]
- Despite understanding these limits and a 2009 guideline[9] as well as a 2012 review of equianalgesic conversion practices[10] aimed at addressing these gaps, physicians, nurse practitioners and physician assistants, and pharmacists still report potentially important variability in application of conversion methods within and between health care disciplines.[11]

Summary and Implications: Cancer-related pain is common both during and after treatment, including for those receiving curative-intent therapy and palliative treatment. This study provides a useful contribution to understanding of how to apply opioid conversion ratios for patients with cancer-related pain.

CLINICAL CASE: CONVERSION FROM HYDROMORPHONE TO OXYCODONE CONTROLLED-RELEASE

Case History

FJ is a 70-year-old male with stage IV prostate cancer metastatic to bone. He has a history of stage III colorectal cancer, which has since been cured, but he has an ongoing chemotherapy-induced neuropathy to his lower extremities due to previous platinum-based therapy and chronic pain to the lower abdomen from related surgeries, including a temporary ileostomy, which was reversed 7 years ago. He complains of moderate abdominal pain. The neuropathy is not bothersome, but he also has severe bone pain to the bilateral ileac crests and moderate pain to the thoracic spine and sternum, all of which are confirmed to have lytic lesions. He has hypercholesterolemia and Hashimoto thyroid disorder. He is currently receiving goserelin 3.6 mg subcutaneously every 4 weeks, bicalutamide 50 mg by mouth daily, simvastatin 40 mg by mouth every night at bedtime, levothyroxine 75 mcg by mouth every morning, dexamethasone 2 mg by mouth twice a day, gabapentin 800 mg by mouth 3 times a day for neuropathy, and hydromorphone 2 mg by mouth every 4 hours. While in the hospital, his oral hydromorphone was switched in 0.25 mg/hour IV. His prostate cancer is stable at present with no new lesions observed and reduction in lytic lesions to bone. He was noted to have diminishing bone density and has osteopenia. He was admitted to the hospital for computed tomography scan, magnetic resonance imaging, updated ultrasounds, and uncontrolled end-of-dose pain, especially to the thoracic spine. He has a planned discharge within 72 hours.

Suggested Answer

There are several medication considerations. The dexamethasone is not desirable because of the osteopenia if the bone pain can be controlled with opioids plus nonsteroidal anti-inflammatory drugs (NSAIDs). A taper of dexamethasone with a slow escalation of an NSAID would make sense; however, he will need protection against gastrointestinal bleeding with a proton pump inhibitor. His hydromorphone can be switched to an extended-release opioid. He was admitted with a daily oral hydromorphone dose of 12 mg/day. His IV dose was 6 mg/24 hours. If we use a conversion of IV to oral hydromorphone of 1 mg to 2.5 mg, his current oral equivalent dose is 15 mg. His pain is relatively well controlled within the hospital, but with IV use there are no peaks and troughs. Consideration therefore should be given to an oral extended-release opioid. The patient's insurance carrier does not cover extended-release hydromorphone. Potential options based on the insurance provider are oxycodone controlled release, morphine extended release, or oxymorphone extended release. We do not have any pharmacogenetic profile on this patient. Since we want to make this conversion quickly while the patient is hospitalized, conversion to morphine or oxymorphone makes the most sense because neither depends on phase I metabolism. Oxycodone, on the other hand, depends on CYP3A4 for conversion to the inactive noroxycodone metabolite and CYP2D6 to the oxymorphone active metabolite. The doctor nevertheless would prefer oxycodone controlled release because the provider is more comfortable maintaining this patient on oxycodone, especially since there has been some diminished kidney function and knowing the 6-glucuronide metabolite could accumulate if the creatinine clearance drops below 30 mL/min.

According to the authors, they used a conversion ratio of 2 when converting from IV to oral hydromorphone, and a rotation ratio of 1.5 when converting from morphine to oxycodone. An opioid rotation ratio of 10 when estimating morphine equivalent daily doses was suggested, assuming that hydromorphone is approximately 10 times more potent than oral morphine on a milligram-to-milligram basis.

Using this logic, the current IV hydromorphone daily dose of 6 mg is equal to 12 mg of oral hydromorphone, which is equivalent to oral morphine 120 mg/day or 120 mg/1.5 = 80 mg oral oxycodone per day. The presumed dose of oxycodone controlled release, then, would be 40 mg by mouth every 12 hours. Because of cross-tolerance and no genetic profile, it was decided to start at a lower dose with an option for breakthrough medication.

While in the hospital, the patient's IV hydromorphone drip was discontinued and he was started on oxycodone controlled release 30 mg by mouth every 12 hours plus oxycodone immediate release 5 mg by mouth 4 times a day as needed. To avoid gastrointestinal bleeding from prostaglandin inhibition with dexamethasone or an NSAID that might replace it, he should be started on a proton pump inhibitor. Omeprazole is less desirable compared to some other options because it can inhibit CYP3A4, which is responsible for the conversion of oxycodone to its inactive form. Therefore, esomeprazole at 20 mg by mouth every morning can be used since it does not inhibit CYP3A4 like racemic omeprazole. When the patient is home, we will recommend a slow taper of dexamethasone and the introduction of a low-dose NSAID of the primary care provider's choice with careful escalation.

References

1. Reddy A, Vidal M, Stephen S, et al. The conversion ratio from intravenous hydromorphone to oral opioids in cancer patients. *J Pain Symptom Manage.* 2017 Sep;54(3):280–288. doi:10.1016/j.jpainsymman.2017.07.001.
2. Berens MJ, Armstrong K. State pushes prescription painkiller methadone, saving millions but costing lives. *Seattle Times.* 2011-12-10. https://www.seattletimes.com/seattle-news/times-watchdog/state-pushes-prescription-painkiller-methadone-saving-millions-but-costing-lives/.
3. van den Beuken-van Everdingen MH, Hochstenbach LM, Joosten EA, Tjan-Heijnen VC, Janssen DJ. Update on prevalence of pain in patients with cancer: systematic review and meta-analysis. *J Pain Symptom Manage.* 2016 Jun;51(6):1070–1090.e9. doi:10.1016/j.jpainsymman.2015.12.340.
4. Strassels SA, Moss KO, Mallow PJ, et al. Hospital admissions associated with cancer pain in older adults with and without dementia. *Pain Manag Nurs.* 2021 Mar 16. doi:10.1016/j.pmn.2021.01.018.
5. Souter K, Fitzgibbon D. Equianalgesic dose guidelines for long-term opioid use: theoretical and practical considerations. *Semin Anesthes Periop Med Pain.* 2004;23:271–280.
6. Reddy A, Heung Y, Bruera E. Authors' response. *J Pain Symptom Manage.* 2018 Sep;56(3):e3–e5. doi:10.1016/j.jpainsymman.2018.05.012.
7. McPherson ML. *Demystifying Opioid Conversion Calculations. A Guide for Effective Dosing.* American Society of Health-System Pharmacists; 2010.
8. Foxwell AM, Uritsky TJ. Hydromorphone conversion dilemma: a millennial problem. *J Pain Symptom Manage.* 2018 Sep;56(3):e2–e3. doi:10.1016/j.jpainsymman.2018.05.014.
9. Fine PG, Portenoy RK. Establishing "best practices" for opioid rotation: conclusions of an expert panel. *J Pain Symptom Manage.* 2009;38(3):418–425. doi:10.1016/j.jpainsymman.2009.06.002.
10. Webster LR, Fine PG. Review and critique of opioid rotation practices and associated risks of toxicity. *Pain Med.* 2012 Apr;13(4):562–570. doi:10.1111/j.1526-4637.2012.01357.x.
11. Rennick A, Atkinson T, Cimino NM, Strassels SA, McPherson ML, Fudin J. Variability in opioid equivalence calculations. *Pain Med.* 2016 May 1;17(5):892–898. doi:10.1111/pme.12920.

45

Guideline-Driven Versus Single-Agent Antiemetic Therapy in Patients With Advanced Cancer

SARAH STAYER AND PAUL TATUM

> The use of low cost anti-emetics currently available can achieve good symptom control in many cases. Other more expensive antiemetics with little or no evidence of benefit in this setting should only be used in those with refractory nausea or in the context of a clinical trial.
>
> —HARDY ET AL.[1]

Research Question: Does using an etiology-based, guideline-driven approach improve nausea better than single-agent treatment (haloperidol) in patients with non-chemotherapy-induced cancer-related nausea?

Funding: The trial was sponsored by the Palliative Care Clinical Studies Collaborative and funded by the National Health and Medical Research Council of Australia.

Year Study Began: 2010

Year Study Published: 2018

Study Location: 11 inpatient sites across Australia

Who Was Studied: Patients at least 18 years old with a diagnosis of cancer and average nausea score ≥ 3/10 (scale 0–10) on nausea rating scale who were not receiving antiemetic therapy

Who Was Excluded: Patients with a short-term iatrogenic or reversible cause of nausea, those who had a definite contraindication to any of the study medications, or those with poor performance status that rendered them unable to complete study requirements

How Many Patients: 146

Study Overview: This is an open-label randomized controlled parallel-arm trial that was conducted in 11 sites. Adult patients with cancer and nausea with an average score ≥ 3/10 were randomized in a 1:1 ratio to either the treatment or control group (Figure 45.1).

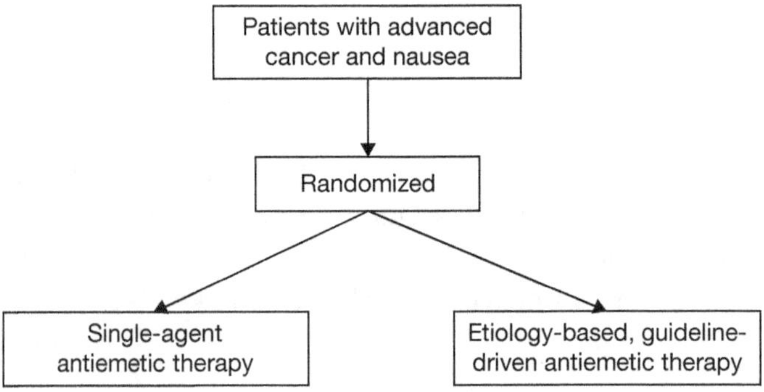

Figure 45.1. Study design of patients randomized in a 1:1 ratio of intervention versus control.

Study Intervention: Clinicians were trained on the various mechanisms of nausea and how to determine the primary cause. Potential causes were recorded and a mechanism of nausea defined when possible. Those in the treatment arm received antiemetic therapy based on practice guidelines developed by an expert panel.[2] These guidelines delineated common mechanisms of nausea and appropriate first-line treatment, and subsequent lines of treatment in a stepwise fashion if nausea was not well controlled after 24 hours. Participants in the single-agent group received haloperidol 1 mg/24 hours, escalated to 2 mg/24 hours and finally 3 mg/24 hours if nausea was not controlled. Metoclopramide was used as the rescue antiemetic.

Follow-Up: 72 hours

Endpoints:

Primary outcome was defined as a reduction of average nausea score to below 3/10 at 72 hours in response to anti-emetic therapy.

Secondary outcomes included average nausea score, best and worst nausea scores, number of patients at each dose level, rescue doses delivered, episodes of vomiting, and global impression of change and adverse events.

RESULTS

- At 72 hours, response was seen in 53% of the single-agent arm and in 49% of the guideline-therapy arm, with no significant difference between the 2 arms.
- At 24 hours, response was seen in 32% of the single-agent arm and in 49% of the guideline-therapy arm, a statistically significant finding.
- Approximately one-third of participants required a rescue antiemetic each day.
- Adverse events occurred in 50% of participants and included fatigue, gastrointestinal upset, anorexia, or anticholinergic effects.
- Greater than 80% of the participants in both arms reported an improvement in their global impression of change (GIC).
- There was a single episode of extrapyramidal symptoms.

Criticisms and Limitations:

- The follow-up for this study was only 72 hours; it is unclear if the 2 arms continue to perform the same over time for persistent nausea.
- Blinding for the study was not possible due to the complicated nausea regimen with multiple different medications in the intervention group.
- Nearly all of the medications used in the intervention arm were dopamine antagonists, similar in the mechanism of action to haloperidol, with the exception of dexamethasone for central nervous system–associated nausea.
- An etiology of nausea was only identified in 54% of patients, which is lower than in other studies and therefore may underestimate the effect of an etiology-based treatment protocol.

Other Relevant Studies and Information:

- Systematic reviews of the literature and expert opinion panels continuously update practice guidelines for cancer treatment–related nausea and are risk stratified. In the most recent update to the American Society of Clinical Oncology (ASCO) antiemetic guideline, olanzapine was added as recommended for hematopoietic stem cell transplantation, while no routine antiemetic was recommended for checkpoint inhibitors. These guidelines do not address non-treatment-related nausea, however.[2]
- A well-designed prospective open-label uncontrolled study of haloperidol for non-treatment-related nausea in cancer patients estimates that 61% of patients respond overall with a 95% confidence interval of 44%–77%.[3]
- In a systematic review for the Cochrane group, 65 studies of haloperidol for nausea and vomiting in palliative care failed to meet inclusion criteria for Cochrane standards, although the review did conclude that topical haloperidol is ineffective.[4]
- A new study was published in 2020 showing that olanzapine to treat chronic nausea in cancer patients unrelated to treatment was highly superior to placebo in ways that "no other drug studied in this situation has been reported to decrease nausea/vomiting more than what was observed in this study." However, there have never been head-to-head trials of olanzapine versus haloperidol or metoclopramide comparing the effectiveness of the various medications.[5]
- A second randomized study compared methotrimeprazine with haloperidol. The response to treatment at 72 hours was 75% in the haloperidol arm and 63% in the methotrimeprazine treatment arm. Rescue metoclopramide or domperidone was used by 40% and did not differ between treatment arms. Drowsiness was the common side effect, which occurred in 12% of the haloperidol-treated patients and 20% of the methotrimeprazine-treated patients. There are no differences in other side effects. The authors concluded that both haloperidol and methotrimeprazine are effective antiemetics in patients with advanced cancer and nausea.[6]
- A randomized controlled trial compared the combination of netupitant/palonosetron (NEPA) with placebo and metoclopramide rescue. NEPA and placebo have the same within-group improvement in nausea with no between-group differences.[7] There has been no randomized trial that has demonstrated a benefit to the use of 5-HT3 receptor antagonists except for tropisetron.[8]
- Based on Multinational Association of Supportive Care in Cancer (MASCC) guidelines for antiemetic choices for cancer-associated nausea and vomiting, metoclopramide and haloperidol are first-line antiemetics,

olanzapine and methotrimeprazine are second-line antiemetics, and levosulpiride and tropisetron are third-line antiemetics based on the level of evidence and quality of the trials.[9]

Summary and Implications: Nausea not acutely related to anticancer therapy can be quickly and effectively controlled for the majority of patients with inexpensive, widely available medications. Dopamine antagonists such as haloperidol and metoclopramide are safe and effective medications for nausea. While fatigue, dry mouth, and dry eyes were common side effects, extrapyramidal symptoms were very rare. Other more expensive antiemetics in this setting should only be used for refractory nausea.

CLINICAL CASE: APPROPRIATE FIRST-LINE TREATMENT FOR CANCER-INDUCED NAUSEA AND VOMITING

Case History

A 62-year-old female with metastatic cervical cancer reports to the emergency department with nausea, rated 7/10, and vomiting 2–3 times per day for the past 2 days. She has decreased appetite and fatigue and reports depressed mood. She continues to pass gas, and her last bowel movement was yesterday. She has not had chemotherapy for the past 3 weeks, and workup is negative for central metastases or bowel obstruction. What medication should be recommended as a first-line agent to treat her nausea?

Suggested Answer

The Hardy study demonstrates that a widely available, affordable, antidopaminergic medication such as haloperidol or metoclopramide could be considered as a first-line agent for treating her cancer-related nausea.[1] This study demonstrated that either medication was very effective in decreasing the symptoms of both nausea and vomiting and improving overall well-being.

The patient in this case has nausea unrelated to chemotherapy and no central metastases that might cause increased intracranial pressure. If the patient had received chemotherapy, then following the ASCO chemotherapy-induced nausea/vomiting guidelines[2] would yield better results than single-agent nausea medications. Likewise, if increased intracranial pressure is discovered, procedures that could relieve the pressure should be pursued. With these causes excluded, medical providers can confidently treat nausea with a first-line agent as above and use ondansetron or olanzapine as a second-line agent for refractory nausea.

References

1. Hardy J, Skerman H, Glare P, et al. A randomized open-label study of guideline-driven antiemetic therapy versus single agent antiemetic therapy in patients with advanced cancer and nausea not related to anticancer treatment. *BMC Cancer.* 2018 May 2;18(1):510. doi:10.1186/s12885-018-4404-8. PMID: 29720113. PMCID: PMC5932901.
2. Hesketh PJ, Kris MG, Basch E, et al. Antiemetics: ASCO guideline update. *J Clin Oncol.* 2020;38(24):2782–2797. doi:10.1200/jco.20.01296.
3. Hardy JR, O'Shea A, White C, Gilshenan K, Welch L, Douglas C. The efficacy of haloperidol in the management of nausea and vomiting in patients with cancer. *J Pain Symptom Manage.* 2010;40(1):111–116. doi:10.1016/j.jpainsymman.2009.11.321.
4. Murray-Brown F, Dorman S. Haloperidol for the treatment of nausea and vomiting in palliative care patients. *Cochrane Database Syst Rev.* 2015;(11):CD006271. doi:10.1002/14651858.CD006271.pub3.
5. Navari RM, Pywell CM, Le-Rademacher JG, et al. Olanzapine for the treatment of advanced cancer–related chronic nausea and/or vomiting: a randomized pilot trial. *JAMA Oncol.* 2020;6(6):895–899. doi:10.1001/jamaoncol.2020.1052.
6. Hardy JR, Skerman H, Philip J, et al. Methotrimeprazine versus haloperidol in palliative care patients with cancer-related nausea: a randomised, double-blind controlled trial. *BMJ Open.* 2019;9(9):e029942.
7. Hui D, Puac V, Shelal Z, et al. Fixed-dose netupitant and palonosetron for chronic nausea in cancer patients: a double-blind, placebo run-in pilot randomized clinical trial. *J Pain Symptom Manage.* 2021;62(2):223–232.e221.
8. Mystakidou K, Befon S, Liossi C, Vlachos L. Comparison of the efficacy and safety of tropisetron, metoclopramide, and chlorpromazine in the treatment of emesis associated with far advanced cancer. *Cancer.* 1998;83(6):1214–1223.
9. Davis M, Hui D, Davies A, et al. MASCC antiemetics in advanced cancer updated guideline. *Support Care Cancer.* 2021;29(12):8097–8107.

46

Safety of Morphine Delivered via Patient-Controlled Analgesia Devices in the Pediatric Population

SOPHIA S. URBAN AND ELIZABETH A. HIGGINS

> This study suggests that morphine administered via PCA is at least as safe, or maybe even safer, compared with conventional IV-only administration in this pediatric patient cohort.
>
> —Faerber et al.[1]

Research Question: Is the delivery of opioid medication, specifically morphine, via patient-controlled analgesia (PCA) devices as safe as delivery via the intravenous (IV) route in pediatric patients?

Funding: Agency for Healthcare Quality and Research, Comparative Effectiveness and Safety of Hospital-Based Pediatric Palliative Care

Year Study Began: 2007

Year Study Published: 2017

Study Location: 42 children's hospitals in major metropolitan areas across the United States, representative of 85% of all free-standing children's hospitals in the country

Who Was Studied: Hospitalized pediatric patients aged 5–21 years who received opioid analgesic therapy with morphine.

Who Was Excluded: Patients in the IV group who received PCA during their hospitalization; patients who experienced cardiopulmonary resuscitation (CPR) or mechanical ventilation (MV) on a hospital day preceding morphine exposure; patients who received opioids other than morphine via PCA

How Many Patients: 34 500

Study Overview: This is a retrospective cohort study in which propensity score analysis was used to create matching cohorts of patients who received either PCA morphine or IV morphine in the inpatient setting. Cohorts included both nonsurgical and surgical patients who had been identified through the Pediatric Health Information System (PHIS) database. Using the information stored in this database, the study examined whether PCA utilization was associated with increased risk of analgesia-related adverse events using 2 proxy variables: CPR and/or the need for MV. Outcomes were analyzed on days 1–3 of opioid administration (Figure 46.1).

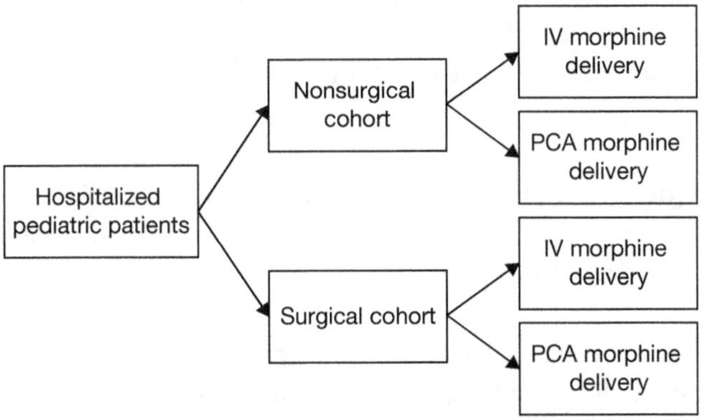

Figure 46.1. Summary of study design.

Study Intervention: Patients received morphine doses via 1 of 2 delivery methods: IV or PCA device.

Follow-Up: 3 days

Endpoints: Main outcome: Analgesia-related adverse event using 2 proxy variables: need for CPR or MV.

RESULTS

- In general, hospitalized pediatric patients who received morphine via PCA versus IV were not significantly more likely to experience an adverse event when propensity matching was used to control for confounding factors.
- Although the absolute reductions in the probability of analgesia-related events was very small when comparing PCA to IV, the data suggest that morphine administered via PCA devices may offer protective benefits in both nonsurgical and surgical patients (Table 46.1).

Table 46.1 SUMMARY OF FAERBER ET AL.'S KEY FINDINGS

Opioid-Related Adverse Event	**Period After Starting Opioid**	**Delivery Method**	**Nonsurgical Cohort**		**Surgical Cohort**	
			***P*[a]**	**OR[b]**	***P*[a]**	**OR[b]**
CPR	Day 1 events	IV	.0100	0.80	.0058	0.56
		PCA	.0081		.0033	
	Day 2 or 3 events	IV	.0024	0.99	.00012	1.81
		PCA	.0024		.00022	
MV	Day 1 events	IV	.0026	1.40	.0307	0.86
		PCA	.0036		.0276	
	Day 2 or 3 events	IV	.0027	0.98	.0038	0.74
		PCA	.0026		.0027	

Abbreviations: CPR, cardiopulmonary resuscitation; IV, intravenously; MV, mechanical ventilation; PCA, patient-controlled analgesia.
[a] Probability, with 95% confidence interval.
[b] Odds ratio, with 95% confidence interval.

  - In both cohorts, PCA use was significantly associated with 20%–44% lower odds of same-day CPR, with a slightly larger reduction in the surgical group versus the nonsurgical group.
  - Surgical patients administered analgesia via PCA had up to 24% lower odds of requiring MV up to 2 days after initial opioid exposure, although this finding was not statistically significant.

Criticisms and Limitations:

- First, and most importantly, this was not a randomized trial, and unmeasured factors may have confounded the findings.
- The lack of detailed information regarding PCA administration—including bolus and basal dosing, dose limits, and lockout

intervals—makes it difficult to translate study findings into comprehensive practice guidelines for PCA use in children.

- Conclusions regarding the safety of PCA devices in pediatric patients may have been overestimated based on the use of proxy variables representative of the most severe adverse drug events; however, it is the less severe adverse effects, such as constipation and pruritis, that tend to be more common with opioid use. Therefore, more information regarding the milder reactions seen with PCA administration could be explored in future studies to better assess the safety profile.
- The window for adverse outcome analysis was limited to 2 days after initiation of analgesic therapy. While this may be an appropriate timeframe given the short half-life of IV morphine and the usually rapid onset of adverse effects after its administration, this narrow window may have excluded adverse events that occurred later than day 3 from analysis.

Other Relevant Studies and Information:

- In 2001, McDonald and Cooper reviewed PCA use in children in their article entitled "Patient-Controlled Analgesia: An Appropriate Method of Pain Control in Children."[2] In the article, they describe PCA devices as not only well tolerated among pediatric patients but also a safe and effective method of analgesic delivery when close monitoring and appropriate device parameters are employed. Moreover, they highlight the widespread adaptability of the analgesic technique to diverse clinical scenarios including postoperative, oncologic, and palliative.
- The Improving Pain Management and Outcomes with Various Strategies (IMPROVE) PCA trial[3] attempted to compare PCA dosing strategies in hospitalized adults and children with sickle cell disease across multiple academic centers. Although the trial was ended prematurely due to low enrollment rates, its design provides a template for future large-scale randomized controlled trials and may help guide the development of strategies for treatment implementation and standardization.
- Despite the safety, efficacy, and tolerability of pediatric PCA device use supported by this study,[1] other investigators such as Dancel et al.[4] suggest that a multimodal approach to acute pain management may be more appropriate than opioid therapy in children given the low risk of adverse effects and long-term dependence. Their research indicates that inventive uses of older nonopioid medications, such as sublingual ketorolac or inhaled methoxyflurane, may represent a paradigm shift away from opioid use and highlights the need to integrate nonpharmacological, multidisciplinary pain management interventions,

Summary and Implications: This retrospective analysis comparing treatment of hospitalized children experiencing pain with either IV morphine or morphine delivered via PCA suggests that PCA device usage is safe. It is the largest and most generalizable study of its kind to date and cleared the path toward future development of clinical practice guidelines regarding PCA administration among pediatric patients.

CLINICAL CASE: WHO SHOULD RECEIVE A MOPRHINE PCA FOR PAIN MANAGEMENT?

Case History

A 14-year-old boy presents to the emergency department (ED) with 8/10 right knee pain. He had been having knee pain at night, which he attributed to a fall during soccer practice 2 weeks prior to presentation. When the pain worsened and his mom noted swelling, she took him to the pediatrician. The pediatrician noted an antalgic gait and was concerned by the amount of pain, so she sent him to the ED. X-rays of the tibia obtained in the ED showed a diaphyseal sunburst lesion of the tibia with sclerosis, cortical destruction on the posteromedial side, and new bone formation in the soft tissues consistent with a suspected osteosarcoma. The patient was given 1 dose of IV morphine on arrival with improvement in his pain to 5/10, but it only lasted a few hours. The pediatric team admits the child for biopsy and pain management and orders a morphine PCA.

This patient's mother is concerned about the safety of a morphine PCA. What should you tell her?

Suggested Answer

The Faerber study supports the use of a morphine PCA and demonstrates that PCA device usage is safe and preferred by patients themselves for its ability to provide a sense of control over one's symptoms.

The patient in this case falls within the age range included in this study and would benefit from morphine PCA. It is possible that he will require surgery and will need analgesia postoperatively; accordingly, he will benefit from a morphine PCA for postoperative pain as well. You can reassure this patient's mother that PCA device use has been found to be a safe and effective method of analgesic delivery when close monitoring and appropriate device parameters are employed. For example, you could explain to the mother that the PCA orders will be written to include a maximum morphine dose per hour with lockout intervals built into the device that limit the amount of medication patients can self-administer within a specified fraction of each hour (e.g., 15 minutes). Additionally, you can also reassure her that the bedside nurse will be frequently monitoring her son's vital signs, especially respiratory rate, to ensure that the morphine dose is not causing respiratory depression or excessive lethargy.

References

1. Faerber J, Zhong W, Dai D, et al. Comparative safety of morphine delivered via intravenous route vs. patient-controlled analgesia device for pediatric inpatients. *J Pain Symptom Manage.* 2017;53(5):842–850. doi:10.1016/j.jpainsymman.2016.12.328.
2. McDonald AJ, Cooper MG. Patient-controlled analgesia. *Pediatr-Drugs.* 2001;3(4):273–284. doi:10.2165/00128072-200103040-00004.
3. Dampier CD, Smith WR, Wager CG, et al. IMPROVE trial: a randomized controlled trial of patient-controlled analgesia for sickle cell painful episodes: rationale, design challenges, initial experience, and recommendations for future studies. *Clin Trials.* 2013;10(2):319–331. doi:10.1177/1740774513475850.
4. Dancel R, Liles EA, Fiore D. Acute pain management in hospitalized children. *Rev Recent Clin Trials.* 2017;12(4):277–283. doi:10.2174/1574887112666170816151232.

47

Efficacy and Safety of Valproic Acid Versus Haloperidol in Patients With Acute Agitation

Results of a Randomized, Double-Blind, Parallel-Group Trial

VINCENT JAY VANSTON AND ALYSSA LANGI

> In the clinical practice setting of emergency psychiatry, intravenous valproate is as effective as haloperidol in reducing agitation, with a better safety profile.
>
> —Asadollahi et al.[1]

Research Question: How does the efficacy of valproate compare to that of haloperidol for patients with acute agitation in the emergency department?

Funding: There was no funding source specified in the paper.

Year Study Began: Patients were enrolled between April and July of 2014

Year Study Published: 2015

Study Location: Emergency department of Imam Hossein Hospital, a metropolitan university-affiliated hospital with an average of 65,000 patient visits annually

Who Was Studied: Adult patients (age range 18–65 years) who were acutely agitated and required emergency parenteral pharmaceutical intervention. Acutely agitated patients included those with violent, controlled, or uncontrolled muscular movements that placed both themselves and hospital staff in danger because of severely disruptive behavior.

Who Was Excluded: Patients with any of the following:

- Readily amenable causes for the agitation (e.g., hypoxemia, hypoglycemia)
- Known hypersensitivity to either study drug
- Hypotension defined as a systolic blood pressure of < 90 mmHg
- Pregnancy
- Breastfeeding
- Known history of liver disease
- Known history of uncontrolled diabetes
- Visible or suspected head trauma
- A previous history of neuroleptic malignant syndrome
- A seizure disorder

How Many Patients: 160

Study Overview: This study was a randomized, double-blind, parallel-group trial in which participants were assigned to receive valproate or haloperidol treatment (Figure 47.1).

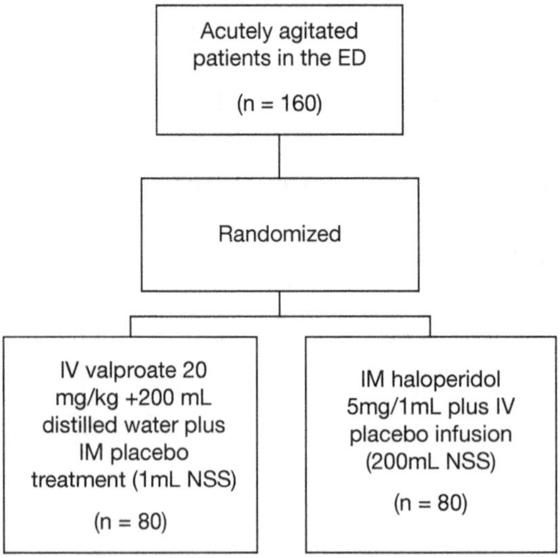

Figure 47.1. Study design and randomization for valproate versus haloperidol treatment.

Study Intervention: Peripheral intravenous (IV) access was established for all enrolled patients to collect serum glucose and standard hemodynamic monitoring as well as a toxicology screen. Vital signs were recorded both before and after the administration of medication and 30 minutes after the intervention. Patients were allocated to either the intramuscular (IM) haloperidol plus IV placebo infusion or the IV sodium valproate solution plus IM placebo treatment. Infusions were given over 10 minutes. If patients continued to be agitated after the study drug was administered, a second dose could be administered at the discretion of the attending. Adverse events were reported directly to the principal investigators, who then decided whether the assigned intervention should be unblinded or if the patient should be removed from the trial.

Follow-Up: All patients were followed until the time of discharge from the emergency service or upon transfer to a psychiatric department.

Endpoints: Primary outcome: The level of agitation was assessed at baseline and at 30 minutes after the administration of drugs using the Agitated-Calmness Evaluation Scale (ACES), Positive and Negative Syndrome Scale-Excited Component (PANSS-EC), and Agitated Behavior Scale (ABS) scores.

RESULTS (TABLE 47.1)

Table 47.1 Endpoint Change in Efficacy Measures at 30 Minutes After the First Injection (Intention to Treat, N = 160)

Characteristics	**Valproate (*n* = 80)**	**Haloperidol (*n* = 80)**	***P***
ACES score (means +SD)			
Baseline	1.64 + 0.75	1.821 + 0.76	.132
Endpoint	4.73 + 1.93	5.45 + 2.09	.028
PANSS-EC score (means + SD)			
Baseline	25.38 + 5.80	24.21 + 5.59	.207
Endpoint	12.47 + 3.47	13.97 + 6.61	.080
Difference	−11.74 + 7.18	−11.41 + 7.21	.649
ABS total score (means + SD)			
Baseline	27.29 + 4.40	28.28 + 4.56	.177
Endpoint	21.70 + 4.44	22.38 + 5.14	.381
Difference	−5.58 + 3.46	−5.89 + 3.31	.651
Second close [*n* (%)]	13 (16.2)	17 (21.2)	.418

Abbreviations: ABS, Agitated Behavior Scale; ACES, Agitated-Calmness Evaluation Scale; PANSS-EC, Positive and Negative Syndrome Scale-Excited Component.

- The baseline agitation scores for patients in the valproate group were not significantly different from those in the haloperidol group.
- Before-treatment and after-treatment mean (±SD) changes in the ACES score of the valproate group did not differ significantly from the haloperidol group.
- A larger proportion of patients in the haloperidol group experienced intense sedation (36.2%) and extrapyramidal symptoms (8.7%) compared with the valproate group (2.5% for intense sedation and 0% for extrapyramidal symptoms).
- The incidence of vomiting was more frequent in the valproate arm compared with the haloperidol arm.

Criticisms and Limitations: One of the major limitations of this trial is that there was no placebo control group. Another limitation is that there may have been bias toward use of IV valproate treatment because of the potential delay in action of IM haloperidol administration.

Other Relevant Studies and Information: A number of case series and retrospective studies support the efficacy of valproate for acute agitation in the critical care setting.[2–5] In regard to patients with dementia, however, a Cochrane review[6] concluded that valproate preparations are probably ineffective in treating agitation in people with dementia.

Summary and Implications: This is the first randomized, double-blind clinical study comparing the use of valproate versus haloperidol for tranquilization of acutely agitated patients in the emergency department. The analysis found that valproate was just as efficacious as haloperidol, with lower rates of intense sedation and extrapyramidal side effects. Though it may be useful in patients with agitation, it does have noteworthy side effects, including headache and vomiting.

CLINICAL CASE: USE OF VALPROIC ACID IN THE MANAGEMENT OF ACUTE DELIRIUM

Case History

A 68-year-old female arrives at the emergency department suffering from acute agitation. She has a history of cervical cancer, hyperlipidemia, and coronary artery disease. As per her husband, she had become increasingly agitated at home over the last 3 days, refusing to take her medications, bathe, or carry on normal conversation without becoming angry or paranoid. He denies any recent falls or injury. She is verbally aggressive toward the emergency department staff and has paranoid delusions and restless behavior.

Her vital signs are as follows: blood pressure 117/65, heart rate 90, respiratory rate 20, temperature 98.0, SpO_2 97% breathing room air.

Is this patient a candidate to receive IV valproate?

Suggested Answer

The Asadollahi et al. study was the first of its kind to suggest that, as compared to haloperidol, valproate therapy may be equally effective in the management of acute agitation. When considering this patient, she does not have any of the exclusion criteria for therapy outlined in the study: pregnancy, hypoxemia, hypotension, liver disease, uncontrolled diabetes, suspected head trauma, seizure, or a history of neuroleptic malignant syndrome.

Based on her current symptoms and medical history, she would be a good candidate to receive valproate therapy to help improve her agitation. Given the incidence of vomiting and risk of aspiration with its use, careful monitoring is warranted. Physical restraints may need to be considered if the patient is unable to remain cooperative for peripheral IV placement, as the valproate cannot be administered intramuscularly. Dosing for valproate would start at 20 mg/kg with the addition of 200 mL of distilled water, given over 10 minutes.

References

1. Asadollahi S, Heidari K, Hatamabadi H, et al. Efficacy and safety of valproic acid versus Haldol in patients with acute agitation: results of a randomized, double-blind, parallel-group trial. *Int Clin Psychopharmacol.* 2015;30:142–150.
2. Sher Y, Miller AC, Lolak S, Ament A, Maldonado JR. Adjunctive valproic acid in management-refractory hyperactive delirium: a case series and rationale. *J Neuropsychiatry Clin Neurosci.* 2015;27(4):365–370. doi:10.1176/appi.neuropsych.14080190.
3. Bourgeois JA, Koike AK, Jamie Simmons ME, Telles S, Eggleston C. Adjunctive valproic acid for delirium and/or agitation on a consultation-liaison service: a report of six cases. *J Neuropsychiatry Clin Neurosci.* 2005;17. http://neuro.psychiatryonline.org. Accessed February 24, 2021.
4. Gagnon DJ, Fontaine GV, Smith KE, et al. Valproate for agitation in critically ill patients: a retrospective study. *J Crit Care.* 2017;37:119–125. doi:10.1016/j.jcrc.2016.09.006.
5. Crowley KE, Urben L, Hacobian G, Geiger KL. Valproic acid for the management of agitation and delirium in the intensive care setting: a retrospective analysis. *Clin Ther.* 2020;42(4):e65–e73. doi:10.1016/j.clinthera.2020.02.007.
6. Baillon SF, Narayana U, Luxenberg JS, Clifton AV. Valproate preparations for agitation in dementia. *Cochrane Database Syst Rev.* 2018;(10). doi:10.1002/14651858.CD003945.pub4.

48

Ketamine

A Toxic Adjunct in Pain Management for Cancer?

LARA WAHLBERG AND NAVENDRA SINGH

This large randomized control trial demonstrated a strong placebo effect and failed to show any additional clinical benefit for ketamine when delivered subcutaneously in a dose-escalating regimen over 5 days, while significantly increasing toxicity.

—Hardy et al.[1]

Research Question: Does the administration of subcutaneous ketamine as a coanalgesic provide clinically significant pain reduction in chronic cancer pain?

Funding: The Australian Government provided funding and had no role in study design or analysis, aside from oversight of the Palliative Care Clinical Studies Collaborative Management Advisory Board

Year Study Began: 2008

Year Study Published: 2012

Study Location: A range of metropolitan settings across Australia

Who Was Studied: Hospitalized patients aged 18 or older with chronic cancer treatment–related pain as defined by a Brief Pain Inventory average score of 3 or greater, despite treatment with opioids and coanalgesics

Who Was Excluded: Patients who had received ketamine for chronic pain within 6 months; had any treatment, including radiotherapy, that could affect pain during the trial therapy; or had contraindications to ketamine

How Many Patients: 185

Study Overview: See Figure 48.1.

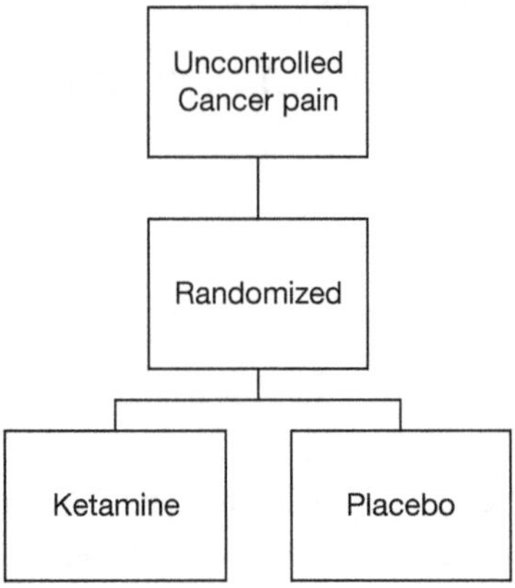

Figure 48.1. Study overview.

Study Intervention: The treatment and control group received subcutaneous ketamine or saline infusion at 3 dose levels (100, 300, or 500 mg) over the course of 5 days. Pain and side effects were measured every 24 hours. If at least 80% of medications were received and pain score improved by at least 2 points with < 4 breakthrough doses of pain medication, the ketamine/saline dose remained the same. If not, the dose was titrated to the next highest level (either 300 or 500 mg). Dose reduction happened if intolerable side effects occurred. The study drug was discontinued if there was no response after 24 hours at 500 mg.

Follow-Up: 5 days

Endpoints: The primary outcome sought was pain improvement, defined by a reduction in pain of 2 or more points on the Brief Pain Inventory by the end of the study period. Secondary outcomes were pain scores on days 2 and 5, as well as adverse events including psychomimetic specific events.

RESULTS (TABLE 48.1)

Table 48.1 SUMMARY OF THE STUDY'S KEY FINDINGS

Outcome	**Ketamine Group** ($n = 93$)	**Placebo Group** ($n = 92$)
Pain scores (BPI)	Mean (SD)	Mean (SD)
Average	5.43 (1.3)	5.21 (1.4)
Worst	8.08 (1.5)	7.64 (1.6)
Least	2.47 (1.7)	2.37 (1.9)
Total number of adverse events	172	103

Abbreviation: BPI, Brief Pain Inventory.

- There was no difference in pain for participants who completed the study at 5 days.
- The number needed to treat for 1 additional patient to experience a beneficial effect of ketamine was 25 (95% CI: 6 to ∞), whereas the number needed to harm was 6 (95% CI: 4–13).
- Neither pain type, nociceptive or neuropathic, was a predictor of response to ketamine.
- There was almost twice the occurrence of adverse events in the ketamine arm versus placebo.
- Those in the ketamine arm were more likely to experience psychotoxicity than those in the placebo arm, and those who did experience this did so at increasing rates every day.

Criticisms and Limitations: The sample was heterogenous and it was underpowered to detect clinically meaningful benefits; the study period was short and there was no long-term follow-up.

Other Relevant Studies and Information:

- A Cochrane review[2] found that evidence on the use of ketamine as an adjunct to opioid therapy for uncontrolled cancer pain is of poor quality. The review cites this study, showing that rapid titration shows no clinical benefit and may be associated with adverse side effects. More studies are needed.

- A small, randomized, placebo-controlled study[3] supported the use of ketamine in treating neuropathic pain syndromes, with adverse effects noted at increasing doses. This study involved only 10 patients in a crossover design and pain was assessed for only 3 hours after administration of ketamine.
- A double-blind randomized clinical trial of oral ketamine versus placebo involved patients with cancer-related neuropathic pain that was poorly responsive to adjuvant analgesics. Starting doses were 40 mg/day to a maximum of 400 mg/day. Of 214 patients randomized, most (160 patients) had cancers in remission and had chemotherapy-induced neuropathic pain. Patients were opioid naive. Analgesia was seen in 31.8% of ketamine-treated patients and 36.4% of placebo-treated patients on day 4. At day 16, 22.4% of ketamine-treated patients and 25.2% of placebo-treated patients had significant analgesia. There is no difference between treatment arms.[5]
- Ketamine mouthwash was used as the active arm of a randomized trial of children with cancer and mucositis. Numerical rating scale (NRS) assessments were repeated for 4 hours after oral administration. The mean pain level by NRS was reduced by 1.64 points with oral ketamine and by 1.32 points with placebo. There were no differences between the arms.[6]
- A randomized controlled trial of topical amitriptyline plus ketamine versus placebo for cancer neuropathic pain found no effect on 6-week pain scores.[7]
- Despite the conflicting evidence, the American Society of Pain and Neuroscience (ASPEN) interventional guidelines for cancer pain published in 2021 stated: "Ketamine therapy for cancer pain should be considered on a case-by-case basis for refractory neuropathic, bone, and mucositis-related pain."[9]

Summary and Implications: Case studies have supported the use of ketamine at subanesthetic doses as an adjunct to opioids for the treatment of uncontrolled cancer pain.[4] This randomized, placebo-controlled study failed to demonstrate a benefit of ketamine for pain, and toxicities incurred in the ketamine group were significantly greater than in the placebo group. Despite the conflicting evidence, guidelines recommend consideration of ketamine on a case-by-case basis for refractory neuropathic, bone, and mucositis-related pain in patients with cancer.

CLINICAL CASE: ADDING KETAMINE FOR POORLY CONTROLLED CANCER PAIN

Case History

You have been caring for a patient with locally advanced prostate cancer. His cancer has invaded his sacral plexus and is causing him excruciating pain, now poorly controlled on a high-dose hydromorphone patient-controlled analgesic (PCA) (12 mg basal, 6 mg demand, 10-minute lockout, 12 mg clinician bolus) after rotation from morphine and fentanyl. His pain has not significantly decreased with aggressive titration. He is on adjuvant treatment with acetaminophen and duloxetine. Methadone is contraindicated for him given an elevated QTc of 510. The primary medical team asks about the potential for using ketamine for pain management. Is ketamine a good option to use here?

Suggested Answer

Based on our current fund of knowledge, ketamine is not an additional medication we would try for pain management if there are other therapies available.[8] This patient may benefit from methadone, but his QTc precludes its use. Increasing the PCA settings would likely not offer improved pain control and would be risking more side effects. Intravenous or subcutaneous ketamine should be considered with close monitoring and slow titration, understanding that it may need to be discontinued if it does not decrease this patient's pain or if toxic side effects are too burdensome. Ketamine could be considered prior to more invasive pain management therapies such as an intrathecal pump.

References

1. Hardy J, Quinn S, Fazekas B, et al. Randomized, double-blind, placebo-controlled study to assess the efficacy and toxicity of subcutaneous ketamine in the management of cancer pain. *J Clin Oncol.* 2012;30:3611–3617.
2. Bell RF, Eccleston C, Kalso EA. Ketamine as an adjuvant to opioids for cancer pain. *Cochrane Database Syst Rev.* 2017;(6):CD003351. Published 2017 Jun 28. doi:10.1002/14651858.CD003351.pub3.
3. Mercadante S, Arcuri E, Tirelli W, Casuccio A. Analgesic effect of intravenous ketamine in cancer patients on morphine therapy: a randomized, controlled, double-blind, crossover, double-dose study. *J Pain Symptom Manage.* 2000;20(4):246–252. doi:10.1016/s0885-3924(00)00194-9.

4. Cohen SP, Bhatia A, Buvanendran A, et al. Consensus guidelines on the use of intravenous ketamine infusions for chronic pain from the American Society of Regional Anesthesia and Pain Medicine, the American Academy of Pain Medicine, and the American Society of Anesthesiologists. *Reg Anesth Pain Med.* 2018;43(5):521–546. doi:10.1097/AAP.0000000000000808.
5. Fallon MT, Wilcock A, Kelly CA, et al. Oral ketamine vs placebo in patients with cancer-related neuropathic pain: a randomized clinical trial. *JAMA Oncol.* 2018;4(6):870–872.
6. Prakash S, Meena JP, Gupta AK, et al. Ketamine mouthwash versus placebo in the treatment of severe oral mucositis pain in children with cancer: a randomized double-blind placebo-controlled trial. *Pediatr Blood Cancer.* 2020;67(9):e28573.
7. Gewandter JS, Mohile SG, Heckler CE, et al. A phase III randomized, placebo-controlled study of topical amitriptyline and ketamine for chemotherapy-induced peripheral neuropathy (CIPN): a University of Rochester CCOP study of 462 cancer survivors. *Support Care Cancer.* 2014;22(7):1807–1814.
8. Thota RS, Ramanjulu R, Ahmed A, et al. Indian Society for Study of Pain, Cancer Pain Special Interest Group guidelines on pharmacological management of cancer pain (part ii). *Indian J Palliat Care.* 2020;26(2):180–190.
9. Aman MM, Mahmoud A, Deer T, et al. The American Society of Pain and Neuroscience (ASPN) best practices and guidelines for the interventional management of cancer-associated pain. *J Pain Res.* 2021;14:2139–2164.

49

American (Wisconsin) Ginseng for Cancer-Related Fatigue

CRYSTAL A. WRIGHT AND CHENG ZENG

> Data from this study support that American ginseng has activity against cancer-related fatigue but that clinically meaningful results may not be realized until 2 months after starting ginseng.
>
> —BARTON ET AL.[1]

Research Question: Does American ginseng improve cancer-related fatigue (CRF) without significant toxicities?

Funding: National Institutes of Health and the Breast Cancer Research Foundation

Year Study Began: 2008

Year Study Published: 2013

Study Location: 40 sites; mostly community cancer centers

Who Was Studied: Adult cancer survivors receiving or having completed curative-intent treatment with CRF scores of 4 or more on a scale of 0 (no fatigue) to 10 (as bad as it can be). The fatigue was present for 1 month or more before study entry.

Who Was Excluded: Patients with brain cancer or central nervous system lymphoma; cancers diagnosed more than 2 years before enrollment; those using opioids, systemic steroids, or other agents for fatigue; those with current or previous use of ginseng; or those with pain or insomnia rated as 4 or more on a scale from 0 to 10.

How Many Patients: 364

Study Overview: This was a multicenter, double-blind trial in which participants were randomized to either the treatment or placebo arms. Participants were stratified according to baseline fatigue score (4–8 vs. 8–10), disease characteristics (initial vs. recurrent disease, hematologic malignancy vs. solid tumor), type of current treatment (radiation, chemotherapy, other targeted therapy), and lifetime duration of all prior cancer treatments (none vs. ≤ 180 days vs. > 180 days) (Figure 49.1).[2]

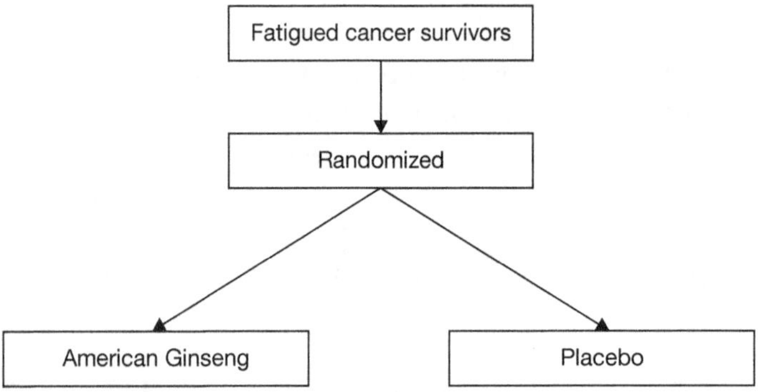

Figure 49.1. Summary of study design.

Study Intervention: The intervention was supplied as either 500-mg capsules containing Wisconsin ginseng with 3% ginsenosides or 500-mg capsules containing rice powder. The treatment arm received Wisconsin ginseng 2000 mg/day, administered as 1000 mg (2 capsules) around breakfast and 1000 mg (2 capsules) around lunch or noon.

Follow-Up: 4 weeks and 8 weeks

Endpoints:

Primary outcome: Change in fatigue (Multidimensional Fatigue Symptom Inventory-Short Form [MFSI-SF] general subscale) from baseline to weeks 4 and 8.

Secondary outcomes: Change in other fatigue measures (MFSI-SF physical, mental, emotional, and vigor subscales; Brief Fatigue Inventory [BFI]) and change in mood (Profile of Mood States vigor-activity [POMS-VA] and fatigue-inertia [POMS-FI] subscales) from baseline to weeks 4 and week 8; grade 2 to 3 toxicities with 1% or greater incidence (Common Terminology Criteria for Adverse Events [CTCAE] version 3.0) from week 1 to week 8.

RESULTS

- The primary outcome (change in the MFSI-SF general subscale at 4 weeks) improved in the American ginseng arm but did not achieve statistical significance. It became statistically significant at 8 weeks (Table 49.1).

Table 49.1 SUMMARY OF STUDY'S KEY FINDINGS

Outcome[a]	**Ginseng 4 Weeks**	**Placebo 4 weeks**	***P* Value**	**Ginseng 8 Weeks**	**Placebo 8 Weeks**	***P* Value**
Change in MFSI-SF						
General subscale	14.4 + 27.1	8.2 + 24.8	.07	20 + 27	10.3 + 26.1	**.003**
Physical	1.6 + 15.9	−0.4 + 14.7	.39	3.0 + 17.9	−1.7 + 18.2	**.004**
Mental	2.0 + 15.2	0.6 + 16.1	.41	2.8 + 16.5	3.4 + 15.2	.80
Emotional	0.5 + 16.1	0.5 + 16.7	.99	3.0 + 17.4	2.3 + 17.4	.68
Vigor	1.8 + 19.0	0.4 + 15.5	.70	4.6 + 20.5	2.5 + 17.6	.71
Total score	4.1 + 13.4	2.1 + 12.9	.21	6.7 + 14.0	3.7 + 14.6	**.02**
Change in POMS						
Fatigue-inertia	14.5 + 25	7.7 + 23.6	.08	18.6 + 24.8	10.2 + 26.1	**.008**
Vigor-activity	5 + 18.7	3.9 + 17.3	.79	8.2 + 19.8	6.4 + 19.8	.47

Abbreviations: MFSI-SF, Multidimensional Fatigue Symptom Inventory-Short Form; POMS, Profile of Mood States.

[a] Scores for all outcomes were converted to a 100-point scale in which a higher number indicates less fatigue. A difference of 10 points was considered clinically meaningful.

- The benefit of American ginseng on CRF was greatest in participants receiving active cancer treatment. Participants taking American ginseng during cancer treatment had statistically significant improvement in the MFSI-SF general subscale at both week 4 and week 8 compared to placebo.
- There was no statistically significant improvement in the MFSI-SF general subscale at 4 or 8 weeks for participants who took American ginseng after completing cancer treatment.

- The secondary outcomes MFSI-SF physical, MFSI-SF total, and POMS-FI were statistically significantly improved in the American ginseng arm over placebo at 8 weeks (Table 49.1).
- There was no significant difference in the incidence of toxicities between groups.
- There was no significant difference between arms in POMS-VA or BFI.

Criticisms and Limitations:

- The primary outcome did not reach statistical significance but did favor the ginseng arm at 4 weeks.
- The study was not long enough to assess long-term (> 8 week) safety and efficacy.
- The authors excluded subjects with pain or insomnia rated as ≥ 4 on a scale from 0 to 10. This helps eliminate confounding variables but also limits the generalizability of the results.

Other Relevant Studies and Information:

- A prior dose-finding pilot study reported that American ginseng 1000 to 2000 mg daily in 2 divided doses appeared to improve fatigue (BFI) more than placebo, whereas a 750-mg total daily dose did not.[3]

Summary and Implications: In this randomized, double-blind, multicenter study involving cancer survivors with CRF, American ginseng treatment led to significant symptom improvement after 8, but not 4, weeks compared to placebo. There were no significant toxicities identified. Based on this and other research, American ginseng treatment is appropriate to consider for patients with CRF.

CLINICAL CASE: WHAT CAN HELP WITH CANCER-RELATED FATIGUE?

Case History

Ms. G is a 70-year-old female newly diagnosed with stage IV breast cancer. She is on palbociclib and letrozole and tolerating therapy reasonably well with an Eastern Cooperative Oncology Group (ECOG) score of 1. She had a recent history of adjustment disorder with anxiety and loss of appetite leading to 15-pound weight loss, which is much improved with mirtazapine. She takes

Tylenol occasionally for mild lower back pain. She has a past medical history significant for coronary artery disease and nonsustained ventricular tachycardia. Her most recent routine lab work including complete blood count, basic metabolic panel, thyroid panel, and albumin was within normal range. A few months into the treatments her biggest complaint is fatigue, which she ranks 7/10. After dinner she can hardly stay awake for things she used to enjoy, such as watching TV or playing cards. She is already working on a balanced diet and gentle exercises such as yoga. She wants to know if there is anything that can help with her fatigue, preferably naturopathic medicines.

Suggested Answer

The Mayo Clinic trial showed that fatigued cancer patients can benefit from American ginseng after an 8-week period. The trial included patients whose other causes of fatigue were ruled out, with pain and insomnia rated lower than 4 out of 10, and who were not on other agents for treatment of fatigue. The trial also did not find any toxicities that were statistically significant.

The patient in this case scenario meets the criteria for the Mayo Clinic trial and could benefit from American ginseng. Given her recent history of anxiety and abnormal weight loss (though treated and controlled at this time), as well as history of coronary artery disease and arrythmia, American ginseng can be a better option due to its low side effect profile compared to a psychostimulant such as methylphenidate. The patient's preference for naturopathic medicines is also taken into consideration.

Thus, it's reasonable for the provider to start a conversation about American ginseng, specifically 1000 mg twice daily with breakfast and lunch. The provider should set the expectation that it may take between 4 and 8 weeks for full benefits.

References

1. Barton DL, Liu H, Dakhil SR, et al. Wisconsin ginseng (Panax quinquefolius) to improve cancer-related fatigue: a randomized, double-blind trial, N07C2. *J Natl Cancer Inst.* 2013;105(16):1230–1238. doi:10.1093/jnci/djt181.
2. American Ginseng in Treating Patients With Fatigue Caused by Cancer. ClinicalTrials.gov identifier: NCT00719563. https://clinicaltrials.gov/ct2/show/NCT00719563. Updated February 9, 2017. Accessed March 9, 2021.
3. Barton DL, Soori GS, Bauer BA, et al. Pilot study of Panax quinquefolius (American ginseng) to improve cancer-related fatigue: a randomized, double-blind, dose-finding evaluation: NCCTG trial N03CA. *Support Care Cancer.* 2010;18(2):179–187. doi:10.1007/s00520-009-0642-2.

50

Management of Intractable Hiccups

AMBEREEN K. MEHTA AND DAVID S. WU

> There was a consistent and statistically significant (p=0.03) improvement in hiccup severity with Baclofen, both subjectively (p=0.03) and by hiccup-free periods (p=0.003). The actual frequency of hiccup was not significantly altered by the medication.
>
> —Ramírez and Graham[1]

Research Question: What is the efficacy and safety of baclofen for patients with intractable hiccups?

Funding: General Clinical Research Center, Division of Research Resources of the National Institutes of Health, Department of Veterans Affairs, Grant RR00350

Year Study Began: Not specified

Year Study Published: 1992

Study Location: Clinical Research Center, The Methodist Hospital, Houston, Texas

Who Was Studied: Adults with intractable hiccups defined as daily hiccups for 6 months or longer, unresponsive to medical therapy.

Who Was Excluded: Patients with depression or renal insufficiency.

How Many Patients: 4

Study Overview: This was a double-blind, randomized, controlled, crossover study in which 4 patients were randomly assigned to receive baclofen or placebo. Patients were admitted to the hospital, observed for 2 days without receiving any study drug (baseline period), and then received either baclofen or placebo for 6 days total. Patients were then discharged with 1 week of tapering to zero dose followed by 1 week of "washout" without any study drug. Patients were then readmitted to the hospital and the protocol was repeated as a crossover.

Study Intervention: Patients received either baclofen 1 tablet (5 mg) or placebo 1 tablet, orally, crushed and mixed in lactose powder, administered every 8 hours for 3 days (total 15 mg/day and 30 mg/day, respectively). The dose was increased to 2 tablets (baclofen 10 mg) of each study drug for another 3 days. After the washout period, patients received crossover intervention.

Follow-up: None

Endpoints: Hiccup frequency was documented by a nurse for 10 minutes 9 times within a 24-hour window and audio recorded for 1 hour 3 times within a 24-hour window. The objective response to the study drugs was counted as the number of 10-minute intervals patients had no hiccups as recorded by a nurse. Hiccup severity was graded on a 4-point scale (0 = no hiccup perceived, 1 = mild, 2 = moderate, and 3 = severe). Patients self-reported a hiccup severity score between 0 (none) and 10 (worst ever experienced) once daily while hospitalized. The hiccup frequency was also manually counted from the audio recording.

RESULTS

- As assessed by a blinded nurse, the hiccup-free period increased by 69% with baclofen 15 mg/day (P = .08) and by 120% with baclofen 30 mg/day (P = .003) as compared to the baseline period, while it remained the same with placebo 15 mg/day and worsened by 16% with placebo 30 mg/day.
- A dose-dependent improvement in subject-reported severity of hiccups was noted: mean improvement of 22.5% ± 3.4% for baclofen 15 mg/day dose and 31.4% ± 4.8% for baclofen 30 mg/day dose as compared to placebo. The effect for the 30 mg/day dose was statistically significant (P = .03).

- However, the actual number of hiccup-free intervals did not significantly increase as measured by audio recording.
- The authors speculate that the discrepancy in findings between nurse observations and manual count from audio recording reflected the different sensitivity of measurement techniques to detect less severe hiccups.
- No side effects from baclofen were reported in this study.
- This randomized, double-blind, crossover study showed that baclofen reduced subjective hiccup severity but did not eliminate intractable hiccups when compared to placebo.

Criticisms and Limitations:

- This study is significantly limited by its small participant number.
- The underlying cause of hiccups is not reported, which limits generalizability.

Other Relevant Studies and Information:

- A Cochrane review published in 2013[2] included controlled clinical trials of adults treated for persistent or intractable hiccups (defined as lasting > 48 hours) and excluded studies with < 10 participants or no assessment of change in hiccup frequency or intensity. Only 4 studies met criteria, all studying acupuncture techniques, and all 4 were deemed high risk of bias. The authors concluded that insufficient evidence is present to guide pharmacological or nonpharmacological treatment of persistent or intractable hiccups.
- A systematic review of oral baclofen in the management of hiccups was published in 2020. In total, 22 patients have been reported in the literature. The doses ranged from 10 mg once only to 20 mg 3 times a day with the duration ranging from 1 to 24 days. The author concluded that it was difficult to draw strong conclusions about the use of baclofen for hiccups as the overall quality evidence was low and recommended more randomized controlled trials for evaluation.[3]
- A systematic review of 5 randomized trials involving acupuncture found that acupuncture used as an adjunctive treatment did improve hiccups (relative risk 1.59) but not when used alone.[4]
- A small 2014 randomized placebo-controlled trial of baclofen for treatment of persistent hiccups (defined as 48 hours to 1 month) in 30 post-stroke patients suggests potential efficacy of baclofen.[5]

- A 2014 randomized placebo-controlled trial of metoclopramide for treatment of intractable hiccups (duration > 1 month) in 36 patients due to cancer, stroke, and cerebral tumors suggests potential efficacy of metoclopramide.[6]
- Dexamethasone, commonly used as an antiemetic during chemotherapy, is the most common drug to cause hiccups. In a randomized study, patients with cancer maintained on dexamethasone had recurrent hiccups (84.8%), while patients rotated to methylprednisolone had a reduced frequency of hiccups (62.5%). The intensity of hiccups was significantly less with methylprednisolone. Interestingly, the authors noted that dexamethasone-induced hiccups appeared to be a male-predominant phenomenon.[7]
- There are multiple case reports and case series using gabapentin for intractable hiccups, with findings suggesting that gabapentin is a promising treatment for severe hiccups in patients with advanced malignancy.[8,9]
- Chlorpromazine was the only US Food and Drug Administration (FDA)-approved therapy for the treatment of hiccups,[10] but due to concern for long-term neurological side effects along with hypotension, urinary retention, glaucoma, or delirium, the FDA withdrew this approval.

CLINICAL CASE: SHOULD THIS PATIENT BE TREATED WITH BACLOFEN?

Case History

A 67-year-old man presents with a 6-month history of intractable hiccups, refractory to a variety of behavioral maneuvers (e.g., holding breath, Valsalva maneuver) and a 3-month trial of a proton pump inhibitor. His medical history is notable for stroke 8 months ago that has left him with residual right-sided weakness and severe dysphagia. He has lost 15% of his body weight since the stroke and is now bedbound. The hiccups are extremely bothersome.

Should this patient be given baclofen?

Suggested Answer

This patient's hiccup symptoms likely fall within the parameters of this trial. Consideration of baclofen is reasonable, especially given his symptom burden and advanced illness. Informed consent with the patient about baclofen is recommended, including discussion of benefits and risks, off-label use, and evidence base.

Summary and Implications: This small, double-blind, randomized, controlled, crossover study suggested that baclofen reduced the severity of hiccup periods but did not decrease the actual number of hiccups. A paucity of strong evidence exists to guide treatment decisions for intractable hiccups.

References

1. Ramírez FC, Graham DY. Treatment of intractable hiccup with baclofen: results of a double-blind randomized cross-over study. *Am J Gastroenterol.* 1992;87(12):1789–1791.
2. Moretto EN, Wee B, Wien PJ, Murchison AG. Interventions for treating persistent and intractable hiccups in adults. *Cochrane Database Syst Rev.* 2013;(1):CD008768.
3. Adam E. A systematic review of the effectiveness of oral baclofen in the management of hiccups in adult palliative care patients. *J Pain Palliat Care Pharmacother.* 2020;34(1):43–54.
4. Yue J, Liu M, Li J, et al. Acupuncture for the treatment of hiccups following stroke: a systematic review and meta-analysis. *Acupunct Med.* 2017;35(1):2–8.
5. Zhang C, Zhang R, Zhang S, et al. Baclofen for stroke patients with persistent hiccups: a randomized, double-blind, placebo-controlled trial. *Trials.* 2014;15:295.
6. Wang T, Wang D. Metoclopramide for patients with intractable hiccups: a multicenter randomised, controlled pilot study. *Intern Med J.* 2014;44:1205–1209.
7. Go SI, Koo DH, Kim ST, et al. Antiemetic corticosteroid rotation from dexamethasone to methylprednisolone to prevent dexamethasone-induced hiccup in cancer patients treated with chemotherapy: a randomized, single-blind, crossover phase III trial. *Oncologist.* 2017;22(11):1354–1361.
8. Porzio G, Aielli F, Verna L, Aloisi P, Galletti B, Ficorella C. Gabapentin in the treatment of hiccups in patients with advanced cancer: a 5-year experience. *Clin Neuropharmacol.* 2010;33(4):179–180.
9. Menon M. Gabapentin in the treatment of persistent hiccups in advanced malignancy. *Indian J Palliat Care.* 2012;18(2):138–140.
10. Reichenbach ZW, Piech GM, Malik Z. Chronic hiccups. *Curr Treat Options Gastroenterol.* 2020;18:43–59.

INDEX

For the benefit of digital users, indexed terms that span two pages (e.g., 52–53) may, on occasion, appear on only one of those pages.

Tables and figures are indicated by an italic *t* and *f* following the page number.